# Appreciation & Praise

*"Dr. Tefft brings us to the final frontier of nutrition, where complete wellness and greater longevity are the status quo...where diet-related disease is absent...where each and every one of us can be our healthiest, our fittest—our best.... I have always believed in the power of personalized nutrition—so should you.... To detoxify and to super-nourish the body according to our personal genetic/metabolic standards is the route we can take to root out the causes of our health problems....* **Your Personal Life** *is a personal reference to nutrition testing and guides you through the most powerful medicine in the world—the inner you—for the rest of your life.... Use it wisely!"*

—**Jorge Monastersky, M.D.; cardiologist; task force board member of the American Heart Association**

*"I was suffering from a lack of energy in the afternoon and poor sleep at night.... My trainer recommended personalized nutrition.... As a result, I did a test and within about seven days it was the first time in two years I slept through the night.... I'm currently worlds better..."*

—**Michael Clark, PGA Tour Pro, 2000 Rookie of the Year**

*"As with snowflakes, no two humans are the same. Each individual possesses a unique biochemical terrain reflecting his or her identity and physiologic status. In spite of this known individuality, allopathic medicine persists in treating patients as representing generic 'norms,' all with disastrous results. In* **Your Personal Life,** *Greg Tefft introduces the reader to the healing efficacy of individualized healthcare offered through (Ortho) Molecular Medicine. Tefft's clinical research on creating optimum ecological environments in the body through personalized nutrition therapy will help define how dysfunctions and disease will be assessed and treated in the future."*

—**Bruce H. Lipton, PhD; Cell Biologist; lecturer and Best-Selling author of** *The Biology of Belief;* **What the Bleep Do We Know? – Conference Speaker**

"About 1960 when my research group and I discovered a substantial protein that all schizophrenic patients excreted...it became clear to me that this might be the beginning of a new paradigm...or what Dr. Tefft calls "real." Using accurate lab methods and orthomolecular medicine, the whole new paradigm is now wide open. Dr. Tefft's book, **Your Personal Life**, is a comprehensive account of how to use the lab analysis we now are familiar with and how to use the correct nutritional or orthomolecular methods for repairing biochemical damage. The information is outlined in detail; the clinical description of the treatment and the responses is impressive. I fully endorse his book for everyone interested in maintaining good health, for providing comprehensive and simple early treatment and for helping even the chronic failure from modern schizophrenia drug-only treatment."

—**Abram Hoffer, M.D.; PhD; medical researcher, editor-in-chief of the** *Journal of Orthomolecular Medicine*

"Thank you again for your contribution to the XXIII Olympiad and your professional representation of the sports medicine field."

—**Peter V. Uberroth, president, Los Angeles Olympic Organizing Committee**

"The best nutrition program ever."

—**Gordon Michaels, owner of Malibu Health and Rehabilitation Center**

"Thanks for all your help with my body."

—**Danny Inosanto, karate stuntman, actor, Bruce Lee's original partner**

"Congratulations on providing the world with a quantum leap in health and fitness technology."

—**Rosalene Glickman, PhD, author of the #1 international Best-Seller, *Optimal Thinking*, president of the World Academy of Personal Development, Inc.**

"Dr. Tefft is America's leader in personalized nutrition."

—**Bill Berger, M.D., Southern California Allergy Research Institute**

"*Health and Awareness Award* to Dr. Gregory H. Tefft, 'In recognition of outstanding community service and dedication to the Chiropractic Oath by supporting the *Reader's Digest* campaign to bring important information to the general public.'"

—**Reader's Digest**


"*As Dr. Tefft points out, the worse the gene-to-environment antagonism, the greater the susceptibility to illness and the shorter the lifespan. This is not merely an academic observation. Acid rain and the misuse of fertilizers are resulting in a global selenium deficiency that is encouraging the spread of the HIV, hepatitis B and C and the coxsackie B viruses. Together, these pathogens have already infected more than one third of the world's population and are killing some 7 million people each year. They are still rapidly diffusing. It is no coincidence that the physical and chemical destruction of the Earth's environment is being accompanied by exotic new illnesses like SARS, CFS, autism, and the explosive rebirth of old foes such as tuberculosis. Your Personal Life contains crucial insights on how we can best help ourselves in the midst of these real health threats.*"

—**Harold Foster, PhD; professor of geography, University of Victoria; International Society for Orthomolecular Medicine's Orthomolecular Doctor of the Year, 2004–2005; board member, Canadian Schizophrenia Foundation**


"*The information in Dr. Tefft's book underscores the importance of recognizing metabolic individuality. Emphasis on uniqueness of the individual will substantially impact health, prevention of disease, longevity and genetic potential in a positive manner. Treating the individual instead of just their symptoms will, in the long run, result not only in better health for Americans, but will also aid in the reduction of the ever-growing health care costs of the nation. I highly recommend this book to anyone who is serious about taking the best care of themselves using the science that will soon be recognized as the future health.*"

—**David L. Watts, PhD; F.A.C.E.P.**


"*An academic's brain + a world class athlete's body + a small town doctor's heart = Dr. Greg Tefft.*"

—**Pavel Tsatsouline, Best-Selling author of *The Russian Kettlebell Challenge*; *Rolling Stone*, 2002 Trainer of the Year, International Elite Special Forces Trainer**

# Your
# Personal Life

# Your Personal Life

*Measuring What Your Specific Body Needs*
*to Live Lean, Long, Strong & Better*

## DR. GREG TEFFT
*with* BILL QUATEMAN

1st Edition


International Standard Book Number: 0-9729866-2-6

Library of Congress Control Number: 2005935611


Published by

Angel Mind

5776-D Lindero Canyon Drive

#123

Westlake Village, CA 91362

818.424.2619

www.Angelmind.net




*Book design and text composition by Bill Fate*


Printed in the USA

# Foreword

## The New Medical Philosophy

### By Jorge Monastersky, M.D.

Modern medicine is at a crossroads. Are pharmaceuticals or "nutraceuticals" going to counteract disease in the future? Or is there going to be a synergistic combination of both forces against disease? Maybe a more precise application of existing "nutra-" and "pharma-" ceuticals is called for. After all, these two types of biochemicals come from the same place–our environment-and we may just need them all to some variable degree in accordance with our most critical and specific needs up to the moment. Yes, nutraceuticals are more considered to be fundamental nourishment by the body than symptom-relief-oriented pharmaceuticals; the controversies persist and the debates go on and on. Perhaps a greater precision in both their applications to each individual truly is the weakest link in the healing process.

In actuality, all health-related science is now focused upon understanding the first, most important link–individuality–as priority over and above the pharmaceutical versus nutraceutical controversy. Once the unique wellness needs of an individual are precisely established, the therapeutic application of nutra- and pharmaceuticals (or both) comes into play subject to a broader interpretation of need using a more multifactorial deductive process. This process should result in the highest benefit-to-risk ratio (highest body benefit/least risk of damaging side effects) in the application of nutra- and pharmaceuticals and furthermore have greater implications to the entirety of lifestyle for a more holistic integration.

Of course the pharma/nutra debate will always be a very heated topic from a capitalistic/political viewpoint when really, more precise diagnostics should be considered the first priority along with closely matched personalizing algorithms which therapeutically match remedial protocols according to one's uniqueness. Nonetheless, the final extinction of one-size-fits-all in the science and application of better health promotion is upon us. Let's just let's not get confused on the priorities of what is most and least important in this process.

The use of more anti-sickness bio-tools in a strictly individualized manner simply makes sense. We already possess many potent "nutra-" and "pharma-" ceuticals. Using them in precise accordance with one's given genetic and metabolic constitution will optimize their positive effects while minimizing undesirable side effects. Consequently, certain "pharma-" and "nutra-" ceuticals may only be used by a small percentage of people whereas other "ceuticals" will have to be substituted in for those people who aren't as compatible. Of course, there may be some nutra-/pharmaceuticals that work well across the board.

Either way, the application of anti-disease intervention is fast becoming more individualized than ever before. However, we must not only individually apply remedial nutra-/pharmaceuticals to the extremes of genetic and metabolic compatibility, but we must also expand and faithfully apply this individualizing process to every aspect of our lives. Everything we eat, inhale, and drink, everything we think and do in the immediate environment that we experience counts and should always be complementary to our wellness and should therefore be customized to our personal uniqueness. This is the only way to eradicate disease potential from our lives. Detoxifying and super nourishing the body according to our personal genetic/metabolic standards is the only route we can take to root out the causes of our health problems.

"Nutra-" and "pharma-" ceuticals should be individually applied only in conjunction with, not as a substitute for, a health-promoting lifestyle in a health-promoting environment that is perfectly holistic. This is the new medical philosophy: leave no stone unturned, nothing taken for granted from the food we eat to the things we do for the most perfect lifestyle possible. And, when it comes to choosing pharma- or nutraceuticals, they are chosen with the utmost care so as not to upset the balance of our life. This is where the controversy resides; balance. The more balance we have, the less we'll need to debate nutras and pharmas because our need for them will be minimal and our control over our health destiny will be at a maximum.

*Your Personal Life* allows you to personally take control of the entirety of engineering your own balanced wellness destiny. It's your personal reference for transcending through all the aspects of being balanced and staying well. From doctor's office to dinner table, nutra to pharmaceutical, to home and work environments, to recreation and exercise pursuits–it's all there. Now you can better connect yourself to the real you at the very core of the wellness world. This is holistic health at its very best, no stone left unturned and nothing taken for granted. This personal reference guides you to the most powerful medicine in the world–the inner you–for the rest of your life. Use it wisely!

*Dr. Jorge Monastersky*
*American Heart Association,*
*Task Force Cardiologist*

# Preface
## Let's Be Real

*The truth dazzles gradually, or else the world would be blind.*

—Emily Dickinson

## Reality Diet and Nutrition

People are hungry to be real, to find out and know what's **really true**. Every day, the popularity of reality TV shows how we want to see and know how people live their lives. These shows, however, are *really* more of the same regular TV, staged presentations designed to get our attention in large numbers to be able to sell advertising time at a premium. Fair enough, we buy into it every day; endless hours, by the tens of millions. And every day, we hear the same question coming from our clients and our colleagues: "With the blizzard of information about vitamins and alternative health care, with our conventional doctors who are good people but just don't have anything for me beyond serious crisis intervention and symptom suppression, how do we know the best way to heal or create wellness and vitality for ourselves?"

The answer is: reality nutrition. What does that mean? The core definition is truth. We think truth is real; what is real is what is true. Statistically, people prefer true stories over fiction. The thinking is, "How do I compare with the hero in that story? Could I do that?" People crave in-your-face-real. We want to know the truth, even though we hardly admit it. We need it more now, especially in light of the confusing and overwhelming information explosion. There are conflicting reports, and support from many big money sources, including agencies that are meant to guide people. Of all the epidemics we now face, there is an epidemic of dirty politics and exaggerated egos, never-ending corporate deceptions and a "profits first over safety" attitude throughout the wellness and health-care industries. In light of this, "real" and "true" are very welcome realities. The ancient wisdom that "the truth shall set you free," is clearly most important in regard to your personal health and well-being than any other area of concern. The truth of this is evidenced by such a huge division in the scientific community: one part devoted to better health, and the other, the accounting, where health care costs are a large component of our economy (approximately 25% of our Gross National Product). Yet the truth about our birthright of wellness seems to be evading us when we consider that illnesses, diseases and obesity have never been more various or virulent. We do live longer, some of us from pill to pill, yet what is the quality of life?

This epidemic phenomenon is intensifying. If the truth were known, all disease, energy and fatness syndromes would be shrinking from view, drug use would diminish and life's quality would be on the upswing—not the opposite, as it is now. The keyword and health reality is, and will always be, truth. Knowing the truth about exactly where your unique body stands in relation to what you do, eat, drink, breathe, and absorb will inevitably set you free. Free to be healthier, slimmer, more energetic and productive and "harder living" than you ever dreamt possible. Down deep, it's the real thing that we all want. And thanks to a specialized arm of science the truth about yourself in this regard will prove to be stranger than fiction, as you shall see. But this deeper truth once revealed will truly set you free from self-health mistakes like never before. In our uncovering of the nutritional truth, the reality of one's body/mind/spirit in relation to wellness leaves no room for error because one's very life is at stake. Guesswork, inappropriate or unproven theory, fads, gimmicks, political manipulations, god complexes amongst health-care specialists, repeated negligence, so-called cures that are actually worse than the original problem, an emphasis upon symptom relief instead of true cause relief, false beliefs, nonaccountability, inaccurate assumptions, toxic environments going unnoticed, intentional or unintentional mistakes, magic-pill potions, lotions, etc, all these have no place in our personal wellness reality, as they threaten our very life. Yet it is these influences which are creating health mediocrity and a culture of unwellness. Especially in light of new technology, this thinking appears simply foolish and actually dangerous to health and well-being. It is truly no longer necessary.

Unfortunately, the saddest part of our current self-healthcare nightmare is that the outright majority of people haven't the foggiest notion about what's measurable and real about their own bodies at the levels that count the most, nutrition body chemistry. These are the deepest levels which reflect the very stuff that we are made of and made from—from inside to outside: atom to molecule to chemical to cell to tissue to organ to system—to the most genetically pure integration of the whole organism. Standard medicine is not at all focused on this most vital healing dimension—this nutritional reality is effectively eluding the conventional professional medical group. To most of them, it's not a central factor. For many standard medical practitioners, the "Galileo dilemma" is apparent. Simply, the world has always been round but it still took scientists hundreds of years to finally all agree with Galileo's original finding. Similarly, today's standard healthcare practitioner is blind to the latest clinical nutrition science revelations. To these practitioners, the world is still flat when it comes to a truly round nutrition reality.

Measurable reality and ongoing scientific accountability is the outright clinical focus of orthomolecular nutritional medicine. This practice uncovers the deepest physiochemical relationships of nutrients, toxins, metabolic and genetic function. This special scientific focus has filled the reality gap between the superficiality and the built-in limitations of routine medical attentions and the exciting revelations provided by the most critical information that we must have about the body.

This then enables us to reduce, eliminate or control all diet-related disease (which, according to governmental/scientific authorities is all disease including that initiated by germs) along with over-fat and under-energy syndromes, diminished lifespan, stunted growth and development in children, psychological imbalances, mediocre fitness and all "metabolic syndrome disorders.*"

Many of us, repeatedly told by our doctors that we have tolerable, little, persistent, to-be-expected problems, can now know for sure that they are not all in our heads or because we are getting older. Orthomolecular nutritional medicine (called biomedicine by the FDA) allows us complete clarity about our nutritional biochemistry and how it correlates to the health

*(the new medical catch-phrase for anything wrong with you not easily called an outright disease)

issue—that's its only job. This job is in direct opposition to standard crisis relief medicine because when this self-care approach is instituted correctly, the body heals itself and illness and disease issues are transformed. In effect it can be considered, (in order of priority), pre-standard medicine or better yet, prevention, the finest complementary medicine available to anyone. As a scientific matter of fact, it is certain primary nutrient and toxic relationships which make all the healthy difference in the world and these "little things" are exactly what standard medicine categorically ignores, doesn't have time for, de-prioritizes or doesn't care about. Who among us really cares all that much about pre-standard medicine? Few do! As a result, do not expect your neighborhood M.D. to understand what we are talking about on the highly specific levels that need to be attended to. They, like each of us, must be reoriented in order to see this clearly as the critical priority that it is, before it is too late for us all.

Consequently, the superficial prevention of pharmaceutical cover-ups; faulty, fragmented research; incomplete or conflicting medical perspectives; symptom-relief shortcuts; therapeutic shortcuts and downright health and nutrition nonsense which commands the attention is literally killing us—unnecessarily.

If the same energy and effort expended upon routine health ideologies was being put into the measurable reality and ongoing scientific accountability that orthomolecular science so effortlessly affords us, there would be no out-of-control diet-related disease epidemic upon us, no epidemic of drug and stimulant dependencies, better quality and length of life, less over-fat, fatigued, depressed unfitness, doctor visits, lower insurance premiums, fewer dangerously overmedicated children and fewer psychological disorders. Measurable health truthfulness and on-going accountability may come to be seen as the greatest gift that science has ever given to humankind. Thanks to a renewed focus on science, the answers to all wellness problems beyond where routine medicine leaves off can quickly become self-evident and effectively controlled to transform our health. We don't have a moment to lose. The real health reality check is upon us. Can we use it wisely?

# Reality Check
# Deeper Than Medicine

## How to Wake Up &
## Take Your Health on a Turn for the Best

- All disease (lifespan, mediocre fitness, mental disorders, over-fat and fatigue syndromes) is diet-related.
- You are *not* what you eat.
- Your body does *not* automatically take only what it needs from food and leave the rest.
- Using pharmaceutical drugs to treat nutrition problems only weakens the body further.
- Diet and nutrition have completely different meanings.
- Any given fresh organic vegetable or fruit is not necessarily good for you.
- MDRs (Minimum Daily Requirements), RDAs (Recommended Daily Allowances), and DVs (Daily Values) have absolutely nothing to do with the nutritional status of your body.
- A once-a-day multiple vitamin/mineral supplement statistically will worsen your nutrition condition; it will not improve it nor provide nutrition or health insurance.
- Muscle testing, Ayurvedic, Chinese, Greek, Egyptian, blood typing, metabolic typing, food-zoned diets, questionnaires, body typing, constitutional typing and/or any popular diet system today cannot properly personalize nutrition for you.
- Genetics have very little to do with your body's up-to-the-moment nutritional state and what to do about it.
- Losing body fat does not guarantee better health.

- You *cannot* make the right food and supplement choices by instinct, nor singularly think yourself well.
- All vitamin and mineral supplements vary tremendously.
- You damage your own genes by not eating right.
- More exercising does not guarantee better health.
- Pharmaceutical drugs do not guarantee better health.
- Doctors do not understand or prioritize nutrition in their practice of medicine.
- The U.S. is the #1 worst in the civilized world for diet-related diseases.
- All that happens to you affects your body/brain chemistry.
- Routine medical tests do not reveal nutritional disturbances.
- Cutting-edge science and leading health authorities do *not* recommend the indiscriminate use of diet and supplements to preserve and maintain wellness.
- The government is *not* concerned about your best health interests when it comes to foods and supplements and environmental considerations.
- Your one-of-a-kind body can never be its best without accountable personalization.
- If the wellness approach in *Your Personal Life* was in general use, all directly-diet-related disease would no longer plague the human race.

To disregard any of the above reality check statements is to miss the core truth about how to use nutrition and all external environmental forces, the most powerful medicine of all, for creating meaningful, healthy, long-lasting, energetic life a quantum leap beyond the superficial influence of traditional medicine. *Your Personal Life* proves each of these indisputable statements and many more as the new starting point and the basis for creating lasting radiant health.

# Contents

# Introduction

# Your Personal Life

*All truth passes through three stages. First, it is ridiculed; second it is violently opposed; and third, it is accepted as self-evident.*
—Arthur Schopenhauer, Philosopher

## Reality Check #1
### You Are Not What You Eat

At this very moment, in the U.S. and similar "technologically advanced" countries like the U.K. and Canada, there is an overwhelming epidemic of degenerative disease. Better known as one or another of over 223 diet-related diseases, these serious yet common health problems include:

- weight gain
- chronic fatigue
- serious health crises
- those who suffer continuing, "tolerable" discomfort
- those who just can't seem to manage a few excess pounds
- those who are morbidly obese and at extreme medical risk

The specific illnesses, the names of which we all know too well, are: heart disease, cancer, arthritis, obesity, high blood pressure, osteoporosis, diabetes, MS, Alzheimer's, premature aging and many more. Nobody can argue against the high incidence of these illnesses, but there is a continuous controversy regarding how best to quickly and healthfully turn this serious problem around for the best on a countrywide—even a worldwide—basis.

1

The worst part of this situation is that the overwhelming majority of conventional wellness/energy-promoting fat loss/antiaging approaches that are the most popular today are based on exceedingly imprecise beliefs and methodologies. These incomplete ideas are far too theoretical and presuming to be considered scientific. In fact, our generalized one-size-fits-all approach to health (or any) issues could not be more unscientific or outdated – and it is to our greatest detriment. It is, in fact, an embarrassment, in the face of scientific truth. Some call this problem "anti-science" or "junk science."

Our society has benefited and is so advanced scientifically yet when it comes to diet, nutrition and weight loss we routinely practice "non-science"—or "nonsense." If this weren't true, ours would not be a nation of degenerating, tired, stressed, fatsos, holding the number one position in the world for diet-related diseases and widespread drug dependence. As always, the statistical facts speak for themselves. Until we wise up about the core truths of why we are becoming uncontrollably fatter, less energetic, depressed and sicker, nothing will change for the better, it will only get worse. At this writing, 50% of North Americans suffer from one illness or another and the problem is growing exponentially.

The best news is that there really is a better way already in place – a definitive scientific reality check—waiting for each of us.  It goes so much deeper than just generic one-size-fits-all wellness and fat-loss information. This new approach is in total alignment with the proven science of the disease and fat issue, and is dedicated solely to exposing the most inconvertible and indisputable facts about your own body's fat-gain, disease-fostering malfunctions—with no bias, no imprecision, no theoretical stretch, no meaningful controversy attached to it whatsoever!

Persisting to disregard the enormous benefits of **Your Personal Life's** fat loss/health-gain reality check technology would be like continuing to insist that the world is flat when direct scientific measurement and practice shows us it is elliptical and rounded. Dismissing this proven scientific research will leave us where we already are, the sickest, fattest country on earth. Other confusions include health care as a strictly commercial enterprise with a total disregard to any benefit. Rest assured that the phenomenon of health politics and profit is not at all uncommon in today's wellness marketplace.  Politics should be considered an epidemic in itself. There can be a very fine line between personally usable science and generic junk science that few people are aware of. When it comes to effectively losing fat and promoting health, discriminating between personally usable and generic junk science makes all the difference in the world—the difference between *lasting* complete success and total failure. Junk science represents information that has no direct connection to your fat loss/health gain needs, whereas personally usable science is directly connected to your most exacting needs with no guesswork, no doubts, no misconceptions. Success is based on numbers. The most common denominator for success is based on where we must start—the fact that despite all our similarities, we are each unique in many ways.

Our own nutritional measurement is the one place that we are most unique and from which to reliably start the fat loss/health gain process for each and every one of us. Starting at this point of real knowing and at this point only grants each of us complete control over excess fat accumulation, energy crises and hundreds of diet-related diseases—all based on personally applied science and completely individualized assessment. All generic junk science, theoretical stretches, fads, gimmicks, rhetoric, propaganda, confusion or nonsense (non-science) is forever surpassed once you have grasped this primary fat loss/health basic concept. Applying this most fundamental information to our personal intakes of food and supplements, we then have the most control and the most impact on all of our health and healing. We can all agree—it always pays to know what we want, know what we're doing and have a specific plan before taking any action, and that is the essence of the real diet secret described in *Your Personal Life*. This means in effect, for guaranteed best results, you must be educated and aware. Look before you leap. *Your Personal Life's* essential nutrition secret is based on the same precisely scientific 100-year-old approach for fat loss/health gain benefits as established historically in farming, livestock and medical science. Now, to best ensure control over fat and degenerative/diet-related disease and symptoms, all we must do is show you how *this same proven approach now applies to each of us personally.*

### A Closer Look

The most underlying undeniable scientific fact is that you must see for yourself that: YOU ARE ABSOLUTELY NOT WHAT YOU EAT and that YOUR BODY DOES NOT merely take from food ONLY what it needs and dump the rest.

This overtly outdated idea is a completely obsolete tribal theory totally out of place in a mega-diversified, rapidly changing world. What all the research has proven over and over again after measuring millions of people's nutritional chemistry is: *you only are what you __retain__* from what you eat, drink, breathe and absorb. This baseline digital measurement is where all wellness begins and ends and it varies greatly from person to person. Once you finally see this clearly for yourself – on your own body— all else will seem like nonsense. Once you finally see this you'll understand just how diet and supplements are the most precisely therapeutic instruments: fully accounted for, measured and complete instead of an overtly generic, fragmented, one-of-each "throw it against the wall and see if it'll stick" proposition as generic non-science maintains. After what you learn here, you'll never look at diet or supplementation in the same way again.

Based on your own specific nutrient and toxic retention profile, *Your Personal Life* allows you to engineer a new metabolism for yourself – accelerate a slow metabolism or slow down a fast—one that effectively burns every bite of food like never before and in turn creates an abundance of energy. You can create a metabolism that you will precisely understand and control for maximum fat burning and health and energy gain - achieved at the same time - without any guesswork. Furthermore, your new metabolism is then based upon a direct measurement of up-to-the-moment metabolic efficiency in its relation to nutrient imbalances and toxic infiltrations. Every one of us can easily control this nutrition/toxic phenomenon once we know what our actual numbers are, when we've taken a measurement. What's going on inside your body cells is really all that matters, and being its own unique design, it describes a metabolic fingerprint of exactly what nutrients and toxins your body is actually retaining from the foods that you consume - a baseline from which the possibilities for a better body and life are limitless.

Herein lies the secret to health results every time, no longer to be ignored by the conventional diet and supplement market and its clearly outdated philosophies. The nutritional insights in *Your Personal Life* go light years beyond the already obsolete metabolic-blood-sensory-constitutional-endocrine-oxidizer-acid/alkaline-parasympathetic/sympathetic-genotrophic-organ-soma and bio-typing nonsense promoted in a large number of best-selling books. These books do not personalize nutrition according to the "you are what you retain" principles. We'll examine their surprising shortcomings further for comparison's sake in the upcoming chapters. *Your Personal Life* actually updates Ayurvedic, Chinese, Egyptian, Greek (Hippocrates) medicine – and all others, before or after, with cause-and-effect science well beyond the comprehension of any who've come before in the entire history of medicine.

## Reality Check #2
### The Dream is Real

It's a dream come true. Thanks to the orthomolecular science behind the information in *Your Personal Life* you are going to learn how to feed your genes perfectly and quickly repair faulty, fat-and-disease building/energy-robbing metabolism like never before by using precise nutrient measurements and proven lifestyle manipulations as your guides. The personalized nutrition plan specifically outlines foods and food families along with accentuated therapeutic supplements as your wellness tools – for your body only.

We all know that the world is round and not flat. With the same scientific insight, a huge paradigm shift is upon us as we quickly move into the final mega-trend of health, energy, and fat control ultra personalized to the most discriminating levels. Now you will understand why the over-fat, disease-ridden, degenerative body/mind epidemic can become a thing of the past—thanks to the same science and technology that has made other aspects of life so much better in so many other ways. Now, because of the most recent user-friendly technology, it's time for the frustration of fat loss and disease prevention to be released and traded in for guidance and self-control. *Your Personal Life* is a "do" book – get ready to take positive action and change your life. You will change the way you think about how to create complete health. You will be given a step-by-step plan and reality checks along the way. What you will learn is based completely upon the medical nutrition scientific root idea of self-knowledge unique to each person and integrates all that is known about naturalism (understanding and applying the perfect dynamic synergy between one's genetic set and one's available environment). This is our map in our quest for the healthiest, fittest, leanest, longest, highest quality life possible. Although *Your Personal Life* correlates all known physics, chemistry, genetic and metabolic science as applied to humans, we bring it to everyone in the most easy to understand, commonsense, graspable terms imaginable.

**6**

Say goodbye to make-believe health. ***Your Personal Life*** introduces a reality check in the final mega-trend of nutrition-based, high energy, low-body-fat, age-inhibiting wellness. It's time to change what we think we know about health – it's time for a better way to be well.

Dr. Greg Tefft
Founder, Personalized Nutrition Consultants
November 2005

# Chapter I

## Real Health is Scientifically Proven

*We often spend so much time coping with problems along
our path that we only have a dim or even inaccurate
view of what's really important to us.*
- Peter Senge

### Reality Check #3
### The World is Changing so Rapidly,
### We're Leaving Our Good Health Behind

### Everything has changed

Our routine way of life is so different from just a decade ago, especially
in the U.S. The way we go about our 21st century day to day survival,
the pace, the electronics and the actual environmental conditions under
which we live are moving further away from our ancestors' way of life
and natural environment than ever before in human history. Our parents, grandparents and great grandparents *never* experienced the rapid
rate of lifestyle changes that we do today, aside from natural disasters. We
call this change "progress," and it has accelerated so rapidly that the typical way of life of just a short time ago is already old-fashioned, inconvenient and even primitive to many in our current generation. No cell
phones, computers, Internet, frozen food, fast food, cars, digital movies,
microwaves; young and old alike wonder, "How did we live without
them!?" We need to ask, "How do we live **with** them?" As professor of
medicine at the University of Massachusetts Medical School, Jon Kabat-
Zinn says, "Our whole society has ADD."

We've rapidly shifted away from a close relationship to the land, to our families (there are more families falling apart now than ever before) and to the natural order of life, into a more progressively compartmentalized version of living. This shift began as we've gone from a more family oriented and originally tribal micro rural existence into a macro urban one – all made possible because of big advancements so easily accessible through technology and conveniences. We've become quite capable of creating a very comfortable disconnection from ourselves, each other, the land, our food, our environment and our higher purpose. We've inadvertently disconnected ourselves from our roots. Technology and social progress has ensured that we now effortlessly have shelter, food, drink, clothes, transportation, and communication with others – all at our fingertips. Once upon a time, we had to grow, raise or hunt our own food, prepare food from scratch in appliance-free kitchens, build and repair our own houses, hand-clean our clothes (sometimes in a nearby stream), go to the family or community well for water, walk or ride our horse or wagon to our destinations, make our own clothes, and have to be very physically active in order to even accomplish the most basic tasks. The mail was central to communication, small town meetings and social gatherings were big news, home doctor visits (virtually unheard of now) were common and operator-assisted phones were few and far between. These days are often called the "the good old days." But a proper comprehension of even some of our most recent past is being buried by the current information overload. Today, accomplishing these same basic living tasks (shelter /food/communication) is almost spontaneous, requiring little or no physical effort at all, just money, oil and electricity. Walking is almost a thing of the past as we sit forever driving cars, in our workplaces and then vegging out while eating fast food in front of our computer and the TV, instead of farming the soil, hunting for dinner, hands-on raising our families, hauling water, feeding the horses and other livestock, composting garbage, bartering service and products, participating at community gatherings or helping our neighbors pick the latest apple harvest or build a barn.

Regular exercise is now easily thought of as a high-tech product that you have to purchase, since our schools no longer offer adequate physical education. Typically we travel to a special exercise place or perhaps it can be done at home in front of the TV again, with special equipment that we buy. Of course, enough free time to exercise is another rarity in the **over-busy, overweight** ADD world we've created. As we've shifted so quickly into a new fast-paced electronic convenience lifestyle, we've also created a harmful and toxic natural environment. There are more man-made toxic residues to be found everywhere than ever before, including in our bodies. The water found in the open wilderness, what little wilderness is left, is no longer safe to drink, it's tainted just like the air and soil. This **toxic explosion** has been magnified because of our **technological advancement.** A profits-above-all-else mentality and how-do-we-makes-ends-meet reality has turned our free time into work at home. We don't make time for ourselves or our families and loved ones, we're living in a pressure-cooker world of 24/7 connectivity in an unprecedented era of information overload.

### *Where Does This Leave Us?*

The air we breathe, the water we drink, pressure we labor under, the neighbors that we try to keep up with, and the foods we eat are very different from generations before. We've become such a fast-paced, convenience first, instant gratification, limited free time, throw away obsessive ADD society that we've barely noticed the subtle changes in our lives that are turning into big problems. We're creating throw away lives to go with these lifestyle choices and we don't realize that we're undermining our health at its very core – until we're already ill.

Some of us have taken notice and are in fact aware of the toxic environment, improperly nourished/synthetically infused farming topsoil, additive-laden food processing, the hyper fast-living pace, overwork, fast food, and the overall emphasis of convenience-centered quantity as the priority over quality of life. Few of us realize the true and total impact of these things on our basic ability to be healthy. There are many ideas and opinions, but few people have ever made the direct connection between these stresses and their own measured core health status at the most meaningful level: their own bodies.

### *Healthier? Wealthier? Wiser?*
### *We Might Live Longer, but How Do We Feel?*

Are we really becoming healthier, wealthier, and wiser than our parents and their parents? Maybe we know more about more things, but cancer is now the #1 killer of human beings, second to heart disease. The #1 cause of preventable death is smoking, #2 is obesity and #3 is the regular use of properly prescribed prescription drugs. More people die each year in hospitals from illness they contracted while there than in the entire Vietnam war.

And when our overall health is compared to previous generations, no matter what authority is consulted, today the average person is fatter, more fatigued, less fit, less physically active, is ultimately suffering more physical and psychological symptoms and illnesses, has less patience and more attention-deficit disorders, is more dependent on prescription and nonprescription drugs than ever before! We are overly stressed and in the midst of an outright epidemic—an epidemic due to a bombardment of time-sensitive survival requirements we're entangled in to rush through and keep up with a very complicated daily existence. As a society, we are losing our perspective on the importance of a properly balanced life as we strive to negotiate the exceedingly complex pitfalls of a modern pressure cooker society gone technologically wild. Ultimately, we are literally blindsided by a media system that commercializes everything including prescription drugs, and we've given birth to an entertainment culture that has taken the place of good reading habits. We have all inadvertently participated in creating an explosive modern way of life which at the most primal human levels is causing the intensive accumulation of progressively harmful stress—which has largely gone unnoticed. But now *it must be addressed on all levels*—physical, chemical, and emotional— before we damage ourselves even further.

## Reality Check #4
### Is The "O" Factor Getting to You?

The overriding problem still stubbornly persists: we are stuck on **Overwhelm**— just too much to do and process, delivered too fast— a powerfully disruptive stress in itself which day by day, week by week, month by month and year by year is dramatically confusing our understanding of what it really takes to be disease-resistant and radiantly healthful. We're constantly being bombarded and distracted from all angles and as a result, our subsequent ability to make good or informed decisions is either seriously impaired or compromised. There is a blizzard of information and endless demands on our attentions and time. No wonder people hunger for some kind of guideline or other clear-cut reality. The real truth that too many of us find out too late or the hard way is that good health is worth more than all the rest of our wealth and wisdom concerns combined. At every turn we are being commercially seduced away from real and healthy common sense by a huge onslaught of disconnected fragments of substitute, modernized information bombarding us from every conceivable direction. The generalized information promoted has little direct connection to our most important needs at the most fundamental biochemical levels and is an illustration of the dramatic limitations of standard medicine. These limitations are at the core of peoples' hunger for more reality. We tire of undesirable side effects and new and improved. We want real and we want it now.

Now more than ever, we desperately require *the real most specific truth about our innermost selves* in order to make the right decisions in many areas, but most importantly our health.

## Reality Check #5
### Take Control
### No One Can Take Care of You but You

The simple truth remains: you and I must take responsibility for our states of mental and physical health in order to elevate our human health condition. We must never unquestionably depend on others to meet these needs properly, nor make our choices for us. Contrary to what most eager-to-sell-one-of-each and overly seductive media would have us think, there is no special diet, exercise, pill, shot, potion, lotion or surgery which dependably ensures you the kind of health and wellness control that each individual requires. There is no one right way or pill for everyone.

- We're stuck in a country where sickness and drug dependency provides a mammoth profit incentive for the medical/pharmaceutical industry.
- We constantly reward these two groups with progressively more medical visits and drug sales—the sicker and fatter we become the more money they make.
- Unquestionably, medical miracles such as infection-fighting antibiotics, vaccines, and some very special lifesaving surgeries have benefited us, but they truthfully cannot be a substitute for the type of non-germ and non-accident-related health control we truly require for maximum self-assured wellness.

- Most of our most natural good health controls were automatically built into the lifestyles and environments of the past in terms of better food, less toxic environments, more physical activity, less stress and so forth, but now they must be clearly and carefully redefined in an entirely new world where the old fashioned ways of living have been so drastically displaced, left behind and replaced.
- These good health practices are now fancifully referred to as preventive medicine, and this premedicine focus is based on monitoring our health at the most influential levels before we become seriously ill, and then working with our health care guide as a prevention team member—instead of a focus upon multiple doctor visits, drugs, and surgeries after we fall into a serious health crisis.

The medical consequences of our widespread inattention to our own preventive health control focus are embodied in just about every statistic-compiling agency from the Center for Disease Control to the National Institute of Heath. Even the Department of Agriculture and a host of university and congressional reports state:

*We are collectively suffering from a modern epidemic of preventable degenerative disease, which is also referred to as diet and lifestyle-related disease.*

*The U.S. is #1 in the world in health-care spending and no better than $16^{th}$ in positive medical outcomes.*

*40% of people - over 1 in 3 - will contract cancer in 2006 according to the American Cancer Association. In 1912, only 3% had cancer in America.*

*The number of overweight kids in the U.S. has doubled in 20 years.*

This type of slow-acting, progressively building disease exceeds the capacities of conventional life-sparing, infection-fighting medical instruments, which flatly fail to correct these problems at their very source.

### Diet and Lifestyle Disease

Diet and lifestyle is where our "dis-ease" problem exists. It is epidemic in proportions. It's something that *we can control*, with food and nutrition. It is something that *modern medicine* in its present form *does not address.** Some say that these medical instruments – mostly drugs—are a case of the cure being more of a problem than the cause, especially when you consider the vast array of side effects present. Drugs cannot repair nutritional problems. Only nutrition can. We regularly neglect our food and nutrition options until last, or until we are suffering painfully.

Here is the core idea: *diet and lifestyle related disease.*† Something each one of us really can control precisely, an area that modern conventional medicine in its present form cannot control with drugs and/or surgery. And, because we are distracted and overwhelmed by everything else that is pressuring us we ultimately seem to place as a lowest priority.

†*Some simple definitions:*

*DIET-RELATED DISEASE*: Any disease (illness, sickness, uncomfortable symptomatic state, etc.) which is affected by or originally caused by the nutritional and toxic balance found in a given body.

There are two types of diet-related disease:

1. **Indirect diet-related disease**: Diseases primarily caused by an infectious or parasitic process whose severity is affected by the nutritional constitution of the body.
2. **Direct diet-related disease**: Diseases primarily caused by developing nutritional/toxic disturbances, also known as degenerative or chronic disease. Note: there are some **degenerative infectious processes** but the original causative agent in these cases is considered to be more infectious than nutritional, although the outcome is always highly nutrition-related.

---

*Pfizer Corp. said it most obviously in a recent TV ad saying "we're here when a healthy diet and regular exercise aren't enough."

14

**All diet-related disease is affected by:**

*LIFESTYLE-RELATED DISEASE*:  Any disease affected by or caused by the way one lives in terms of work, leisure, play, posture and diet.
*ENVIRONMENTAL DISEASE*:  All of the above variables of diet and lifestyle in conjunction with a consideration of the overall impact of air, water, food, soil, farming/processing/storage methodology, climate, living/working environment, stress, social structure on disease and/or genetic structure.
*GENE-RELATED DISEASE*:  Any disease directly caused by weaknesses in one's genetic structure and/or any/all aspects of diet, lifestyle and environment which exceed the capacity of the genes to metabolically maintain wellness.

For those who consider diet-related disease as a higher priority in life and do really want to take decisive anti-disease preventive action, there is an overwhelming onslaught of media-obsessed self-help information to sort through, information that is supposed to help us to eat and supplement better, exercise more efficiently and control our lifestyle more appropriately. Some of this information is very useful, but much of it is categorically what scientists refer to as "non-science" or nonsense. This non-science, fads, fantasies, unproven theories, junk science, magic pills/potions/lotions/gimmicks and downright delusional fiction, overwhelmingly permeates the self-help, fitness and wellness world. Self-help information technology is changing as rapidly as the rest of our lives, forcing us to try to keep up with the latest trend in the hopes of attaining superior health and fitness results. Still, the majority of people trying to help themselves, other than those using some generic seemingly beneficial guidelines, really are not sure without a scientific doubt—measurably and proven—that they are really making the right choices when it comes to the most discriminating specifics of diet, detoxification, supplements, stress management and of course, exercise. The *right choices* in these preventive areas will ensure independence from drugs and doctors without question. It's now time to stop being distracted from the truth, time to stop feeling like we're always playing catch up to the latest wellness developments.  It's time to stop relying upon and guessing about inappropriate medical and commercial approaches to solving our purely nutritional, toxin and lifestyle dilemmas. There really is a better way to be sure about the choices you make in the pursuit of superior health. There is a better way to be well.

## A New You in a New World—Genes versus Environment
### The Whole Story

*Reality Check #1 Revisited*: The introduction section of this text gently touches upon what each of us can actually do about our modern wellness dilemmas in order to decisively catch up with the biochemical truths about the deepest disturbances within our body from which all demonstrable health problems arise. In effect, we can pick up where standard medicine actually leaves off. And having this knowledge, we can then know exactly what to do about these problems in ways that we can take action ourselves. Simply put, these problems can easily be solved with new developments in human-direct science and technology. But *first we must make a total paradigm shift* in our perception of these fundamental problems. Secondly, in order to see exactly how these problems can be efficiently resolved, *we must graduate to a purely scientific procedure*, with all guesswork eliminated, once and for all. Anything less and we'll never overcome our modern diet-related disease plague – it will just intensify further. To reach our own starting points from which all modern wellness reformatting begins, we first have to truly understand two central scientifically validated concepts. First and foremost: *you are __not__ what you eat, drink, breathe, and absorb.*

In modern society, it has been scientifically determined that your body simply does not take what it needs most from food and drink and then simply dumps the rest as previously believed. This tribe-only idea has been scientifically proven to be a completely outdated philosophy in modern melting-pot societies due to the presence of more *diverse* genetic pools, radically *changed* environment (including food availability) and drastically *altered* ways of life—with *intensified stress* levels to contend with.

Instead, science has indisputably determined that *you are what you ultimately retain* from what you eat, drink, breathe once it's inside—if it's good or bad, nutritionally synergized or not, chemically balanced or unbalanced, healthy or very unhealthy. The best news regarding this newer, updated scientific truth is that, in fact, there is a mammoth system of clinical science and technology devoted to completely uncovering the deepest nutritionally environmental and lifestyle-correctable problems. Then, as we are presented with the most scientifically valid solutions the world has ever seen, we are more capable than ever of making the right choices based on this data. The existence of this science, called orthomolecular medicine, is predicated upon a hidden conflict that we've taken for granted, until now.

In essence, Orthomolecular Medicine contends that the greatest health-robbing conflict we face is that *people are not efficiently retaining* and utilizing perfect proportions of the essential nutrients from food needed to maximize lifespan and minimize disease anymore. Mistakenly, we've been led to believe that our genes through their biochemical processing instrument, known as metabolism, automatically sort nutrients and toxins for perfect wellness. But this is simply not the case as statistically demonstrated person by person, time and time again. The ultimate reason for this undesirable phenomenon can clearly be found when you consider the role of genes, the environment and the overall process of natural selection.

Politically, the open diet, nutrition and wellness market conveniently chooses to ignore these scientific facts and will continue to do so as long as you and I let them get away with this deception by continuing to buy supplements and fad diets indiscriminately. Subsequently, all of our ills are directly connected to this one truth about human life: the less conflict between one's genes and their chosen environment, the greater the health potential. The more correct environmental choices (food, drink, etc.) that one makes which are keeping in alignment with the genetic design, the greater one's health potential or ability to survive as the naturalist Darwin said. Conversely, the fewer correct choices we make, the less chance for good health. Simply put, your own genetic set is inherited from your ancestors as directly shaped and conditioned by the forces of nature, in other words, the impending environments we will subject ourselves to. What exactly your ancestors ate, drank, breathed and did—such as work-play-family, etc., is programmed into your genes.

Unfortunately you cannot go back to their way of life so that your genes can automatically receive the influences that they're most used to historically—the actual food, drink, air, climate and so forth. However, the more that you can re-create these most perfect conditions for your own genes – the more perfect your life and health will be.

Natural Selection, also known as (healthy) survival of the fittest, has two variables:

1. How well your genes are transmitting your ancestor's blueprinted life experiences to you as your own specific and innate constitutional strength.

2. To what degree your particular environment and lifestyle choices are synergistic (matched) or conversely—antagonistic (mismatched) to your genetic design. Exceed your ancestor-given genetic capacity to adapt to a changing environment and you will degenerate into mediocre health and disease very rapidly as your body's operational status rapidly declines.

**This means that when there is greater gene-to-environment antagonism you will be more susceptible to sickness; a shorter, unhealthier lifespan; and less energy. In fact, too much antagonism between environmental influences and genetic set can actually damage the genes themselves and DRAMATICALLY shorten lifespan to boot.** In fact, the ones who survive the best are those who have the strongest genetic constitution* to begin with, and who do not conduct their lives (eat, drink, work, play, etc.) or expose themselves to environmental influences that their genes simply cannot handle due to antagonistic mismatching.

GOOD GENETICS + SYNERGISTIC INTERNAL/EXTERNAL
ENVIRONMENTS
is the direct road to the **Healthiest/Longest Survival Rate**

### *Genetic Signature VS. Genetic Expression–The Inside Story*

Genetic Signature (genotype) is what your body actually wants (defined as specifically as possible) from the environment for total health perfection. Genetic expression (Phenotype) is what your body actually receives from the external environment and is able to functionally sort out successfully or unsuccessfully (adaptation). In more technical terms, genetic signature is called genotype whereas genetic expression is called phenotype; *the greater the difference between signature and expression, the lesser the chance for survival.*

Genetic expression should be considered as your up-to-the moment internal environment based upon what it is exposed to from the external environment. The more one exposes his/her body to constant imbalances of food, drink, emotional stress, body management (hygiene), toxins, and

*least-inherited genetic flaws

activity which it cannot perfectly adapt/adjust to, the more genetic expression will be different than genetic signature. Your gene's fixed ability to adjust your body to what is exposed to it is the limitation. *The larger the difference between genetic signature and expression, the greater the chance for all illness, premature aging, energy deficits and lower quality of life to set in.* This occurs simply because the body's actual operational state becomes dysfunctional from too much environmental antagonism which it cannot healthfully itself to. The stressful imbalances of environment that it has been exposed to are just too much for it to handle healthfully. A state of maladjustment or maladaptation is the basis for natural selection. Those who cannot adapt properly always die younger and are more diseased. Those who achieve the greatest synergy between what their genes ideally want and what the environment actually delivers always enjoy the longest, most energetic, healthiest lives possible. The operation of their bodies are always able to be functionally adaptable because *genetic limitations are never exceeded.*

Natural selection contends that only the strongest survive, and those who are strongest and therefore most likely to survive have two redeeming features:
1. A genetic set with the fewest flaws (self-induced or inherited) or what we sometimes call mutations.
2. The least difference between genetic signature and genetic expression or, in effect, are making the most genetically compatible environmental choices in the pursuit of life.

Example: Building a better house is like building a better body.

When you compare a house to the human body it becomes plain to see what genes, environment, and natural selection are all about. Building a house takes several steps:
1. Architect designs the house.
2. Builders assemble the house according to the building materials suggested and the way shown to fit them together by the architect.

### Best House
Most-proven architectural design
Highest-quality construction materials
Assembled closest to plan

*Result*
Beautiful, comfortable, earthquake-fire-flood-lightening-resistant/weatherproof/low-upkeep house that lasts and lasts.
*Worst House*
Least-proven design
Lowest-quality construction materials
Assembled in a shortcut sloppy manner
*Result*
The money pit, or a house that falls apart/breaks down constantly and collapses with the first earthquake or physical stress.

**Body comparison:**

*Better Body*
Most-proven (over time) genetic design
Highest-quality nutrients taken in the right proportions exactly according to design
*Result*
A body that lives longer, resists disease and fat buildup better and reliably provides maximum energy release over time
*Worst Body*
Least-proven or most-flawed genetic design
Lowest-quality nutrition with the least adherence to genetic design*
requirements from the environment and the pursuit of life
*Result*
Short life, increased fat deposition, fatigue and sickness

### The Source of All Disease—The Secret Unfolding

*Reality Check #1* revisited yet again: According to geneticists Crawford and Marsh, food is king over all.

### Human Extinction Caused From Eating Wrong—Is it Possible?

Our most serious ongoing problem of a debilitating modern-day diet and degenerative disease epidemic only persists and intensifies because our genetic designs from the past cannot cope with the amount or rate

*not eating or living the way your genes require

of current environmental changes (especially diet), that we are exposed to which are less than perfect for each one of us in the present.

For example, if we were building a house, it would be like changing all of the building materials available to the house builders and designers *overnight* without fully discussing the differences or consequences for everyone concerned. Until the house builders and designers are able to catch up with these changes and their meaning to the total design, the houses that they build at first will fall apart more easily, until the passage of time allows them to better analyze, experiment with or experience the perfect combination of new materials to again ensure the most durable houses. But time may run out before the earthquake hits.

In human terms, this means that when you change the environmental influences or construction materials (food, water, air, lifestyle, etc.) too quickly for the genes to catch up or keep up (adapt), your only reward is deviation of genetic expression from the primal genetic design, which in turn leads to human earthquakes, aka more sickness, fatness, shorter life spans and a notably lower quality of life. This is happening in the U.S., unrelentingly. Additionally, geneticists and anthropologists completely agree repeatedly in distinguishing *food* out of all the other external environmental variables as **the most impacting and controllable environmental force overall.**

As a poignant example of this, two prominent geneticists – Michael Crawford, PhD, and Michael Marsh PhD, compiled a book: *The Driving Force – Food, Evolution and the Future,* which clearly conveys this point. After an extensive review of all pertinent genetic, social, anthropological and evolutionary research, they postulated that "food is the driving force that has molded the shape of the species as well as the limiting force that has fixed lines of selection." They also observed that today, in our society, food is of such a commonplace nature that it is taken for granted and its qualitative relationship with long-term biological considerations is overlooked. They additionally expressed the concern that the historical changes in disease patterns, the contrast in disease incidence from country to country, and the socioeconomic contrast between countries definitively demonstrate that we are witnessing a signal of the **power of food as <u>the</u> most dominant factor in all evolution.** This means that all other environmental considerations take a back seat to food.

## *Food is King*

According to Beatrice Trum Hunter from the *Townsend Letter,* Crawford and Marsh's findings "pose serious questions as to the impact of present-day food and agricultural policies on immediate and future generations." Crawford and Marsh believe that "among other follies, agricultural practices have emphasized yields stressing quantity rather than quality." *Nutrition has not been a prime goal.*

A good example can be seen in animal feeding practices. Both the protein and nutrient values of farm animal food products have been diluted by fat as compared to free-ranging wild animals who categorically have lower body fat values. These geneticists and many others have noted that food has always been a crucial factor in shaping life's evolutionary processes on this planet from the very earliest time when life first emerged on Earth up to the present, and that this will continue into the future. According to these scientists, food, nutrition, and diet can no longer take a back seat in the creation of good health. In fact, it already occupies the front seat whether we acknowledge it or not. In reference to the human body, there is one additional factor, which compounds this inferior construction food-first dilemma problem even further: Our widespread lack of attention to the finer points of our genetic blueprint at the most critical and controllable points of nutrition has been philosophically covered up by the one-size-fits-all, convenience-first philosophy of buy-today-discard-tomorrow wellness achievement being massively promoted by the media and the open market.

Our failure in providing human bodies with their exact environmental needs, especially qualitative nourishment on the most discriminating levels according to person-specific degrees (personalization), what we need to become our healthiest and maintain each body that way, has been completely ignored in favor of the idea that "what's good for you is good for me." This commonplace practice is most easily seen in the current wave of diet and supplement sharing among people. According to the marketplace, you are supposed to be convinced that what seems to work for one person will work equally well for you. Our genetic pool diversity is simply too great to support this notion and it shows in all our illnesses. As a result, generic one-size-fits-all nonsense (or non-science philosophy) pervades the diet, supplement and even medical industries. Personalization as represented by these sources is only superficial at best and not valid at the most critical levels. To a house-builder, one size fits all is as if we were treating all of our bodies as though we were the same set of tract houses. We each are far too unique (as are non-tract houses) to accept this unresourceful idea, but the average person just doesn't know it yet or mistakes what they are led to believe about generic nutrition as personalization and the real thing. It clearly is not. You are truly unique, no two people are perfectly alike, and this must be addressed precisely on the levels of nutrient retention because nowhere else matters.

**The following table represents all the ways that we have been scientifically determined to be different:**

## TABLE OF UNIQUENESS

### EXTERNAL DIFFERENCES

Height, weight, hair distribution on body, hair texture and color, degree of baldness, skin thickness, skin activity, skin color, skin oil content, body shape, head and face shape, muscularity, bone size, retinal image, eye color, size of eyes, size and shape of teeth, finger and toe shape and size, length and proportion of limbs and torso, fingerprints, aura, and body odor.

### PSYCHOLOGICAL DIFFERENCES

Mental and emotional activity levels, emotions, beliefs, values, attitudes, personality, intelligence quotients (IQ), interests, likes and dislikes, behavior and energy levels, quickness of thought, intuition, and dream states.

### INTERNAL DIFFERENCES

Size and shape of all internal organs including brains, bones, muscles, glands, stomach, intestines, etc.; quantity and composition of enzymes, hormones, vitamins, minerals, amino acids, fatty acids; blood type, composition and pressure; pulse rate; systemic and organic strengths and weaknesses; pain threshold; taste reactions; pH; digestive, absorptive, utilization; detoxification and elimination patterns; anabolism and catabolism rates, toxin presence; number of body cells; cell division rates; cellular metabolism; chemical composition of tissues and tissue amount, oxidation rates and efficiency; genetic structure (DNA); fertility rates; and menstrual cycles.

Understanding the above information as it relates to nutrition is a development of Dr. Roger Williams' original research and is the primary focus of orthomolecular medicine. In the case of the house, without knowing exactly what the original blueprints says or exactly which level of quality and material integration was put into effect, we can literally disassemble the house to find out what's present. But when it comes to the living human body it's simply not so easy to figure things out because it's much more difficult to see what the genes actually say or what the body's building materials are actually made of at the atomic/molecular/biochemical level. It's even more difficult to find out exactly how it's all functioning together before a medically diagnosable disease or recognizable condition actually appears.

Obtaining and therapeutically implementing this foundational scientific information is the primary focus of *Your Personal Life* and is something that standard medicine and diet/nutrition/lifestyle practices have completely glossed over. It begins with revisiting *Reality Check #1*—you are *not* what you eat, drink, breathe and absorb. *You are what you retain* from what you eat, and this differs from person to person. No two people are exactly the same outside or inside at any given moment – ever.

*Example:* Two people can both eat one half of the same orange. The actual amount of vitamin C and potassium found inside their body after eating and metabolizing (digesting, absorbing, utilizing and eliminating waste) will be different for each person and it will have a different effect upon their health.

Why? Because the nutrients that go in may or may not stay in and be used by the body properly due to:

1. Variable nutrient deficiencies, excesses, antagonisms and toxins already present in the body, which have an effect on how food is utilized.
2. The relationship of one's genetic expression to his or her genetic signature; in other words, retention depends on exactly where your genes stand at the moment in relation to nutritional and health outcomes.

These two preceding scientifically validated facts clearly dismantle the notion of one-size-fits-all nutrition and diet. But there is a much deeper relationship to disease that needs to be clarified in order to demonstrate the source of directly diet-related disease.

## The Source of Disease

After nutritionally examining literally millions of already medically diagnosed sick people using comparative statistical clinical science to closely compare results with the help of geneticists, chemists, physicists and mathematicians, a startling revelation was discovered. Each diet- related disease has its own unique nutrient/toxic profile. In other words, highly specific nutritional and toxic disturbances have been identified, which then were associated with each and every disease. But which came first, the nutritional disorder or a particular disease?

## The Chicken and the Egg

Which came first, the nutritional and toxic disorder or the disease disorder it's actually associated with? A simple guess—the nutritional disturbance itself always precedes the disease, even in gene-related disease, which it's associated with. From this clinical truth we have derived two ultimate reality checks. The first one is:

### Ultimate Reality Check #1
**Nutritional disturbances progressively intensifying over time create and promote all degenerative/chronic disease and hamper the healing process from infection or injury.**

Whether we refer to *Benefits From Nutrition,* (a 21-year-long government study), any journal of applied nutrition, the latest laboratory diagnosis book or leading health authority on this subject, it is scientifically proven that:

- All disease is diet-related and there are specific associations between nutrients, toxins and diseases.
- As stated on page 1–2 of *An Evaluation of Research in the United States on Human Nutrition—Report No. 2 Benefits from Nutrition Research:* "The solution to illness can be found in nutrition."
- Most importantly from the study above and multitudes of others, when you precisely correct the pertinent nutritional disturbances found, "you can defer or modify the development of a disease state."

- The Report also states, "Better health, a longer lifespan and greater satisfaction from work, family and leisure time are some of the benefits from improved nutrition."

In effect, our leading scientists are convinced that nutritional disturbances come first, disease comes second. The sooner and more accurately we correct nutritional disturbances, the more diseases are prevented or resolved by natural healing processes. Even if we've inherited a genetic defect, we can still improve upon it or even prevent it if we've created the defect in our own lifetime.

Clinical science and technology has provided two steps to this natural process:

1. The exact detection of all nutritional and toxic disturbances.
2. The precise correction of all nutrition and toxic disturbances.

These two steps applied in conjunction with only one theme—scientifically proven on the individual," not someone else or averaged from statistics. This brings us to "Ultimate Reality Check #2":

*Ultimate Reality Check #2*
**All that really matters to your health is measuring
the particular nutritional and toxic
disturbances in their totality, found in your body only,
and the exact plan to correct imbalances found
in each individual case.**

*Fatter, Weaker, Sicker, Stressed, Shorter Lives—Who is
Accountable?*

A generation of fatter, lower-energy, shorter-living, more stressed out, less physically fit, sicker, more fast food and drug dependent, toxin-infested humans is what we have, all due to hyper progress. This is complete with substandard human physical makeup and inferior philosophies in a "sell first, ask questions later" sales environment. Compounding this is a one-size-fits-all mentality and enough high turnover fads to last many more generations—especially as they're found in diets, supplements and other highly influenced lifestyle variables.

All this goes on with no true understanding about what it actually takes to correctly choose the proper external environmental input—especially food or to reliably balance the internal environment with full accountability – instead of guesswork. The overall wellness market provides no true accountability, no real assessment for the human condition at the levels where accountability counts the most: external environmental considerations. This market has no before-and-after measurement of what their products and services do to your unique inner environment, good or bad, truly healthy or not. Is it any wonder people can't seem to stay well and be fit even when they really want to? orthomolecular medicine is so powerful because it provides the most comprehensive accountability available. And, it puts each person in the driver's seat for their own success.

### *The Tug-of-War Begins*

Experiencing the fastest healing process and the healthiest, fittest, longest life possible is totally based on a tug-of-war between what's inside of you and what choices you are exposed to and make from the outside.

***Food is always the most dominant variable.*** It adds up to either a more balanced or imbalanced metabolism. The more balanced, the greater one's health, the less balanced, the greater the illness that is inevitable. Good or bad health is always in the balance:

**What's outside    ← TUG →    Health    ← TUG →    What's inside**

Radiant wellness is all about a better self-understanding and the precise choices which must be made in the name of well-being, person by unique person. The less guesswork, faddism, false presumptions, unproven theory, corporate sales rhetoric, politics and even incorrect instincts we expose ourselves to, the more scientifically correct our choices will be. We always start with nutrition which is the dominant factor in making or breaking our health and how well we will be in this life. When we are true to our genes, our genes will be automatically true to us. We're guaranteeing a better life of radiant health and longevity. We will survive as the ***strongest and fittest*** under these inclusive and ***most vital*** circumstances.

The implications of these ultimate reality checks and just how willing you are to enter the tug-of-war for supreme health are the secrets to radiant health in modern-day society and provide the essence of this book. Medical testing has taken the guesswork out of medicine. Now, nutritional testing takes the guesswork out of nutrition. Welcome to the most important and real diet secret of *Your Personal Life*.

# Chapter II

## A Good Life or a Painful Premature Death
## A New Movie Script for Life

*There are no riches above a sound body.*
—Apocrypha

We need a new vision of how we create health. Now, the movie we see in our head is: "I'm sick. I go to the doctor. He fixes me."

The new version of how to see our health is: "I'm well. I go to the doctor. We work together and I do more to help myself because the doctor really can't.

We need to replace old thinking with new thinking, old doing with new actions.

You are what you eat must be changed to: You are what you *retain* (hold onto) from what you eat.

It's what's inside that counts must be changed to: It's *knowing* what's inside that counts.

Survival of the fittest must be changed to: Survival of the *most inclusive*.

We need to include new ideas and new more effective ways of doing things if we want new and better results, especially when it comes to our health and wellness.

28

### *What Do You Want?*

Do you want to live long? Do you want to lose weight? Do you want more energy? Do you want to be beautiful? Do you want to build your body's muscles? Do you want better digestion? Do you want lower cholesterol or blood pressure, cleaner arteries, better mental clarity, more sleep?

What have you been doing to achieve these health results? How are they working? How can you tell if they're working? Or not?

### *How Do You Know What You Need to Get What You Want?*

When we start to ask these basic questions, we realize with thundering truth, we don't know how illness or health is created for each individual person. We have never scientifically measured (we can't, if we don't know what they are) these mystery pieces to know our health status and most importantly, what we biochemically and nutritionally need to heal or create health.

### *Where Do You Get What You Need?*
### *What Garden are You Eating From?*

So, what do you need then, to be your most radiantly healthy and long-lived? Do you subscribe to a health newsletter to find out? Do you read books on diet and health? Do you take a multivitamin? If so, why? Who recommended your health products? Why did they recommend them? Have you ever measured what was in those products? Can you tell if they're helping you or not? How can you tell?

### *Is It Worth the Effort?*

You'll pay for your health now or you'll pay for your health later. This is part of the new vision of creating health we want to be aware of. We can either continue eating what we eat, taking the vitamins we think are good for us and sifting through the confusion of all the health information, or we can do something different. Doing something different always takes some effort, at least to start. Maintaining any routine takes some effort to keep it going but in the end it's entirely worth it. Creating radiant health is no different and we need to know that this effort is part of how we will be successful at living longer, losing weight, having more energy, lowering our blood pressure, and avoiding illness and degenerative diseases of all kinds.

If you'd rather not make this effort, and I ask you to consider this very seriously, then I suggest that this book and its suggested plan of action are not for you.

### *The Right Approach is Everything*

The exact way that we approach nutrition and diet will determine the outcomes, desirable or undesirable, but there is one fundamental difference. The essence of this most critical difference can be found simply by taking a closer look at what the words diet and nutrition really mean for us.

### *DIET*

***Definition:*** The science of what you consume with ***no direct accountability*** for what nutrients and toxins are actually in what you \*consume or absorb nor what is left in your body and how it is utilized by the body.

***Approach:*** In order to help organize an eating program, people ***try*** different one-size-fits-all types of diets and supplements based on government MDR, RDA, DV statistical recommendations; Blood Types; Zones; low carb/high fat and protein models (Atkins); modified food fasts; high fiber/raw food/macrobiotic programs; vegetarian plans; questionnaire-based metabolic typing systems, etc.

***Results: Very difficult to determine*** at the deepest metabolic, glandular and cellular levels. Superficially, a few pounds/inches may be lost or gained as measured on a weight scale or measuring tape, some symptoms may diminish or increase perhaps by coincidence only and some energy may be gained or lost as a matter of subjectivity, perhaps.

***Primary Problem: No dependable scientific accountability*** for what is really occurring chemically inside at the core levels of metabolism as to whether or not nutritional rebalancing is really taking place. This means that the ***Scientific Accountability Rating*** or ***SAR*** \*\* is low (or nonexistent)

\*(What you eat, breathe, drink, and even absorb through your skin, nose and mouth and other openings are considered what you consume).
\*\*SAR is used as a classification to assist our understanding of the apparent degree of clinical truth as applied to diet and nutritional systems.

as far as being true to the scientific principle "you are what you retain from what you eat."

*Secondary Problem:* Statistically there are more people with diet-related, degenerative disease, including obesity, than ever before in U.S. history. This is simply because people are not accounting for the most toxic and nutritional variables at their very sources inside and outside of the body.

*Future Prediction:* Persisting in any diet only approach to the way that we eat and drink and breathe will only ensure an increased incidence of 223+ diet-related (direct and indirect) diseases, obesity, bothersome symptoms, allergies, hormonal upsets, psychological dysfunction, genetic destruction, and fatigue. This will include shortened high quality life spans, greater drug dependencies, and perhaps the early extinction of the human race as postulated by the geneticists Crawford and Marsh or if not, very possibly the extinction of a *quality* life.

## NUTRITION

*Definition: The science of what is measured* in a given food, supplement, water, or air as compared to what that particular body actually retains. This is as a function of digestion, absorption, utilization, and elimination from what is consumed. This measurement shows *what a body actually retains from what is consumed.*

*Approach:* People self-apply governmental RDAs, MDRs, DVs, Food Pyramids and other generically averaged diet/supplement statistical guidelines. These are all derived from averages from special nutrition tests performed on test subjects in order to determine what is retained in the bodies of the test subjects after eating certain foods and drink that have also been nutritionally tested for content. Generalized statistical averages are computed from the conglomeration of these tests on others and have been delivered to us by government compiling agencies such as the Food and Nutrition Council.

*Results: Very difficult to determine for any given person <u>not tested directly.</u>* These are much like the exact problems encountered with diet results whereby the statistics that apply to others cannot possibly apply to you because each person is so highly unique in what they nutritionally retain. Plus, nutrient retention in food varies so widely, at an all-time historical high, which further complicates this scientific scenario.

*Primary Problem: Each person is completely unique.* This means that no two people are alike in the way that their body retains nutrients, and therefore these generic statistical guidelines, generated from other people, are not specific enough for any given individual. Plus, there is *no scientific accountability* for results using this information. The *SAR* is not significantly greater than that for diet in consideration of any one particular individual.

*Secondary Problem:* Same problems as diet—more diet-related disease and all the problems that go along with it.

*Future Prediction:* Increased disease and obesity states, greater loss of quality life amongst people, increased drug dependence as time progresses, and much greater confusion about what exactly to do in order to remedy these problems.

### *Personalized Nutrition*
### *aka Orthomolecular Nutritional Medicine*

*Definition*: The science of what *each unique body actually retains* from what is directly consumed by that body.

*Approach: Each person is tested directly* for the nutrients and toxins that their unique body is retaining at the moment. Then a *medically proven*, completely customized diet and supplement program is designed and instituted to correct any metabolic, toxic or nutritional disturbances found.

*Results: Precisely determined every time.* Retests are taken to examine and asses one's progress and to troubleshoot any problem areas found at the deepest cellular levels. The SAR is 100%.

*Primary Problem: None.* Each person is directly tested whereby nutrient and toxic disturbances are detected and nutritionally corrected with full accountability for all results at the deepest biochemical and genetic levels.

*Secondary Problem: None.* Personalized nutrition was specifically developed to end all diet-related disease and obesity for each and every one of us at our own personal levels and pace of life.

*Future Prediction:* The end of nutrition-related problems over time; less disease, more energy, more effective prevention, greater mentality, less body fat accumulation, better sex life, *greater peak performance in all of life's pursuits.*

### *Personalized Nutrition Against Disease*

The seminal book, "Nutrition Against Disease," by Dr. Roger Williams, who's considered to be the Godfather of personalized nutrition, proposes that we use the measurable information about nutrition on the inside of our body in conjunction with what we consume from the outside as a therapeutic weapon against all disease, as well as shortened lifespan, over fat problems and poor quality lifestyle.

Over 55 years ago, at the time Dr. Williams conducted his research and wrote his many books on the subject of biochemical individuality, the technology for applying the principles which he discovered for each individual was not available to the general public. But now it's convenient enough, technologically refined enough, affordable enough, medically proven enough (as a result of the millions of dollars of unrelenting research and cross-referencing that's been done by our most advanced medical laboratories) and simplified enough to positively impact each and every one of us with consistent, measurable readings. Were he alive today to see this wonderful dream of world health coming true, I suspect he would be one of the most fulfilled scientists on Earth. The greatest medicine of all is within arms reach and all we need to know to use this natural gift is to ***first find out*** what's inside of our internal environment and then make the most perfect matches from the external environment. These are the same external to internal environmental matches that synergistically promote our genetic signature for now and future generations. This scientific process brings the concentrated focus and power of physics, mathematics, and chemistry onto our own bodies.

### How Does it Work For Me?

The process one must use in order to achieve this is to first be tested (nutritionally, not medically in as much as the tests are completely different*) in order to reveal exactly where the body stands nutritionally at the moment of measuring. Secondly, these test results are automatically compared against millions of other people previously tested and successfully nutritionally rebalanced over many years. Third, based upon each person's retention similarities, as compared to the most similar people tested (in terms of their initial retention profile) in this huge database, a complete nutritional program is then statistically strategized food by food, vitamin by mineral, milligram by microgram, according to certain

*The critical difference between medical diagnostic and nutritionally diagnostic testing is discussed in subsequent chapters.

scientific principles that we will discuss later. Fourth, the same test is given periodically as a retest in order to closely monitor the progress that an individual makes and to adjust the nutritional program as needed until full nutritional balance and toxic elimination is achieved as demonstrated by only the retest results, not guesswork.

This is personally applied science delivered on the most scrutinized and controlled basis ever seen in the history of nutritional medicine, so that all nutritional outcomes can be highly controlled until full success is achieved person by person, case by case. Since the labs report that 99% of the many millions of people already tested in the U.S. have as Dr. James Bralley states, "multiple, sometimes profound, deficiencies, excesses and toxic accumulation, all of which routine medical test completely ignore," the need to know this and sort these disturbances out to perfection must be crystal clear and the chances that we are out of balance seen as 99 to 1. Although this seems bleak, it is actually good news simply because when we find something wrong nutritionally, our chances of changing that for the better increase dramatically. Based upon the World Health Organization report that the U.S. is number one in the world for measured nutritional/toxic disturbances, number one in the world for diet-related disease at large (not counting Third World countries), number one in the world for medical drug dependencies and now, according to the Center for Disease Control, number one in the world for premature death caused by the "side effect complications of correctly prescribed medications compounding over time," it's scientifically safe to *mistakenly assume that we are attacking nutrition-related disease with side-effect-promoting drugs*, instead of desirable benefit-only-promoting nutrition. And it now appears to most people that the so-called "drug cure" (better read, cover-up) is worse than the problem it addresses. With personalized nutrition applied, there are no problems, only solutions. We owe a debt of gratitude to Dr. Williams. He was absolutely correct as far back as the 1930s, and today his original work is about to blossom. But can this science actually prove any nutrition-to-disease connections?

### Brief Overview of Some Nutrition-to-Disease Associations

Formerly, the best way to determine diet and nutrition's relationship to disease was to put things in reverse by actually nutritionally testing people who were already sick and looking for the obvious associations in both direct and indirect diet-related disease. Then, the idea was to use that information to detect the same nutritional disturbances in healthy people and quickly correct them before they turn into these diseases. The following represents only a tiny fraction of the "As"—3 to be exact—out of the total alphabetized list of these primary and secondary vitamin-and mineral-only associations appearing in scientific literature and repeated in clinical studies that we do:

*Addison's disease*—primary: excess soft tissue retention of calcium; deficiencies of tissue sodium, secondary: deficiencies of magnesium, copper, potassium, selenium, vitamin D, E, A and C excesses of lead, zinc, iron, phosphorous, manganese, sodium, cadmium, vitamin B3, B6 and vitamin A.

*AIDS*—primary; zinc, selenium, vitamin E, deficiencies, secondary; magnesium, iron, phosphorous, cobalt, vitamins – B1, B3, B5, B6, C and excesses of manganese, iron, mercury, thallium, arsenic, silver, fluoride, sulfur, lead, tin, cadmium, B1, B2 and inositol, B12, D, E, A, K.

*Arthritis (osteo and rheumatoid combined)*—primary: magnesium, copper, selenium, vitamin A, vitamin B2, vitamin B3, vitamin B5, vitamin B6, vitamin B12, vitamin C, vitamin D, vitamin E deficiencies, secondary: chromium; and excesses of calcium, sodium, potassium, phosphorous, iron, manganese, cadmium, lead, zinc, mercury, thallium, arsenic, silver, fluoride, sulfur, tin, copper, vitamin B1, vitamin B6, vitamin B12, vitamin B10, vitamin C, vitamin A, vitamin D and vitamin K.

The list of diet-to-disease connections is very long and growing every day as clinical research progresses. The number and intensity of nutritional variables connected to each disease is becoming more refined every day with continuing research. The therapeutic value of this information relative to your own circumstances is increasing astronomically. The complexity of nutritional associations is quite self-evident, but due to the most recent comparative technology research, science can take all of these and many more variables into consideration for each and every person, day by day, step by step, start to finish, before and after, with extreme precision over the rest of our lives.

Nutritional tests are given and very closely and scientifically examined concerning people who are not only sick before the testing but also with those who are overweight, fatigued, prematurely aging, mentally deteriorating, unfit and unresponsive to exercise, sexually dysfunctional, suffering the slowest metabolic rates, under different stages of stress, suffering from allergies, digestive dysfunction, and most every modern lifestyle disease there is. Comparisons are made for future reference through applied comparative data-based laboratory technology. These same nutrition/toxic direct tests were given to the healthiest people with the least amount of body fat problems, those with the highest energy, those who were longer living, clearer in mental function, greatest athletes, lowest stress, fastest metabolisms, best digestive systems, least symptomatic, lowest amount of allergies, if any, to compare against those who were suffering the most, strictly on nutritional/ toxic/medical comparative bases. All known common denominators were noted, clinical trials began and continue and success is now guaranteed when this nutrition information is utilized properly in a highly controlled cause-and-effect outcome scenario.

Finally, we can determine—from applying nutrition tests to those in perfect health and those in imperfect health and then making statistical comparisons from all dimensions of science—the cause and the cure, the source of all disease from the nutritional standpoint. Plus, it has been medically proven repeatedly (on millions of people) that we can use certain principles to correct any nutritional disturbances tested in any individual using a systematic scientific approach known most formally as orthomolecular nutritional medicine. Diet no longer counts in and of itself, guesswork doesn't work, one-size-fits-all and you-are-what you-eat ideologies are now considered dangerous ideas. These obsolete ideas may become illegal someday, just as driving a spike into the base of the skull for headaches, bloodletting, swapping a medical test with another or treating psoriasis with x-rays became illegal.

### *Learn From the Mistakes of Others*

Perhaps the most powerful medicine of all, the ultimate prevention plan of all nutrition-related disease was originated by first testing those who were already sick and then cross-referencing the statistics generated from all identifiable nutritional abnormality patterns or profiles such as those mentioned in the above diseases and many more. Then when a new person is tested, we can compare their test results to that existing database and accurately deduce exactly which diseases are developing in their body and to what extent, long before symptoms may become present or a disease develops as diagnostically labeled by a medical practitioner.

*In effect, we can find out what smaller, undetectable problems are developing before they develop into bigger, overwhelming ones. Knowing long before we are in crisis is the most scientific means of prevention the world has ever seen. This is the real healing power of nutrition.* Additionally, people with already medically diagnosed conditions will heal faster than ever before. We therefore consider ortho-molecular nutritional medicine as complementary-to-all medicine and not as traditional or alternative medicine.

### The Primary Accomplishments of Personalized Nutrition

### Accomplishment I: Detection of nutrients and toxins present.

It reveals exactly what biochemical disturbances are expressed as related to nutrition that each individual's body cells are suffering from.

*How?* By directly measuring fundamental nutrient and toxic retention in the body from appropriate body specimens including hair, urine, blood, saliva, stool, and breath. This includes:

Deficiencies, excesses, antagonistic relationships of and between minerals, heavy metals, vitamins, vitamin-like substances, proteins (amino acids), fats (fatty acids and prostaglandins), enzyme intermediates (organic acids), sugars (including glycoproteins), toxic compounds (including solvents), hormonal synergy, allergies (both hidden and high-histamine allergies). From this baseline of nutrient and toxin retention measurements and their direct or indirect correlations for a given individual, we can then statistically correlate and compute:

- Metabolic type, rate and tissue acidity
- Thyroid and adrenal glands' functional hormonal output along with most other glands
- Autonomic nervous system function and sympathetic or parasympathetic activity
- Diet-related disease tendencies (so very important to prevent problems before they start)
- Nutrition-related symptoms
- Digestive system weaknesses and strengths
- Definitive mineral-related allergic tendencies
- Sensitivities to concentrated sugars and insulin resistance
- Biochemical pathways where the greatest metabolic dysfunction is

occurring which is, in effect, degenerating the health of the entire organism

***Accomplishment II: Correction of all imbalances of nutrients and toxics present.***

The nutritional repair and rebalance any biochemical disturbances found inside each individual's body cells.

***How?*** By laboratory-proven programs of ***completely personalized nutrition eating plans including***: customized supplementation precisely tailored to biochemical uniqueness which will dependably eliminate all test-measured deficiencies, excesses, antagonistic relationships of and between minerals, heavy metals, vitamins, vitamin-like substances, proteins (amino acids), fats (fatty acids and prostaglandins), enzyme intermediates (organic acids), sugars (including glycoproteins), toxic compounds (including solvents), hormonal synergy, allergies (both hidden and high-histamine allergies), using a series of therapeutic principles that have been medically proven over time. This correctional nutrition therapy includes:

- Foods to completely avoid at this moment and those to eat more of every day
- Detoxification procedures to rid the body of poisons and sources of external contaminants to avoid
- Macro and micro nutrient zone recommendations (exact proportions of food and supplemental nutrients for the fastest, most complete results)
- A nutritional and toxic baseline from which to compare all future metabolic improvements of nutrient retention and in function

Literally, to ***make every bite, every drink you take, and every breath count for better health*** and factor in every supplemental nutrient in exact synergistic proportion, for the fastest and most complete results possible as allowed by genetic design (which will be revealed as well in time). (Note: even one's genetic design can be super enhanced over and above perceived genetic/enzyme limitations). This is the way nutrition should have been presented to us, long before wild and crazy fad diets, indiscriminate pill popping, unrealistic drug dependencies, and all other diet and nutrition nonsense that has ultimately doomed us to health failure after unhealthy failure. Personalized nutrition science, a.k.a. ortho-molecular nutritional medicine, is dedicated only to provide the most precise answer to every nutrition-related problem delivered scientifically every time, for each unique body. When this is done correctly, there is no more reason for tricky guesswork, one-size-fits-all absurdities, doubts, confusion, theory, gimmicks, fads, opinions, unfounded beliefs, "throw it against a wall and see if it'll stick" approaches, mega-dosing, extreme diets or any other nutrition nonsense. It is simply the purest science applied only to the individual at hand—no one else.

Most simply, what exactly does the personalized nutrition process do for you?

1. **Reveals** precisely and exactly which of the most fundamental nutrients each body's deficiencies, antagonistic disturbances and excess retentions at the moment of measurement (this is all that matters when it comes to repairing the body).
2. **Demonstrates** toxic levels and other related poisons within the body.
3. **Deduces** scientifically from the above measurements in comparison to a database of millions metabolic type/rate, glandular function, disease tendencies, toxic environmental exposure, symptomatic relationships, nervous system function, stages of stress, and much more.

With the above information in hand, a report of findings efficiently corrects problems found by:

1. Applying diet and supplement corrections in accordance with the **law of opposites.** * In other words, strategically fortifying your body with specific foods and customized supplements which contain the highest amounts of the nutrients that the body has deficiencies in and proportions in the lowest amounts of the nutrients your body is retaining an excess of.

   Example: If your body has been tested in regard to the two fundamental minerals calcium and potassium, and it is found that your calcium is being retained in excess, and potassium is a deficiency, all that needs to be done in order to correct this problem is to feed the

*The law of opposites, what Albert Einstein referred to as relativity, is the key to all nutritional correction.

body according to the law of opposites. This means, more potassium-rich foods and supplements are applied and less calcium rich foods and supplements are given until neither a deficiency or an excess of either one exists and they are in perfect proportion for maximum metabolic efficiency.

Note:Tthe above process automatically detoxifies the body and removes metabolic imbalances simultaneously, while accelerating metabolic rate so that every bite of food creates more energy and less fat and waste. As each body balances out the essential nutrients, all toxins are pressured to leave the body rapidly.

### Future Refinements:
Leaving nothing to chance, we must remeasure the effects of the program with future tests in order to check the body's metabolic response to the program's specialized diet and supplementation. Then, through comparative data analysis, the lab automatically refines the program to perfection as your long-term metabolic pattern, or genetic signature, emerges.

### Expected Outcome (Prognosis):
The end of nutrient deficiencies, excesses, disturbances and toxic infiltration. A faster, more efficient metabolism with less body fat accumulation, elimination of fatigue, slowed aging, dramatically increased immune system, greater mental clarity, less "old age symptoms," improved athletic performance—a higher-quality life altogether.

### Added Special Benefits:
1. The end of guesswork about which foods and supplemental nutrients your body truly needs.
2. Control over the impact of nutrition, environment, and lifestyle on each unique body.
3. Protection from nonsense nutrition or unfounded nutritional ideas that harms health more than helps it.

### Do You Want to be a Diet Gambler or Nutrition Detective What's the Difference? What's at Stake?

The question remains, would you rather gamble with diet and supplements using the current guesswork system that most people are accustomed to by trying to assume that daily recommendations from government statistics have any basis in fact for your unique circumstances? Or would you rather be a personalized nutrition detective and only utilize the most personalized science? This is where you, your body, your mind in effect are the complete nutritional study from start to finish, not someone else in some highly generalized fragmented study who has nothing to do with you in your uniqueness or accountability for the problems found in you and any improvements that you make. It's really a choice that we all must make in light of this most beneficial scientific discovery.

A comparable example in standard medicine would be a have a friend or relative take your annual physical exam with its routine medical lab tests and use those results on yourself. Does that make sense? Of course not and it is actually illegal for medicine and should be illegal for any and all diet guesswork. The resultant health risks are the tremendous multitudes of diet-related diseases, both direct and indirect, that come from making nutritional mistakes. These mistakes are mounting up as our inborn nutritional reserves are rapidly depleted and our highly progressive society is doomed to more diet-instigated and diet-curable disease than ever before. Generic nutrition approaches are obsolete in light of this new science, while individual specificity is now the standard. And there are certain principles of natural law that govern how this works. These include:

1. Comparative Correlated Clinical Research (CCCR)
2. The Law of Opposites (LOO)
3. "Seesaw" Effect of Nutrient Stabilization (SENS)
4. Interactive Antagonistic Nutrient Displacement (IAND)
5. Target Chelation Acceleration (TCA)
6. Mass Action/Enzyme Kinetic Loading Effect Principle (MAEKLEP)

These preceding principles will be further expanded upon in subsequent chapters. They will soon become enlightened society's new common sense. These physiochemical principles itemized above are your tools in the tool chest for making a more healthy life. They are the personalized nutrition weapons against all disease and illness and unwanted symptoms. When put into play properly for a given body they will efficiently correct nutritional and toxic disturbances found. It's all based on foods that you eat more of and those you eat less of, vitamins and minerals to intake more of and those to take less of and tests to distinguish the difference and then monitor the rebalancing process to perfection. Finally, the science couldn't be simpler.

# Chapter III

## Diets Become Extinct
## Personally Applied Nutrition is the Replacement

*Ours is a world where people don't know what they want and are willing to go through hell to get it.*

—Don Marquis

### Diet Patterns

Ongoing research has demonstrated certain patterns in diet among people. Much of this same research has focused on nutrient needs, digestion, absorption and food allergies. Dr. Roger Williams demonstrated that we each inherit unique needs for specific nutrients which are what we refer to as our genetic signature. We inherit these needs from our ancestors; these are similar to their own needs but with our own special combination of unique digestion characteristics, absorption traits, enzyme patterns, and nutrient transport and excretion factors.

Consequently, in such a mixed-up genetic pool as found in the U.S., this variability phenomenon is the primary reason why the government's *one-size-fits-all* Recommended Dietary Allowances of vitamins, minerals, carbohydrates, fats and proteins are inadequate and even improper for many people. It's all due to the nature of our innate Genotrophic (signature) design. Each person uniquely requires more of one nutrient than another. German Army research has identified a distinctive pattern of digestive fluid and amino acids from person to person which further confirms the presence of human digestive patterns. Dr. Richard T. Powers, PhD, and many others before him have found close relationships between food allergies, blood types and immune systems in their research. Dr. David Watts, PhD, has found many relationships between mineral retention and just about everything that goes on in the human body. The process of human uniqueness investigation continues relentlessly in universities, laboratories and amongst independent researchers, as it has been determined by science that this is the primary key to nutrition-related wellness. Furthermore, there is a general research consensus that humans fit into three very basic genotrophic categories of diet: vegetarian, meat-eater and omnivore. There are established sub groupings within these categories. An example of one of these sub-groupings can be found within the vegetarian category where there are ovo-lacto-pesca-vegan types of vegetarians (Ovo = eggs, lacto = milk, pesca = fish, vegan = vegetables). Within these sub-groupings even further distinctions about each specific food and nutrient need can be made using the appropriate laboratory procedure which ultimately culminates in nutritional specificity per person never before possible.

## *The Ongoing Fallacy of Popular Diet Systems*

The greatest short coming and fallacy of popular diet systems is that they simply do not allow enough for human uniqueness from vegetarians to carnivores. They come from a predominately *one-size-fits-all* concept and in some cases are very extreme and one-sided when it comes to nutrient recommendations and other dietary factors. A large number of modern fad diets have been derived from untested personal experience, capitalistic manipulations, trendy logic and/or uninformed advertising. Popular modern diets include high-protein or high-carbohydrate content, low-cholesterol diets, low-fat diets, high-monounsaturated fat diets, low-glycemic index diets, fruitarian diets, raw food diets, alkalinizing diets, detoxification diets, ethnic diets, Zone diets, blood type diets and numerous weight loss diets including ketogenic diets. And the list continues on. But because we are each so unique in so many ways, these diet and supplement plans are generally very limited in their positive benefits and lead to much confusion when it comes to choosing them or determining if they are truly helping. In fact, many of these plans have proven to be dangerous for people because they do not accommodate for individual nutrient needs properly. The mismatching of diets can upset a body's metabolic balance, causing a deterioration of health and well-being. This is exactly why various research authorities, most notably Harvard University, have withdrawn support for the indiscriminate practice of diet and supplementation to promote health and wellness. The FTC and FDA are constantly pulling the plug on products and programs that are actually dangerous for your health such as coral calcium. The

USDA Center for Nutrition Policy and Promotion states on their web site at www.mypyramid.gov that one size doesn't fit all. Considering the widespread use of these common generic diet programs, combined with our *one-size-fits-all* attitudes of what's good for me is good for you, is it any wonder why people are not achieving the health and overall well-being they truly deserve? Are you designed to be more of a vegetarian having to ingest extra vitamin C, iron, copper and B12 and to eat four times a day or a heavy meat eater requiring differing degrees of these nutrients? Maybe or maybe not. This is the real question. Only a person's personalized orthomolecular nutritionist knows for sure, but he or she has to first determine your nutrient retention pattern and its indigenous metabolic profile, type, pattern or body type first to be certain. (These four terms are connected by definition, although "profile" refers more to the lab testing part of typing which in effect determines your actual nutrient and toxic retention, which is most important.)

### *What is Metabolic Typing?*

The art and science of metabolic typing was developed before the technological advances of nutritional testing became apparent. This semi scientific "art" attempts to interconnect genetically predisposed human patterns dividing everyone into distinct physiological categories of similar characteristics. This classification process, once completed, has typically been used as the historical forerunner of nutrient retention tests for nutritional evaluation and therapy. Metabolic Typing analysis has been based on one's blood type, nervous system characteristics, PH, endocrine gland balance, oxidation pattern, body shape, body composition, personality, hair and facial features and more.

### *Where do Metabolic Types Come From and What are Their Implications?*

Metabolic types come from our human genetic pools or more accurately termed Genotypes and Phenotypes. Strictly speaking, **genotypes** reflect the entire genetic constitution of a person distinguished from his/her physical appearance; **phenotypes** reflect the entire physical, biochemical, and physiological make up of an individual as determined both *environmentally* and *genetically*.

Subsequently, we have groups of humans with similar genetic characteristics based on an original genetic set (or pattern) which has been modified over time due to the influences of environment. Simply put, we all come from identifiable ancestral tribe origins (see Ancestral Typing in glossary). Due to environmental variations such as climate, diet, lifestyle, and socialization factors, our genetic set has been further differentiated from its primal origins into other races and body types with certain genetic characteristics indigenous to each race and still others found in all races. What we have had genetically delivered to each of us individually here in modern times is body type variation from more than a 40,000 year line of environmentally affected evolution.

Whether your specific ancestors were hunters, gatherers, farmers, fishermen, savage warriors, peaceful citizens, lived in cold climates, warm climates, high altitudes, low altitudes, etc., all has a pronounced effect on what you are as an individual today and what you require from the environment to be your healthy best. As previously stated, from a purely environmental standpoint, diet is the single most important factor in feeding your genes properly. Stay closely within the path of your genetic origins and their antecedent environmental patterns and you'll physically and mentally thrive. Stray from this path as *one-sizing* would have you do and you'll suffer the consequences of greater diet-related disease. These concepts frame the debate for the environment versus genes.

Additionally, we are rapidly losing the wellness benefit automatically built into traditional lifestyles as we collectively stray far and wide from the essence of our genetic design. There is no question that the U.S., due to extensive multi-cultural variations which cause us to digress from our traditional eating and living patterns moment by moment, is creating diet-related disease statistics which are at an all-time high. We are, in fact, the world's largest melting pot. Where else in the world can you find someone genetically designed to be more of a vegetarian eater wolfing down a beer and burger to be "in" with friends, then having to pop a Tums (with extra calcium, of course) for the severe digestive stress the beer and burger causes? Where else in the world can you find a genetically programmed meat-eater becoming a straight vego-vegetarian due to religious beliefs and then consequently suffer from anemia, parasites, chronic fatigue and premature aging? Where else in the world can you find someone designed to be an omnivore trying out the latest grapefruit diet suffering then from chronic pathological diarrhea but thinking that it's okay because he's been mistakenly told by others that he is in a detoxification process? Where else in the world can you find someone with pronounced magnesium deficiency continuously mega-dosing calcium which only serves to worsen the deficiency? Where else in the world can you find an asian thyroid dominant type (an ethno-endocrine type) subsisting on a 40-30-30 zoned macronutrient proportion (carbohydrate/protein/fat) when they really may require a 70-20-10 proportion for best results? If we were each tested for nutrient retention, none of this would happen and our average combined health status would dramatically improve.

We certainly cannot forcibly change what's been genetically built into our body over the last 40,000 years overnight, but with personalized nutrition we can certainly learn to work with it to make better environmental choices and ultimately improve upon it now and for all generations to come.

### *Religious and Evolutionary Perspectives on Metabolic Types*

Considering religious doctrines, it may very well be that when God officially put man on this earth he placed him in the Euphrates Valley. At that time and still today, this region is semi-tropical by nature. This area had the nuts, seeds, fruits, and vegetables necessary to nourish the type of metabolism man was initially endowed with. At that time in history, man could reach up and pick food from the land whenever he desired it. For the purpose of discussion, let's call this first metabolic type Type 1, since theoretically this was man's first body type on earth (geneticists project that there is 1.8 million years of human DNA on earth).

When man began to migrate away from the Euphrates region, he learned to bring goat's milk and some other foods into the diet. These small modifications in diet altered his phenotype only slightly as he slowly became a Type 1A metabolizer. Over time, through the generations, the Type 1A metabolizer was better able to fully utilize these initial diet modifications more efficiently through the processes of digestion, absorption, assimilation, and elimination. Those people spreading out into Greece and Northern Italy had to learn to add grains to their diet for a lack of other food availability. They could no longer reach up and pick their food year 'round. At first, babies born to this group could not adapt well as they grew. Many became weak, sickly and many died. The stronger children who survived this environmental stress in turn had babies who were a little stronger and better adapted to the new grain-rich diets. Gradually, this tribal line mutated into a Type 2 metabolizer with the ability to efficiently utilize foods that would undermine the health of Type 1 metabolizers, thanks to newly acquired genetic capabilities not found in Type 1s. As people continued to spread out and populated the colder climates to the north and higher altitudes, they had to increase their dependency on grains and stored foods for survival. And, they had to begin consuming small animals to fill the gaps in food scarcity. Further, phenotypic mutation took place over time to form another metabolic type we'll arbitrarily call Type 3. During these difficult periods in history, anyone born with incompatible metabolic types for their respective environment would die prematurely in infancy, childhood or early adulthood. This is called "natural selection."

As civilization moved even further north, the people had to hunt and consume animals like deer and bear to survive. As in the case of Type 3, children born who could not adapt to this diet change died prematurely. Those who were left were quite hardy and thrived on heavy purine (red meat) diets giving rise to our next metabolic category of Type 4.

This same type of mutation pattern occurred as people populated China, India and the Pacific Rim islands. Those born in these particular regions had to become Type 1A metabolizers or remained as Type 1. Numerous religious sects indigenous to these areas forbade meat and animal products so that Type 4s didn't mutate in these groups often. And again, those born into these societies with the wrong metabolic type would not survive. All in all there are at least 8–10 basic types of metabolizers with differing nutrient needs. Notably, East Indian and Asian philosophers and teachers come to America and believe that all Americans should practice vegetarian diets because the peoples of their homeland are predominantly vegetarians. These philosophers completely overlook the fact that we cannot change any metabolic type in one or even two generations, let alone in a person's own lifetime. It takes a minimum of eight or more generations to successfully effect any permanent phenotypic changes.

One should not be frustrated about the type of metabolism you have inherited. You cannot help being what you are other than by learning to environmentally work with metabolism for optimum health results. Ignoring one's metabolic makeup can only cause harmful effects especially when diet is modified for purposes of fitting into someone else's philosophy, fad, or religion. The dietary needs of one's own body, as measured by nutrition testing, are the only real protection from *one- size-fits-*

*all* traps. In ancient days, people died quickly when they were born into a rigid environment mismatched to their genetic set because they had no choice, there were no supermarkets around the corner to supply them with the right foods that their bodies could healthfully metabolize.

Sadly, it's not much different today even with the supermarket around the corner because without first measuring your own nutrient retention profile, there is truly no way to know exactly what you need from that supermarket for best health. As we now know, the direct result of this guesswork problem is our current epidemic of rampant diet-related disease. This nation is simply carelessly overfed yet seriously undernourished. Here we are, attempting to keep people alive, not with the proper nourishment we each require but with nutritional stereotyping, generic, non-nourishing, side-effect-promoting drugs, a huge array of pills, lotions, potions and surgeries which have no direct connection to the root cause of our ailments – nutrition/genes/environment. These quick fixes are just false substitutes for the real thing.

### Abstract: A Contemporary Message about Evolution and Genes

Recently, I actually discovered a best-selling book which blatantly stated that our genes haven't changed in 100,000 years. This is truly an absurd, completely false statement written by somebody who is not a geneticist or anthropologist. This false information has only compounded our widespread *one-size-fits-all* fallacies and beliefs. The real genetic scientists, Michael Crawford, PhD, and Michael Marsh, dedicated their entire research project to food's effects on genes and discovered that food (and secondarily environment) has shaped and continues to genetically shape the species beyond Darwinist gene mixing concepts. As a research scientist, medical school professor and epigeneticist, Dr. Bruce Lipton points out in his book, *The Biology of Belief* the truest genetic perspective actually comes from Darwin's predecessor, Jean-Baptiste Lamarck, who demonstrated that cooperation and community are the foundation of survival.

The primary dilemma that they found is that today, food in the U.S. is of such a commonplace nature that it is taken for granted and its qualitative relationship with long-term biological considerations is overlooked. According to Crawford and Marsh's research findings "...the historical changes in disease patterns, the contrast in disease incidence from country to country and importantly, the socioeconomic contrasts within a country suggest that we are witnessing a signal of the potential power of food as a dominant factor in evolution." In reference to this book, medical journalist Beatrice Trum Hunter says in the research abstracts compilation, *Townsend Letter,* that these factors also "pose serious questions as to the impact of present day food and agricultural policies on immediate and future generations." Crawford and Marsh believe that "among other follies, agricultural practices have emphasized yields stressing quantity rather than quality." Nutrition has not been a prime goal, as, for example, in animal feeding practices; both the protein and nutrient values of animal food products have been diluted by fat. In her analysis of Crawford and Marsh's book, *The Driving Force - Food, Evolution and the Future,* Ms. Trum Hunter states that the authors found that food has always been a crucial factor in shaping life's evolutionary process on this planet, from the earliest time when life first emerged up to the present, and it will continue to do so into the future. If de Lamarck would have been taken seriously, as he is now, we likely would have a fully empowered perspective of nutrition as shaping our phenotypes and perhaps metabolic typing and testing science would have a prominent place in our health concerns today rather than the back seat it currently occupies.

### Genetic Change

An excellent example of how our genes have changed in the last 10,000 years was revealed in an article "Unkind Milk" appearing in the Vol. 18, No. 12, October 1993, issue of *The Harvard Health Letter.* Stephen E. Goldfinger, M.D., et al., stated that "about 10,000 years ago, according to scientists' best conjecture, a genetic mutation occurred among the populations of northern and central Europe that had learned to herd dairy animals and consume milk products." These historically new genetic developments, which lead to the occurrence of Blood Type B, allowed 80% of these people and their descendants to produce ample lactose into adulthood, making them an exception to the human rule for drinking milk. Lactose intolerance is very common among other ethnic groups. For example, milk disagreed with about 50% of all adult Hispanics and with at least 75% of people of African, Asian, or Native American descent in one government study.

In reality, our genes have changed many times over the last 100,000 years and will continue to do so until the end of time, for better or worse, depending on how we deal with them from a food, societal, and environmental standpoint.

## *Origin of Allergies*

Where do most food allergies originate? Straying off your ancestral eating patterns is going to increase the likelihood of causing incidental food allergies and sensitivities. This is a poignant consequence of an incompatibility between your internal and external environment. A given body is simply not used to or can't quickly adapt to certain foods (including a host of new additives and residues in today's food supply). Following sections will go into more detail about the current dire complications and how to eliminate them relative to biochemical individuality and good health. For now, suffice it to say that a properly tested/typed person will know what foods to avoid completely for optimum wellness. The good news about food allergies is that many food sensitivities can be overcome with the correct nutritional knowledge.

## *The Old Way to Individualize Nutrition*

Just like us, the ancients wanted to know what their proper diet should be, especially when taken sick. Today, this holds true especially for Americans. Due to the constant inter-breeding of genetically different populations combined with an ever-increasing rejection of traditional ethnic diets, the new modern diets have emerged. Unfortunately, modern diets no longer correspond to our individual genetic framework of digestive, absorptive, assimilation and excretory capabilities. Everyone, including the ancients and our recent ancestors, wanted a better way to utilize nutrition precisely, without guesswork and without consequence.

The food problem really begins first with digestion and then proceeds on to absorption, metabolic utilization, and excretion. Not everyone's body can efficiently digest every kind of food. Buildups of undigested or partially digested food can lead to a multitude of problems including indigestion; gas; cramps; bloating; constipation; diarrhea; ulcers; headaches; fat and weight gain or loss; cellulite; rashes; liver, kidney and other organic stress; as well as allergies. Digestible proportions of the macronutrients, proteins, fats, and carbohydrates each person needs and can digest is as highly specific to them as is their need for each vitamin, vitamin-like substance and mineral. Absorption into the body of what has been digested is another process that is very individual-specific.

The genetic design of the digestive tract itself and certain abnormalities that might have been created over time directly affect exactly which nutrients and toxins get in and which don't. Then the way the body arranges what is taken in from the digestive tract is a very specific process again based upon multiple biochemical pathways and many enzymes that run them all, which need to be in proper working order for the most efficiency. How the final chemically toxic products of these three processes are broken down and eliminated from the body is then another metabolic matter, very specific to one's internal environmental condition. With all these things considered, science continually proves that if we follow the correct nutritional plan for each unique, up-to-the-moment and long-term metabolism, diet-related disease will vanish from our lives and at the same time, life span and functional energy span will lengthen considerably.

But what about the ancients? They didn't exactly have our diet secret because of their primitive reality. Individuality was no secret to them but their approach was very limited compared to today. However, these rather obsolete approaches to individualization created the provocation for direct nutritional testing.

### *Historic Origins*

The first personalized nutrition began as metabolic typing. This science, really began with Hippocrates, the father of modern medicine and his health-minded followers in Greece. Hippocrates postulated that different sorts of people have different maladies. He diagnosed his patients on the multidimensional basis of what he called "the four humors" (translated: fluids) and sequentially developed a metabolic typing system which utilized four temperaments and two body types. His post-diagnosis nutrition and lifestyle treatments were specific to each of these patient categories. Hippocrates's favorite motto was "thy food shall be thy remedy." To this day Hippocrates's methodology is still well-received.

Ancient Chinese, Egyptians, Buddhists, and Hindus were also body-typers or metabolic typers as represented in the chart below:

## ANCIENT METABOLIC TYPING     CONSTITUTIONAL TYPES

| | |
|---|---|
| Ancient Chinese Medicine and Acupuncture | 5-7 Elemental Types/14 constitutional types |
| Ancient Egyptian Medicine | 7 Organ Systems |
| Ancient Greek Medicine and Hippocrates | 4 Humors, the Liver-Bile Type |
| Ancient Buddhist/Hindu Traditions (Ayurveda) | 7 Energy Center Types and Vata, Pitta, Kapha (5 elements) |

### *Ancient Metabolic Typing Systems*

### Chinese Typing

Ancient and modern Chinese philosophies of medicine focus on the balance of life in relation to each person and require the use of diet, hands-on therapies, exercise, proper rest, and herbs to restore balance. Their healing concepts base therapeutic treatments on the specific nature of each person rather than the nature of the diseases they suffer from. This is the underlying purpose of metabolic typing. People in the West who have undergone Chinese therapeutic experiences can attest to its affectivity, despite a number of its inherent limitations.

The Chinese practitioner subdivides this body typing system according to constitutional Types. Practitioners routinely divide each person to be treated into their specific constitutional type before beginning any therapeutic intervention. The fundamental principles of constitutional therapy originated in 3,000 B.C. and quickly spread throughout Asia, the Middle East, Europe and the West. As a means to properly type an individual, the Chinese healer must closely examine the patterns of responsiveness and creativity that develop during childhood and which persist throughout life. Each individual's constitutional characteristics are not perfectly fixed. They can be slightly modified by environmental factors and internal development. However, metabolic/constitutional types rarely change significantly and never completely become another type. This is related to an ongoing history of behavioral and physical tendencies which began early in life and center on physical, spiritual, and mental development. Therefore, a person's constitution is determined on the basis of present conditions and long-term patterns. It is no wonder that "nature, time and patience are the three great physicians," according to an ancient Chinese proverb. Comparing these to the West, our health practitioners have classified Type As and Type Bs as personality types and also those individuals considered to be at risk or not at risk. Type As are categorically ambitious, very motivated, always productive, highly goal oriented, constantly pushing the upper limits of their abilities, very considerate of working associates, eat too quickly, drink in excess and don't usually get enough rest. Type Bs are generally relaxed, take things in stride, allow for pleasure and leisure, let others worry about deadlines and satisfying work demands, tend to eat slowly and sleep a lot.*

Western health professionals classify patients further, based upon tendencies present during illness into two categories:

1. *At Risk* - persons severely debilitated after contracting common influenza. After becoming infected by the flu, these particular individuals may suffer a secondary infection or a worsening of symptoms. This is due to a chronic degenerative disease state that they already have, or in the case of children, with underdeveloped immune systems. This compromised health status undermines overall resistance to the flu, leading to an increased probability of death or prolonged hospitalization.

At-risk examples: Individuals including elderly people, very young children, organ transplant patients, diabetics, people with ongoing or recent cancer therapies, those with chronic respiratory diseases, and morbidly obese people.

2. *Not At Risk* - people infected by the flu who then suffer only minor symptoms of discomfort, maybe miss a day or two of work or school and ultimately recover in a week or less. These people are considered constitutionally healthy and not immuno compromised with a characteristically normal, healthy response to viral infiltration.

Traditional Western health practitioners may consider these four rough-edged body-types (Type A, Type B, At Risk, Not At Risk) in relation to their giving their patients treatment recommendations. The doctor may

*(Note: It is obvious that not everyone purely fits into either one of these preceding categories, but this type of categorization does help to better clarify and classify differences Westerners see in each other.)

recommend that the Type A slow down a little and let the body heal, or make special therapeutic allowances for At-Risk individuals by very closely monitoring their illness response. Chinese medical philosophy originally utilized five (now seven with modern additions) constitutional elemental types along with the law of yin and yang (opposite forces) to calculate the nature of disharmonies individuals are most likely to suffer from and the total symptomatic progress of any disease for that type. After starting with a balanced diet, Chinese practitioners can utilize special concentrated, mineral-rich foods, called herbs, in order to more quickly resolve underlying constitutional imbalances which, when present, increase a person's initial susceptibility to lack of recovery from disease. The constitutional imbalances that Chinese practitioners focus upon are actually metabolic imbalances which when properly aligned nutritionally, maximize immune function. Chinese elemental types include wood, fire, metal, earth, water, *heat/dryness, and *energy.

Each fundamental type is also further divided into two subgroups, very similar to At Risk and Not at Risk Western types. Each type is far more differentiated beyond Western type As and Bs in terms of behavior patterns. Each of the At Risk and Not at Risk subgroups in Chinese medicine are referred to as either weak or stressed constitution. Individuals with weak constitutions tend to become sick more easily, have more nutrient deficiencies and imbalances or basic energy deficiencies, take longer to recover from ailments, are easily upset or damaged by stressful environmental influences, and require more interventional therapies to nourish and strengthen their bodies. Stressed constitutional (or metabolic) types are far less susceptible to illness. When they do become ill, they recover much faster and with less lifestyle disruption. Stressed types seem to be more resistant to overall environmental irritation. In retrospect, the Chinese system of metabolic types consists of 7 behavioral types and 14 constitutional types and 2 subgroups (weak and stressed) for each of the 7 elemental types (wood, fire, metal, earth, water, heat/dryness, and energy).

Chinese philosophers describe the law of yin and yang. This law divides the universe's opposing forces within each of us, our entire lifestyle and even the entire universe.

**Distinctions of Yin and Yang:** cosmic bodies, temperament, time of day,

*These are more modern-day additions to the five primal elements.

season, magnetic pull, temperature, physical density, speed, relative moisture, heavenly body location, organs, height, distance, sides, light, sexual characteristics, and constitution. The above distinctions are used to reveal the characteristics of movement and energy within each of us and around us due to the natural attraction between yin and yang. Chinese medicine and philosophy have helped to clarify laws of nature for each of us. Given the ancients' lack of understanding about the human body, especially the nervous system and our real diet secret technology, it is quite an achievement.

## Ayurvedic Typing

Ayurvedic was a religious derivation of medicine, initiated by the belief that the god Indra conveyed the knowledge of long life to one of the Hindu rishis or seers. This philosophy originated in the 5th century B.C. Its application is based upon on the Vedas which are considered to be the oldest known philosophical writings.

An Ayurvedic philosopher views health within a universal context where human life is thought to be a direct extension of the life of the creator, also known as the cosmic consciousness. Therefore an individual's health is based upon their exact relationship with the cosmic consciousness. Ayurvedic healers intend to reestablish harmony between an individual and the life of the universe, by balancing the universal forces from without and within which are indigenous to each person. The life-force expression of the cosmic consciousness is termed prana. Prana represents the animate power of life which provides vitality and endurance to each human being and provides the basis for healing. This life-force/energy is classically expressed in terms of five great elements: earth, water, fire, air and ether. These elements are seen as both functions and characteristic aspects of the human body which hold it together in vital synchrony. Then there are three forces or doshas which balance the form and substance of the body: vata, pitta and kapha. These in turn, act on the five Great Elements as their dynamic forces. Vata and kapha types are total opposites while pitta is the mediating force between the two extremes. When all the doshas are in balance, the body functions in optimum synchronicity. When balance is reduced, disease takes over. The doshas uniquely combine in each person giving rise to body types, each of which lean towards one Dosha or the next. These doshas cause tendencies in each person, although one or two doshas will be most dominant through the shaping of personality and constitution. dosha dominance and consequential imbalances provide unique strengths and weaknesses which create tendencies toward certain illnesses and disorders.

Kapha types: prone to lung, heart, stomach, and immune disorders

Pitta types: prone to liver, gallbladder, blood, small intestine, stomach and spleen disorders; also prone to strokes and cancer.

These three doshas affect just how prana (life force) flows through the body in either balanced or unbalanced fashion. This ancient philosophy contends that the prana or life force flows through the body in a specific pattern of meridians or rivers of energy. These rivers of energy roughly correspond to Chinese acupuncture meridians. Like the Chinese, the Ayurvedic practitioner uses pulse and physiognomy for patient diagnosis and treats each individual with foods, herbs, and other special treatments related to each dosha, the five elements, and meridian pattern.

**Greek Typing**

In 460 B.C. Hippocrates was born on the Greek island of Cos. He's credited with creating the first school of medicine dedicated to the scientific approach to understanding health and the body. He and his followers did not consider good health and bad health as gifts or punishment from the gods like other contemporaries but believed states of good and bad health to be consequential to natural and orderly processes which could be understood and effectively treated by man. Because of these beliefs Hippocrates is historically considered a towering and revolutionary figure for his time and is still revered for his insights by modern practitioners to this day.

From his text, *The Nature of Man*, Hippocrates stipulates that the human body contains blood, phlegm, yellow bile, and black bile (the four Humors) which constitute the nature of the body. When any or all of these elements are out of balance (deficient, excessive or unadjusted to by the other Humors) pain is experienced and illness persists. Hippocrates applied the triad of healing to his patients by approaching each patient with specific roles for himself as physician, the patient him or herself, and the controllable aspects of the patient's environment. Treating each patient differently according to their uniqueness, ***Hippocrates used proper and specific foods and drink,*** suitable exercise, and calmness of mind and body during his healing interventions. Also, he believed in certain opportune moments which occurred during the healing process (aside from prevention with its own set of opportune moments) where a crisis could be averted if acted upon soon enough. He called these moments Kairos. This is the root word for crisis where life or death could hang in the balance. Pepsis or "the forces of healing," could be accelerated or left alone according to physician discretion as related to disease timing factors.

Furthermore, Hippocrates believed that properly treated illness could have beneficial effects by helping to create a new order among the four Humors of each individual, and by helping to eliminate poisons and impurities within their specific system.

Ancient Hippocratic methodologies are no longer strictly practiced today but their influences have followed man throughout history from Galen to Paracelsus to Avicenna to many traditional healers in practice at this time. Medical doctors continue to take the Hippocratic Oath. The sciences of naturopathy, chiropractics, homeopathy and osteopathy embody many of the Hippocratic principles. The process of nutritional toxic cleansing or detoxification is still an important part of nutritional sciences to this day, many hundreds of years later.

*Ancient metabolic typing systems* each provide many insights into human differentiations well beyond one-size-fits-all and most importantly, they *considered diet and nutrition the most fundamental pieces of the puzzle.*

Unfortunately, these systems are very limited when it comes to putting the body under the microscope from a nutritionally scientific standpoint. There is no direct measurement provision for "you are what you retain from what you eat." Due to their primitive nature and artistic approach to individuality, they pass over the molecular level distinctions we now comprehend in regard to the human body as discernible through the modernized sciences of anthropology, genetics, epigenetics, physiology, anatomy, neurology, psychology, embryology, biochemistry, Biology, clinical nutrition sciences, barometric, physiatry, genealogy, and physics. Using these modernized sciences now embodied in orthomolecular nutritional medicine sciences, we now have more information than ever before about one's biochemical uniqueness and how to balance it.

**Modern Metabolic Typing**

Since 1900, with the discovery of the blood types by Landsteiner, there have been numerous researchers and research studies which have created the body of knowledge for metabolic typing, metabolic patterning, metabolic profiling, constitutional typing, endocrine typing, sensory typing, soma typing, body typing, or simply typing (our favorite term). Below is a very brief historical overview which includes many of the proponents of personalized nutrition testing. The ones with a "T" at the end have the greatest connection to the orthomolecular medicine of today.

### Modern Typing Overview

1900  **Karl Landsteiner, M.D.** Discovered the ABO blood types.

1925  **Dr. M. Kretschmer** investigated and categorized body types based on the proportion of derma most developed in the embryo (endomorphs, ectomorphs, mesomorphs). Published *ymptoms of Visceral Disease* (1919).

1931  **Dr. Cary A. Reams,** a student of Albert Einstein, began developing The Theory of Biological Ionization and the ability to differentiate thousands of metabolic types. Published *Choose Life or Death* in 1982.  (T)

1940  ABO blood types linked to diet by German Army.

1941  **Charles Stockard, PhD** Animal research demonstrates that endocrine gland hormones form specific body and personality patterns. Human research has confirmed this. (T)

1950  **William H. Sheldon, PhD** Further developed Kretschmer's research and published the *Atlas of Men.* 1954

1952  German research group (state-sponsored) showed that each healthy person has a distinctive pattern of amino acids in their intestinal digestive juices, proving human digestive patterns. (T)

1956  **Roger Williams, PhD** Wrote *Biochemical Individuality* and *Nutrition Against Disease* which demonstrated the true uniqueness of each of our bodies from a physiological and biochemical standpoint. (T)

1960s  **Henry G. Bieler, M.D.** Developed the first endocrine typing system based on European research. Developed the first modern system to match body type to diet; wrote *Food is Your Best Medicine* in 1965. (T)

**Thomas M. Riddick, M. S.** Developed the principles of Zeta Potential in relation to the human body and authored *Heart Disease: A New Approach to Prevention and Control,* 1970. (T)

**E. Abravanel, PhD** Published *Body type Diet and Lifetime Nutrition Plan* which is an updated weight-loss version of Bieler's project.

1970s **James D'Adamo, N.D.** Researched and developed the first blood typing system for diet based on 20 years of research; wrote *One Man's Food*, 1980.

**George Watson, PhD** Developed the first oxidation typing system; wrote *Personality, strength, and psychochemical energy*, 1979, which utilized a five type psychological system based on oxidation rates, pH, psychochemical odor analysis and a personality self-rating; involves diet and supplements matched to each type.

**William Kelley, D.D.S.** Developed the first nerve typing system as an extrapolation of Watson's work and Francis Pottenger's PhD research on the autonomic nervous system; it involved three nerve types with four variable levels of oxidation efficiency and subsequent individualized nutrition therapy.

1980s **James Braly, M.D.** Pioneered the development of food allergy testing and methodologies and related this information to the biochemical uniqueness of each individual; wrote *Food Allergy and Nutrition Revolution*, 1985. (T)

**D.L. Watts, PhD** Linked tissue mineral assays to metabolic type and nutritional needs. (T)

**Gerald Berkowitz, M.D.** Wrote *The Berkowitz Diet Switch* and attempted to match diet to Sheldon's original body types.

**Richard T. Power, PhD, Laura Power, B.A.** Expanded, combined, and refined preceding metabolic typing systems relying heavily on endocrine typing and blood typing methodologies; wrote many articles over a number of years.

1990s **Deepak Chopra, M.D.** Wrote *Perfect Health*, popularizing the ancient system of Maharieshi Ayurveda featuring vata, pitta, and kapha.

Dr. Elliot Abravanel, Dr. Jeffrey Bland (T), Dr. Donald Donsbach, and Dr. Michael Colgan(T) have also contributed a great deal to typing research and information along with Drs. Pauling (T), Pfeiffer (T), Pottenger (T), Hoffer (T), Foster (T), Eijkman (T), Gerson (T), McCormick (T), Szent-Gyoergyi (T), Moerman (T), Shute (T), Klenner (T), Stone (T), Cott (T), Issels (T), Kaufman (T), Cheraskin (T), Horrobin (T), Osmond (T) and Riordan (T).

There are countless researchers and laboratory projects worldwide in the process of further investigating the biochemical uniqueness of each individual and the relationship of diet to that uniqueness. As you can see the (T) is not assigned to everyone above. The ones who get this symbol are those who've truly bridged the gap between merely typing theories versus directly scientifically measuring the retention of nutrients within the body, which is now the formative science basis for orthomolecular medicine. There are new technologies and information breakthroughs regarding nutrient retention which is categorically referred to as the last frontier of nutritional wellness medicine.

The following tables are an extreme condensation of that which has been revealed by metabolic typing, with some degrees of reinforcement from orthomolecular testing.

## TABLE I: NERVOUS SYSTEM, ENDOCRINE GLANDS, and OXIDATION

All the endocrine glands are composed of two parts or types of cells: acid and alkaline. Each of these cells produces distinctly different hormones that balance each other's effects within the body. The nervous system controls the yin yang balance or the calming and stimulating balance of these hormones. The acid cells known as acidophils are controlled by the *sympathetic nervous system* which is the part of the nervous system prepares our bodies for fight or flight. The alkaline cells or basophils are controlled by the *parasympathetic nervous system* which is the part of the nervous system that has a calming affect on the body. Your overall response to stress is a function of the *autonomic nervous system*'s balance. Dr. Kelley's research demonstrated three types of stress response patterns.

**SYMPATHETIC TYPE** - Usually blood type A. Response to stress includes:
1. Effect on the adrenal glands which contracts muscles and constricts blood vessels, which raises blood pressure.
2. Input to the thyroid which speeds up metabolism, heart and pulse rates.
3. Stimulating the pancreas to elevate blood sugar, constrict digestive juices, and suppress hunger.
4. Effect on the thymus which mobilizes the immune system for defense and repair, also known as the "fight or flight" response."

A sympathetic dominant type of person has a weak parasympathetic response. Continuous stress resultantly causes: migraine headaches, nausea, chest pains, diarrhea, rapid pulse, low blood pressure, physical weakness, adrenal crisis, and ultimately suffocation, cardiac arrest, and death.

**PARASYMPATHETIC TYPE** - Usually blood type O. Response to stress includes:
1. Initially weak Sympathetic response followed quickly by an exaggerated parasympathetic response.

2. Muscles and blood vessels relax.
3. Blood pressure and pulse lower.
4. Heart rate and metabolism slow down.
5. Blood sugar falls.
6. Hunger increases and digestive juices flow.

A parasympathetic dominant type when exposed to prolonged stress suffers from obesity, fluid retention, sexual tension, mental fogginess, ulcers, heart arrhythmia, and loss of muscle tone.

**BALANCED TYPE** -Usually blood type B or AB. Response to stress includes:
1. A balanced sympathetic response initially followed by a gentle parasympathetic response.

### OXIDATION PATTERNS

The parasympathetic nervous system conserves oxygen while the sympathetic nervous system burns oxygen.

**SYMPATHETIC TYPES** - Must conserve oxygen by taking greater amounts of antioxidant nutrients including sulfur proteins such as chicken, eggs and shellfish and vitamins A, E, F, C, B5, selenium, and manganese.

**PARASYMPATHETIC TYPES** - Must burn more oxygen by taking oxidants such as iron, phosphorus, copper, B6, iodine, and B12.

Generally speaking oxidants are red in color and antioxidants are yellow - in "old school research."

The following represents a highly simplified representation of six primary Typing systems:

## TABLE II: METABOLIC TYPING SYSTEMS CONDENSED DIET OVERVIEW
I. Sheldon/Berkowitz  II. D'Adamo  III. Bieler  IV. Watson
V. Kelley  VI. Power  VII. Diet Categories

| OMNIVORE (+) | VEGETARIANS (+) | MEAT-EATERS (+) |
|---|---|---|
| **I. Mesomorph** - muscular, great strength and endurance, enjoys physical activity, noisy, callous, competitive | **I. Ectomorph** - tall, thin, small bones and muscles, restrained, self conscious, fond of solitude | **I. Endomorph** - short, round and soft, relaxed, sociable, even-tempered, lethargic |

| OMNIVORE (+) | VEGETARIANS (+) | MEAT-EATERS (+) |
|---|---|---|
| **II. Blood Type B**<br>Medium build | **II. Blood Type A & AB**<br>Trim/lean build | **II. Blood Type O**<br>Large bones/large build |
| **III. Adrenal Type**<br>Strong, muscular, curly hair, large features, energetic, very physical, good digestion, easy-going disposition | **III. Thyroid Type**<br>Small bones, thin, easily fatigued, insomnia, delicate features, high pulse, rashes, sensitive, high-strung | **III. Pituitary Type**<br>Lanky and tall, wide mouth, large forehead, large arms and legs, artistic, creative, flirtatious, sexually oriented |
| **IV *Medium Oxidizer**<br>Balanced blood (pH 7.41-7.46), warm, cooperative, optimistic | **IV. *Fast Oxidizer**<br>Alkaline blood (pH 7.47 +)<br>Irritable and impatient | **IV. *Slow Oxidizer**<br>Acid blood (pH 7.3 - 7.4)<br>sullen and depressed |
| **V. Balanced Nervous System**<br>During stress: sympathetic response first followed by parasympathetic response, then balance, medium blood pressure | **V. Sympathetic Dominant**<br>During stress: high pulse, no hunger, migraines, nausea, muscles constrict, chest pains, low blood pressure | **V. Parasympathetic Dominant**<br>During stress: slow pulse, hunger, relaxed muscles, lethargy, fluid retention, high blood pressure |
| **VI. Adrenal Type B**<br>Muscular, large features, medium bones and build, athletic, high blood pressure, heart strain<br>**Balanced Type AB**<br>Medium bones and muscles, balanced mental and physical orientation, affable, and adaptable | **VI. Thyroid Type A**<br>Thin, quick, small bones, delicate features, high strung, creative, very mentally oriented<br>**Pineal Type A**<br>Domed head in back (occiput), aware, sensitive, dreamer, receiver<br>**Thymus Type** (any ABO)<br>Tall and lanky, long limbs, knobby joints, wide chest | **VI. Pituitary Type O**<br>Large, wide forehead, obsessive, charismatic, "transmitter"<br>**Pancreas Type O**<br>Fat, round, soft, jolly, food-oriented, diabetic tendency<br>**Gonad Type O**<br>Male: baldness, heavy body |
| **VII. 3 large meals**<br>High protein, cultured dairy products, eggs, butter, whole grains, nuts, seeds, almost any vegetables, fruits, all red and white meats, potatoes, yams, bananas, high fiber, (roughage/beans) | **VII. 5 small meals.**<br>High starch, medium fat, raw milk, eggs, cheese, yogurt, kefir, whole grains, bananas, vegetables, fish, poultry, shellfish, acidic fruits, tomato, roughage, no beans, low purine meats, unsaturated fats<br>**Thymus Type**<br>High intake of raw foods, few animal products, rotation diet | **VII. 4 small meals**<br>High protein, no milk, no cheese, no wheat, some grains in limited amounts, alkaline vegetables and fruits all red and white meats, potatoes, yams, squash, medium roughage, high purine meats, saturated fats |

+ SUPPLEMENTS - Some basic supplements do match typing categories. But each persons needs are so unique to their biochemistry - age, disease, genetics, gender, food patterns and sources, lifestyle, etc.— that further differentiation is required for the sake of accuracy. Eating patterns are corrected with appropriate specimen evaluation to precisely differentiate individual needs.

* Not completely accurate due to indigenous discrepancies and limitations.

As you can see in the above, metabolic typing systems have delineated basically three types of diet. Manipulations of these diets have been brought up repeatedly in popular modern diet systems from the Zone diet to Atkins to blood type diets to metabolic typing diet and more.

## *Metabolic Typing Now Converts to Nutrition Testing*

Metabolic typing was intended to be a systematic, constitutional analysis of an individual's physiology to determine a long-term nutritional pattern. But because it did not measure nutrient retention directly, its therapeutic value was eventually found to be very limited and surprisingly inaccurate. At first, clinical science maintained it as a priority in the assessment of a given individual. Then, it was to merely assist designated laboratory tests on body specimens for a (then) very limited amount of body chemicals to further clarify and refine both long-and short-term nutritional needs. Then, as time went on and technology progressed, allowing us to look even more closely at every possible nutrient and nutrient connection in the body, the metabolic typing non-testing process fell into the background as a low or non-priority for the needs of the moment. Thanks to orthomolecular nutritional test-correction medicine, we can now most effectively:

1.) Determine the most metabolically efficient short-and long-term protein pattern for an individual.

2.) Anticipate and measure unusual individual nutrient needs regarding all foods, special forms of foods or supplements and very high or low amounts of certain nutrient factors.

3.) Determine the best long-or short-term diet and supplement pattern for an individual.

4.) Detect hidden or suppressed/antagonized inherent genetic strengths and develop them nutritionally.

5.) Better elucidate any metabolic ramifications reflected from long-and short-term nutritional patterns as measured by nutritional/metabolic deficiency & dysfunction analysis

6.) Design the appropriate macro/micronutrient food and supplement ratios within the diet pattern and monitor results with retests.

Old and obsolete, *metabolic typing has now been replaced by new and improved personalized nutrition.*

## *The Precise Use of Nutrition—Once and For All*
### *A Better Way to Be Well*

<u>Before</u> it was "diets," <u>now</u> it's "dynamically adjusted nutritional programs predicated upon testing and retesting and proven medical therapies" that really work. There always has been a better way to go about your nutrition and here it is. And as you will see, the science of personalized nutrition is designed to go to the most extreme and necessary lengths to "dig out" the facts of the matter when it comes to our own biochemical uniqueness and what is precisely called for when it comes to diet and supplementation strategies for the attainment of superior wellness results.

This process goes light years beyond merely categorizing an individual on the basis of factors such as: blood type, height or weight range, Chinese-Ayurvedic-Egyptian-Greek categorizations, pulse rate, blood pressure, hair characteristics, skin traits, muscle size, shape and tone, bone factors, overall shape, head and face shape, personality, ethnicity, intelligence factors and dream states. It goes deep into the internal environment by using laboratory tests that reveal even more specific information about every genetic, metabolic, and nutrient function we can scientifically measure and understand. Detecting allergies, toxins, nutrient deficiencies and excesses, breakdowns in digestion, absorption, utilization and excretion, pre-and post-disease states is all part of this process. A properly tested individual will know exactly what his or her metabolic and wellness status is, what foods and supplements he or she will thrive on, what foods and supplements to completely avoid and ultimately will have a fully customized diet and supplement program for his or her body type only. In essence, *a properly tested individual will never have to haphazardly guess* about what foods and supplements he or she needs to be in accordance with how they were genetically designed to live. Since each of our bodies were designed from the start to be healthy (the process is termed homeostasis), the precise nutritional program that personalized nutrition yields will ensure wellness in direct accordance with nature. No magical pill, no *one-size-fits-all* supplement or food, no one meditation technique, and no one special exercise can replace this real nutritional secret to true health.

There are 76 minerals, 17 vitamins, many known vitamin-like substances, 47 fatty acids, 12 essential amino acids, 30 non-essential amino acids, hundreds and perhaps thousands of phyto-nutrients and vitamin-like compounds found in nature, still not all understood—all of which the individual chemistry of our body (and mind) is designed to utilize. Along with the physics of life and genetic interbreeding, most of our genetic design is based on the amounts and types of these nutrients found in the specific regions from our ancestral origins. These various nutrient groupings have shaped our bodies, minds and lives for centuries and this process continues. Only in the last 100 years or so have we stepped out of our pre determined nutritional boundaries into our melting pot society. Progressive pursuits have created fundamental problems of incomplete wellness which is cumulatively plaguing us as a current and ever-intensifying epidemic of diet-related disease. This is compounded by a host of debilitating problems such as: synthetic and mass production agricultural methodologies, nutrient-depleted and disappearing top soils, extensive food processing, improper food storage, poisonous food additives, pesticides, herbicides and other environmental pollutants, preparation of enzyme dead foods, and more. We repeatedly mention and will address this "epidemic epidemic" because this phenomenon only serves to further undermine the foods that we consume and add extra toxins to our bodies that were not designed to efficiently handle this overload that has accumulated over the last 40,000+ years of evolution.

Is it any wonder, then, that the science of personalized nutrition should be considered the most important process to retrieve our lost health once and for all? It may be among scientists, but most people are being kept in the dark. Conspiracy?

### The Hidden Conspiracy

Three texts listed in the bibliography, *Innocent Casualties, The FDA's War Against Humanity, Good Intentions and Natural Cures They Don't Wants You To Know About*, go into great detail about political cover ups designed to keep us all in the status quo of health achievement where the powers that be are in control. There are many more hidden agendas afoot here which have mostly to do with the people who make the most money from all markets—health and nutrition alike—wanting to stay on top. It is not within the scope of this book to go into detail on this part of a crucial issue. But suffice it to say that it does exist and not with our best health interests at heart, just their profits. Throughout this book, we make reference to a few of these manipulative politics as a way to better understand the realities of why the nutritional and healthful life we all live isn't better.

In fact, the advertising practices of drug companies, nutrition companies, and doctors are bombarding us with their information in order to manipulate us to become completely immersed with their way thinking and way of treating illness. Because of this perspective, there is great confusion and resistance to change before we even address the issue of the additional problem of socio-cultural lag. This lag is the differential between what cutting-edge science has shown to be true and the time it takes the average the person to comprehend these changes. This lag is, on average, considered to last at least 30 to 40 years.

The mistaken notions of you are what you eat and one-size-fits-all are good for all routine business right now but very bad for good health at any time. As people become aware of the personalized nutrition process, this will completely reverse. There will be a great shift—a new mega trend—to start substituting the nutritional mistakes of the past with the benefits of this new and improved way of participating in superior nutritional practices afforded by and through the real diet secret: testing.

# Chapter IV

## Real Diet Secrets Revealed
## Symptoms Are Obsolete

*Man is a food-dependent creature. If you don't feed him,*
*he will die. If you feed him improperly, part of him will die.*
—Emanuel Cheraskin, M.D., D.M.D.

Aside from the different types of Zone, blood type, and metabolic typing diets and other approaches to organizing nutrition, there is the symptom approach. In this case people attempt to match the physical symptoms they experience to specific nutrients that they then resultantly need. This very bad idea leads to:

## Reality Check #6

*The actual symptoms that one's experiencing*
*cannot be used as a guide for effectively organizing*
*food and supplemental input for improving health.*

Obviously, if somebody has the jitters from drinking too much coffee or is nauseated from drinking too much alcohol, stopping the intake of these substances will automatically help.

There are literally hundreds of symptoms which can plague us, ranging from very mild discomforts to full-blown unbearable pain. From headaches to body aches; fatigue to excessive restless energy; itchiness to numbness; flaky, sensitive dry skin to painful acne-ridden oily skin; constipation to outright diarrhea – there are just so many symptoms possible in the human body. And they all have two things in common: First, they represent the body's attempt to alert us consciously to the fact that something is wrong and second, symptoms are merely the tip of the ice-berg when it comes to the sometimes very complex physiochemical chain of events which take place before the actual symptom is noticeable.

Usually, the greater the intensity of a given symptom, the more serious the body's problem. The more accompanying symptoms we then experience, the more complex and far-reaching the problem is. In either instance, the time it takes for the physiochemical chain of events to occur for a symptom to appear can vary widely. These events can take a few, like those causing the pain of a burn, to many years as in developing the progressive pain and stiffness of osteoarthritis or a sudden heart attack, which is many years in the making.

Faster appearing, more noticeable symptoms can be a blessing in that they let us know when something is wrong quickly so that we can take action to correct the problem before it worsens. Unfortunately, this may not seem like a blessing in the case of some very pathological conditions like a highly malignant cancer where the chances for survival are minimal by the time they're felt. Symptoms which are less noticeable at first, and then become more progressive and eventually chronic in nature, are harder to understand in relation to exact cause. Many things can happen physiochemically before we can really feel something and identifying the initial disturbance which set things into motion may be more difficult. This is a strong provocation for drug cover-ups, what I call a shortcut to thinking. Therefore, these more subtle and hidden symptoms may be more difficult to act on at the core for total relief. A burn hurts long before the symptoms of progressive heart disease are apparent.

Clearly, early detection is desirable for these kinds of progressive problems, but saying that it's all in your head or that they are a function of aging and then quickly covering it up with a drug may not be the best idea. Stresses create the physiochemical events which in turn create the systematic progression of eventually noticeable symptoms. "Eustress" is positive stress such as unbridled happiness or a good exercise session, whereas "distress" is considered negative stress such as that from an injury or the loss of a loved one. Symptoms of Eustress could include a sore abdominal region after laughing so much or sore muscles after exercising. For the most part eustresses are beneficial, whereas in the case of distress there are only negative, health-robbing consequences when left unattended.

Excepting immediate injury like a burn, distresses may persevere and accumulate for years before noticeable symptoms ensue. In either the case of fast-appearing symptoms or progressive onset symptoms, it always pays to reverse, correct or favorably modify symptom-producing physiochemical events along with their instigating stresses, as long before symptoms appear as possible. Correcting these unhealthy events by strengthening the body's nutritional constitution at all cellular levels is where the science of true prevention resides. This helps even in the case of accidental injury whereby any damage sustained is adapted to and repaired more easily. The accompanying physiochemical reaction sequence-to-symptom chain of events following a given accident is significantly improved upon thanks to the body having fewer weaknesses to begin with and a subsequently faster healing physiochemical response rate to counteract the injury. Avoiding a burn is always the best prevention, but a nutritionally reinforced physiochemical healing response is next best thing. This superior healing response inevitably reduces symptomatic intensity and duration which equates with less lasting damage done and more complete healing.

Unfortunately, our entire system of conventional allopathic medicine is centered primarily upon symptoms and not necessarily their preceding, causative, physiochemical events, which are very much harder to notice unless detectable by conventional diagnostics, which has its limitations. Conventional medicine uses diagnostic procedures to briefly look for what's behind most symptoms so that it can group them into a disease or condition with a specific name. This diagnostic approach is essential to help sort out symptoms and impending life-threatening conditions. But many symptoms can be mutually shared by many nameable diseases. Is your headache from too much stress or a brain tumor, leukemia or from lack of regularity? Proper diagnostics can sort this out somewhat in light of the fact that at least 150 different conditions or diseases demonstrate headache as a primary symptom. Most people only enter the doctor's office when enough symptomatic intensity (discomfort) presents itself beyond a specific person's tolerance level. The doctor typically is expected to alleviate the symptom as quickly as possible with a fast-acting pill, lotion, potion, injection or something because it hurts. We're taught to expect immediate relief.

Most before and after symptom-driven conventional diagnostic technology, disease profiling methodologies, and subsequent symptom blocking (quick fix) drug mediated therapy is far too superficial and incomplete an approach to address disease prevention or eradication. There are just too many flaws to this process and the ensuing results can be very misleading, many times confusing and sometimes even dangerous. Maybe that's why the leading cause of malpractice amongst medical doctors is misdiagnosis (not to mention human error in the process, which must be kept at a minimum while diagnostic technology is at a maximum).

Furthermore, this symptom-only medical approach which is then applied to those most (obvious) nutrition-related disorders is even more flawed. People believe that they can connect symptoms to nutrition problems such as a folic acid deficiency in hair loss or zinc deficiency in acne or perhaps essential fatty acids for itchy skin or painful joints. There could be some nutrition-to-symptom connections in these cases but there are many more variables to consider on a case-by-case basis in order to make a proper assessment. Unfortunately, this symptomatic approach to nutrition is highly inaccurate as compared to even less nutrition-direct, more medically complicated or generalized body disorders like headaches.

Even general disorders can symptomatically express themselves in various ways due to nutritional inconsistencies present within the physiochemical systems of the body both directly related to and not directly related to any given disorder. As an example, a person may come down with a headache from eye strain on the computer. The headache is caused from eye strain but this particular person, thanks to a vitamin A deficiency, has suffered blurred vision longer than somebody without a vitamin A deficiency. But how do we know which is which? And due to this vitamin A deficiency, this same person develops a stiff neck and then becomes sick later that evening due to the standing weakness of the immune system, predisposed by the A deficiency. A person without a vitamin A deficiency and with better vitamin C functionalization may not have the blurred vision for more than a few minutes after being on the computer and may never get sick or develop a stiff neck from the same amount of stress. But again, how do we know for sure? This "how do you know what to expect" phenomenon has all to do with biochemical individuality whereby a given problem might have many different manifestations within different bodies leading to various sets of symptoms for each body due to the same stress. Another good example of this is in the case of arthritic pain. The pain experience of one individual with fatty acid imbalances, lead accumulation, and zinc deficiency will be noticeably greater in quantity and quality than a person suffering arthritis—without these same nutritionally fostered physiochemical disturbances. The symptom to-nutrition-connection is closely connected to the presence of inadequate or faulty nutrition only when all the facts are fully known, which of course is impossible without the nutrition testing in play.

Consider the disease scurvy, which indisputably is a direct result of vitamin C deficiency. In 1740, the British sailing ship Anson began a four-year voyage around the world. In four years, 626 out of 920 men died of scurvy. In commenting about the occurrence of this disease on board the Anson, Richard Walter (an officer on ship) commented "this disease, so frequently attending all long voyages and so particularly destructive to us is surely the most singular and unaccountable of any that affects the human body. For its symptoms are inconstant and innumerable and its progress and effects extremely irregular: for scarcely two persons have the same complaints and where there is found some conformity in symptoms, the order of their appearance has been totally different however, though it frequently puts on the form of many other diseases and is therefore not to be described by any exclusive and infallible criterion…"

In effect, our biochemical individuality directly effects our specific nutrient needs and also the symptomatic and non-symptomatic expression of nutrient insufficiency and all symptom-related conditions whether they are directly diet-related or not. In other words, everything you feel has very much to do with nutritional status no matter what problem we're investigating. This scientific fact has been demonstrated in research time and time again and is typified in one favored study by Richard Velazquez which truly discerns this symptom variability phenomenon in depth. However thanks to the "kill symptoms first, ask questions later" approach of conventional medicine and the asymptomatic approach to nutritional disorders, centuries of holistic wisdom has been completely side-stepped. Instead of considering the interconnected roles that essential nutrients play within cellular metabolism and the widespread cell/tissue/organ/system-wide effects nutrient insufficiencies/imbalances can exert upon all physiochemical events, we're focused upon what I refer to as "symptom paradox."

This can be defined as symptomatic ambiguities which become more blatantly apparent in light of the extreme diversity of disease expression from person to person and are exponentially compounded in the presence of a greater number of nutrient deficiencies, excesses or toxicities present; this includes the consideration that any and all body functions can be deteriorated differently in accordance with an individual's specific biochemical expression. Therefore, nutrition-related degenerative diseases typically exhibit **greater symptomatic variations and biochemical expressions** which **increase as the degree of nutritional inconsistencies intensify.** What this means is, the more nutritional imbalance that occurs, the more symptoms and disease that are expressed. This symptomatic variability paradox makes it even more difficult to use any set of conventional medical lab test "markers" to nutritionally define a disease. Unless there is testing for nutritional inconsistencies in the first place (not at all a routine medical practice) before conventional lab tests are used, it's impossible to relate this non-nutritional evaluation lab science to accurately explain the nutritional components of all symptoms and their resultant diseases. In other words, conventional diagnostic profiling for symptoms and the utilization of standard medical tests cannot define the human symptomatic experience as related to nutrition. And because of the body's physicochemical complexity and uniqueness, we cannot directly match a symptom to a nutrient level unless we have direct measurements of the nutrients occurring at the same time the symptoms are being expressed. This is the paradox that is compounding our illness and confounding our health. Symptoms are truly obsolete when you consider that with personalized nutrition technology, one can measure and correct genetic and/or metabolically induced physiochemistries relative to nutrition and the external environment – long before the physiochemical breakdowns which lead to symptoms and disease ever occur. In other words, we can finally get in front of symptoms and correct them before they may even occur long before symptom–focus conventional medicine can. So why don't we?

Furthermore, thanks to the labs comparing nutrition tests with symptoms and diseases, (and even regular lab tests that medical doctors practice routinely), we can now delineate a clearer nutrition-to-symptom-to-disease connection in each and every body perfectly, healthy or not. The greatest health benefit is that after nutritionally testing literally millions of bodies already sick or suffering from a given disease, the labs have found characteristic and highly specific nutritional imbalances which are always connected to each of these diseases and symptoms. These can then automatically and statistically be compared to each individual body once it's tested, in order to look for developing disease states or symptoms that would be related to a nutritional disturbance. This correlational technique provides the ultimate prevention. But again, this statistical process relies on a nutrition test first and cannot be calculated by any other means, even standard medical examinations and tests, and certainly not questionnaires or symptom surveys alone. Symptoms aside, all other conventional and ancient approaches to nutrition are now considered obsolete in light of personalized nutrition, which is testing nutrition disorders directly and then directly applying clinically proven nutritional management to each individual. These two steps are what we must accomplish in order to receive the full wellness benefits that orthomolecular medical science has repeatedly proven are attainable. The entire application of this science is based upon the previously mentioned two-step process below which is necessary in order to accomplish the most targeted nutritional management ever conceived.

### *The Two Primary Accomplishments Personalized Nutrition Realizes with Targeted Nutritional Management*

#### *#1 Detection*

*Targeted nutrition reveals exactly which nutrition-related biochemical disturbances a given body's cells are suffering from.*

**How?** Biochemical disturbances are revealed through direct and indirect measurement of the body's:

- primary nutrient and toxic metal retention profile (deficiencies and excesses of minerals, vitamins, vitamin-like substances, proteins, fats, sugars, toxins, etc.)
- metabolic *type, rate,* and *tissue acidity*
- *thyroid, adrenal and other* glands' functional hormonal output
- autonomic *nervous system* function as parasympathetic or sympathetic dominant

- diet-related *disease tendencies* as correlated from statistical comparisons
- nutrition-related *symptoms* experienced
- *digestive* system weaknesses
- mineral-related and other *allergic tendencies*
- *sensitivities* to concentrated *sugars*
- biochemical pathways where the greatest *metabolic dysfunction* is occurring

### #2 Correction

*Targeted nutrition nutritionally repairs and rebalances any biochemical disturbances found inside your body cells.*

**How?** Laboratory-proven programs of ***completely personalized nutrition*** and customized supplementation are precisely tailored to each individual's biochemical uniqueness as tested. This includes each individual nutrient deficiency, antagonistic imbalance, and toxin and describing:

- ***foods*** to completely ***avoid*** at this moment, and those to ***eat more*** of every day.
- ***detoxification*** procedures to rid the body of poisons and delineate sources of external contaminants to watch out for.
- macro and micro ***nutrient zone*** recommendations (exact proportions of real food and supplemental nutrients for fastest, most complete results).
- a ***nutritional*** and ***toxic baseline*** from which to scientifically compare all future metabolic improvements as measured by retesting (this goes way beyond the welcomed energy gain, symptom-reduction, and fat-loss that most people strive for as positive symptoms).
- how to literally ***make every bite of food count*** by factoring in every supplemental nutrient in exact synergistic proportion, for the best rebalancing results possible as allowed by genetic design.

Personalized nutrition science can provide the most precise nutritional answers every time, for any unique body by taking the two steps listed above. Targeted nutrition management simply means identifying each of the nutrients that are out of balance and restoring them back into balance.

### Why Only Nutrition Testing in Order to
### Target and Manage our Nutrients?

This seemingly repetitive topic may invite impatience for those of you who now understand the value of nutrition testing and correction. But believe it or not, there will be some who still think that other ways of interpreting nutritional status have validity even when using tests is the Center point.

First, let's define what a real nutrition test is.

It is any *direct measurement* of a mineral, vitamin, amino acid, fatty acid, vitamin-like substance (such as CoQ10), phytonutrient (such as indole), enzyme intermediate (such as HMG, which is the metabolic precursor for cholesterol), toxin (such as mercury or pthalates), nutrient ratio (such as calcium/magnesium or Omega-6/Omega-3), nutrition-related allergy, hormone pattern, specific gene direct-test which demonstrates nutrient usage patterns, metabolic rate classification and balascopic overview (nutrient-related disease tendency).

Note—*conventional medical tests don't even scratch the surface of this hidden nutritional domain* where over 223 diet-related diseases can begin to take hold.

This is why we say that these tests go beyond the limitations of conventional medical tests. In comparison, a medical test is like giving an algebra test to a biology class; it's apples and oranges, they're not the same no matter what the problem. Hair, saliva, urine, blood, breath, and even fecal tests reveal this special, specific information directly. In fact, as opposed to medical science, about 80% of nutrition testing specimens are not from blood sources, whereas with medical diagnostics, blood represents about 80% of the test specimen medium. Nothing else can stand up to the scrutiny of a nutrition test. This is exactly how it works for standard medicine in regard to medical tests and this is how it works for nutrition in modern society. Anything less is considered pure guesswork or nutrition nonsense, a fallacy by scientists—therefore, the tests simply provide the nutritional truth. All other information is secondary to an actual test. Future retests will closely examine your therapeutic progress at the sub-cellular level, fast or slow, good or bad. There are stories about people feeling better or losing weight or symptoms that have disappeared that go along with these retests but that's all secondary to the direct measurement of what's actually occurring at the deepest levels of the body that are the most crucial. There's simply no other scientific way to tell how well your body's responding to a nutrition program.

It sounds complicated, but it's simple now due to explosive technological advances which make all of the above a simple, pushbutton, easy-to-use, lab-generated, computer analogue, simplified, non doctor essential, inexpensive arsenal of the most powerful nutrition diagnostic ever seen. This is no exaggeration. Hair, saliva, urine, blood spots, and even fecal tests reveal all.

To test or not to test – that now becomes the question. Scientific research has determined that we can't manage our nutrients without one. From a simple logical standpoint, it makes absolute sense to know whenever possible exactly what foods and supplements your body truly needs, from gene to enzyme to toxin, before you indulge yourself. Any other approach remains guesswork, especially when indisputably **no two people are alike** and therefore have such a very different nutritional needs. This uniqueness phenomenon, **biochemical individuality**, is based on over 640 bionutrient chemicals and 400 toxins that can be accurately measured and precisely repaired. In fact, using this type of nutrition information in regard to Arizonian Biosphere II researchers, UCLA predicted 166 years of disease-free life for the participating individuals if they stayed on their uniquely perfect diets in a clean environment.

So, if a person still doesn't test, what's their alternative?

- One-size-fits-all diet practices where you just eat whatever everyone else says you should eat. The question we need to ask is, would we feed an Eskimo, whose traditional diet is 90% animal and fish, an East Pakistani's traditional vego-vegetarian diet? Or feed a ballerina like a Sumo wrestler or a newborn infant like an 85 year old? Hopefully not, but many people still do.

- One-size-fits-all supplement practices, where we just follow the Daily Values (DVs) or RDAs and take A – Z multivitamins and minerals, etc. and whatever a relative or a friend or the clerk at the health food store says we need. But, would we continue to do this if we knew that the U.S. Food and Nutrition Board who created the MDRs, RDAs, DVs, etc. recently stated that "these recommendations have nothing to do with the specific needs of an individual"? Would we continue one-size-fits-all supplementation if we knew that the Clayton Biochemical Institute at the University of Texas recommends that "each person should be tested and an individualized nutrition repletion initiated" and that Harvard University further backs this up by withdrawing its support for the "indiscriminate use of diet and supplements" (guessing)? In truth, there is no such thing as an all-in-one A – Z multivitamin/mineral that really works.

- We can use symptom questionnaires, blood type, zone, muscle testing, or Atkins diet and supplemental formats. Follow these seemingly more personalized programs and you'll automatically be individualizing nutrition – right? As science has demonstrated, *wrong.* These nutritional formats are still considered one-size-fits-all theory and not the scientifically derived directly measured nutrition facts of only your body. Symptoms have no direct correlation with specific nutrient needs anyway and questionnaires are basically useless because they don't measure a body's biochemicals directly. The straw that breaks the camel's back can be seen when people are nutritionally tested who are on these one-size-fits-all programs, taking their respective supplements, even with medical supervision. Anywhere from 81 to 99% (depending on which study) of these people nutritionally evaluated who haven't ever been tested before show across-the-board, often profound, deficiencies, excesses and hidden surprises like toxins and hidden allergies and even more biochemical disturbances. HANES research shows that 53% of the people that take a multivitamin are in worse health than those who don't. Two-hundred twenty-three nutrition-related diseases, fatness, fatigue, and endless symptoms are the result of these measurable imbalances easily avoided in the first place with the right testing information from the start.

Those who have used nutrition tests as their diet and supplement guide to eliminate nutritional and toxic disorders eventually test out perfectly time and again, with no further imbalances. So why waste any more valuable time and health on one-size-fits-all rhetoric, fads, theories, and non-accountability? Take the tests and become your best. This puts the decisions for scientific health control in the hands of each person to do or not do what is best for them.

*Scientific Laws and Principles Which Ensure Nutrition Success*

# Reality Check # 7
## The Body Acts as it Will, Not as We Want

This particular reality is of extreme significance because in my clinical practice, I can tell you that I have encountered person after person who thinks that they can literally will their body back into balance. Among this group are holy men, yogis, psychics, martial art masters and other assorted strong-willed people. The fact of the matter is, once we start testing them, they tend to have even more nutritional and toxic disorder than others who do not subscribe to this "I can do it all with my mind" idea. It should be no surprise that as testing's proof in your face reality hits these people—and those who believe themselves to have good instinctive sense about nutrition—very hard, it violently shakes the very core of their belief systems as they find that they're completely wrong about this.

People who think that they can instinctively sort out how to mentally and physically nourish their bodies for best performance have no idea about hidden allergies and the subsequent allergy and addiction syndromes that Dr. James Braley discovered in the late '70s and early '80s. In effect, people become addicted to things that they're allergic to, and don't even realize it. They pass off their hidden allergy addictions as instincts. In my clinical work, time after time, I've found patients that are literally addicted to the foods that are the worst for them at the moment and haven't the slightest idea that they are having an allergic reaction. As the old saying goes, you can lead a horse to water but you can't make him drink. In our case of allergic-inspired cravings, this transforms into a new saying "you can lead a human to water, but you can't make him put down his soda pop." Sugar, starch, and fat cravings are all part of this anti-instinctive disharmony between body and environment.

There are three philosophies relating to the mind-body connection; existentialism, epiphenomenalism and dualistic interactionism. The existentialists believe that they can think themselves well. The Epiphenomenalists believe that their body ultimately controls their mind by its exposure to food, environment and experiences. The dualistic interactionists believe that both mind and body affect each other and that the whole has to be taken into consideration in order to achieve the best balance possible for radiant health.

Existentialism says, exactly what you're thinking has nutrition-altering effects on your body. As an example, when we're afraid, we deplete nutrients in an accelerated and disproportionate manner as needed by the endocrine system to adapt to the stress of being scared. Your mind's recognition of fear initiates this entire flight or flight process. Conversely, an epiphenomenalist example would be, if you eat a whole quart of ice cream, chock full of sugar and fat, or perhaps a couple packages of Twinkies (remember the Twinkie Defense), you think and feel much differently than before you ate it. The science of biochemical individuality relates to dualistic interactionism. There are meaningful effects of mind and body on each other that strongly impact on your nutritional status and subsequent health. But we cannot rely on either alone, independent of the other, to achieve our most radiant health. Obviously, the more specifically you can feed your body on an individualized basis, the better for your mind. Also, the better you can feed and fill your head with the most positive and learned thoughts, the better for your body. It's important to work ourselves from both angles, but neither one alone is the secret to perfect wellness. There are certain laws and principles of nature that we have uncovered and can explain scientifically. These phenomena are the underlying causative agents for all that occurs in our special bodies and minds, good or bad, healthy or unhealthy. Orthomolecular science capitalizes upon this information in a very highly targeted manner in order to reliably manipulate the positive impact of nutrition on the entire individual, time after time in person after person.

Once people go beyond the idea that proper nutrition consists of indiscriminately consuming food from the basic food pyramid and understand that real nutrition involves much more than diet, they begin to drop the mistakes of the past immediately. Orthomolecular medicine, or personalized nutrition, has determined that nutrient utilization is affected primarily by the following factors:

1. Individual genetic and metabolic characteristics
2. Nutrient bioavailability in food
3. Toxic accumulation in our body, food, and in our environment
4. Neurological activity
5. Endocrine function
6. Specific dynamic action of food
7. Intestinal absorption efficiency
8. Cellular utilization of nutrients
9. Enzymatic patterns and blocks
10. Antagonism and synergism between vitamins, minerals, aminos, fatty acids, and other nutrients, toxins and hormones
11. Stress (distress and eustress)
12. Disease states present or developing
13. Exercise profiles, rest patterns
14. Age, occupation
15. Drugs

***Which nutrients and toxins actually reach the cell*** and the consequences of "too much" and "too little" is our ***most major concern*** in personalized nutrition.

Technically speaking, the three physics/chemistry principles below are what mostly governs nutritional order in our body in this regard, and what personalized nutrition is manipulating for best health:

> A. Laws of mass action (Albert Einstein and other scientists)
> B. Physical relativity (Albert Einstein) between atoms and molecules
> C. Enzyme and diffusion kinetics (Krebs and others)

The ***Laws of Mass Action, Relativity*** and ***Enzyme and Diffusion Kinetics*** define the nature of and exactly how all chemical reactions take place and can further explain precisely what happens inside and outside of cells and within given pathways of all chemical reactions which take place in a human body. All of these pathways only work in the presence of water, which as we know, is the major constituent of our bodies along with available oxygen. Without oxygen and hydrogen none of this will take place—there is no life. The entire spectrum of these reactive enzyme-mediated biochemical pathways requiring oxygen and immersed in water, from digestion to absorption, to utilization, to excretion (elimination) is called metabolism. This overall biochemical process provides the only means by which we build up or break down all matter once inside the body as well as how it is moved about and/or stored. Within the sum total of metabolism there are only two components; the building up part, or anabolism, and the breaking down part, or catabolism. Both have a specific beginning and ending point for any given pathway or simply a start to finish. Whether breaking a substance down to release energy (like breaking down carbohydrates into ATP—adenosine triphosphate—which is energy) or building up a tissue in the body (like using calcium to make bone tissue), it will all start at a point A (with the starting substance officially called "substrate") and ends after multiple intermediate chemical conversion steps controlled by enzymes* to end at point Z (product). We will look closer at enzymes in subsequent chapters.

---

*enzymes by nature include those found in digestive juices, the food itself and within body cells (enzymes are made of protein's amino acids).

Examples:

***Catabolism*** (Substrate or point A): Sugar in an orange
Step 1: (enzyme)          Step 2: (enzyme)          Step 3: (enzyme)
Step 4: (enzyme)          Step 5: (enzyme)          Step 6: (enzyme)
Product or Point Z in this case is energy (ATP)

***Anabolism*** (Substrate or point A): Calcium in spinach
Step 1: (enzyme)          Step 2: (enzyme)          Step 3: (enzyme)
Step 4: (enzyme)          Step 5: (enzyme)          Step 6: (enzyme)
Step 7: (enzyme)
Product or Point Z in this case is bone cells/tissue

The number of steps taken varies depending on what series of chemical reactions and which pathways we are referring to. Whether we are talking about breaking down a complex protein in the intestine into individual amino acids for use by the liver or a genetic stimulation which causes the RNA—or ribonucleic acid—to assemble individual, previously broken down amino acids into certain proteins that regulate cellular processes such as respiration, there are a certain amount of steps and certain specific enzymes involved. Some enzymes can be shared with other pathways but each pathway has its own characteristics and there are several thousand of them which run the body in all its functions, throughout each of its tissues. Furthermore, these enzymes and their respective pathways predominate inside of cells but are also found on the outside. The body cell's membranes act as specially designed barriers which allow certain substances such as enzymes to stay within a cell and concurrently keep other things out. The membrane will inevitably allow certain things in like sugar (as monosaccharide) and certain things out such as ammonia, depending on what type of cell we speak of. What is available or found on the inside and the outside of a given cell has to do with how well the cell membrane is functioning as well as what is going on inside the cell or around the cell. Either way, the efficiency of the cell membrane can add or subtract to the overall efficiency of metabolism and when functioning properly, allow the life-sustaining biochemical pathways to work efficiently.

***The overriding goal*** of orthomolecular personalized nutrition medicine is ***to create more energy from less food and drink.*** In order to create the fastest or most efficient metabolism, we must arrange the nutrition in our body so that all the biochemical pathways that either break down the food into energy or use energy to build into substance and matter within our bodies run as freely and efficiently as possible both inside and outside of cells. When this occurs at peak efficiency, we simply state the case that "processing be of the most amount of energy from each bite of food as genetically possible, with the least amount of toxic accumulation and excess fat buildup." Automatically we have more energy to fight disease, to maintain youth longer, to subtract excess fat, to keep our minds clear and our body functions working at their peak, all day long while having more of the substances we need to maintain and repair the body for dependable operation as long as possible and under all circumstances of stress. When the nutritional balance is out of order within the body, the opposite occurs. An increase of inert, unnecessary, toxic, and/or antagonistic particles retained and/or functionalized by the body interfere with fast metabolism because they directly oppose the most healthfully bioactive, necessary, nontoxic, synergistic ones, which ultimately results in less chemical-reactive efficiency—or energy. I like to refer to anything that does not belong in nature or is excess or deficient as an "antagonist." In a body with a faster metabolism we're asking for a maximum synergy of oxygen, water and all nutrients for the greatest energy-releasing potential possible. The key points of weakness that antagonistics go after or disrupt are the enzymes, cell membranes, and any or all intracellular and extracellular chemical environments which they can inevitably mix up or disrupt, causing a downslide in the energy gradient (loss of energy). In other words, these antagonistics induce less energy to be made, along with more consequential, health-robbing, physiochemical dysfunction to be present. Excesses of undesirable chemicals such as dangerous toxins like mercury and even essential nutrients which in turn act toxic when they are too high, burden all biochemical pathways but create extra disruption throughout the excretory mechanisms of the body, again leading to many direct and indirect stresses and potential breakdowns in body systems. Too many minerals, not just the heavy metals, can damage kidney membranes in time. A major excess of even a vitamin such as ascorbic acid (vitamin C), can lower the pH of the body which in turn depletes the buffering* systems of the body like those present in the kidney, which

*A buffer is a chemical substance that simply neutralizes a strong acid or alkaline chemical.

Note: in Chapter 5 we will look more closely at enzymes as inspired by Dr. Linus Pauling (under the discussion about organic acids), inasmuch as they are special biochemical places within metabolism that we can directly impact function with precisely synergized nutritional input.

produce bicarbonates and which again lead to kidney stress due to an overload of coenzymes – vitamin C— in this case. At high levels and/or in antagonistic proportions, vitamins and minerals, (formally known as coenzymes or cofactors due to their stimulating effects on enzymes), can be very toxic regardless of whether they are considered to be fat or water soluble. People have been categorically taught to fear fat-soluble vitamins in excess due to the body storage capacity for them, more so than water-soluble vitamins which don't store as easily, but this is not the case. Orthomolecular medicine has demonstrated that water solubles disrupt function as well, in excess and imbalance.

It is the function of applied personalized nutrition to effectively sort out nutrition for the most optimum metabolism possible through the use of only assessment and measurement and proven corrective therapy so that the above principles and chemical dynamics are adhered to every time, in every body for maximum wellness benefits. For the purposes of commonsense simplicity, I have arranged an extreme simplification of this information as follows:

### *The Scientific Power of Customized Diet and Supplementation: Digital Laws and Principles*

The clinical control that we can apply to one's given nutrient retention and functional metabolic status relies on four simplified processes of food and supplement input.

1. *Law of Opposites.* According to quantum-mathematical (digital) formulation, **we systematically apply more of the nutrients that a given tested body is retaining less of and less of what the body is retaining more of.**

*Problem:* After testing, your body exhibits a deficiency of potassium and an excess of soft-tissue calcium.

*Solution:* Utilizing statistically respective foods and food groups, along with quantumized supplemental proportions (in accordance with all atomic and molecular relationships known about interactive nutrient synergism or antagonism), we can supply your body with much more potassium, and its particular synergists and much less calcium and its particular synergists, to the point where no imbalance exists.

2. *"See-Saw" Homeostatic Effect.* Through millions of time-extensive clinical/comparative trials, orthomolecular-focused medical labs have determined that *you cannot reliably affect a desired retention rate of one mineral or associated vitamin without proportionately adjusting the intake of at least 14 other synergistic and/or antagonistic nutrients.* Simply, if you imagine all the fundamental nutrients sitting on a seesaw, if you change the amount of one nutrient, it subsequently affects the balance of all the rest.

*Problem:* A given body exhibits a potassium deficiency.
*Solution:* In order to reliably change this phenomenon, we have to adjust potassium intake to a higher level, plus we must proportionately increase these seven specific synergistic minerals: sodium, magnesium, cobalt, manganese, zinc, phosphorous, and iron. Additionally, we must proportionately reduce these three antagonistic minerals: lithium, cobalt (if in excess), sodium (if in excess) and all inappropriate ratios of the synergistic minerals listed above which in effect will collectively cause antagonism to potassium retention. We must proportionately increase 7 synergistic vitamins: vitamin A, vitamin B1, vitamin B2, vitamin B3, vitamin B5, vitamin B6 and vitamin E as well as proportionately decrease the ease of vitamin antagonists: vitamin D, vitamin B10 and dramatically reduce vitamin B1 if it is in excess.

3. *Interactive Antagonistic Nutrient Displacement (IAND).* Based upon the indigenous atomic properties (such as atomic weight and charge) and subsequent reactivity potential of each element to the next (atomic weight, electric charge, reactivity/action potential differentials etc.), *we apportion target-specific elemental antagonists which in effect oppose each other and subsequently increase the elimination of undesirable excesses along with their relative deficiencies* in an accelerated manner.

Note: certain Phyto- chemicals, amino acids, fats, sugars and vitamin-like substances affect therapeutic outcomes and therefore are statistically correlated in formulistic remedies for a given individual.

*Problem:* Excess calcium retention in soft tissue.

*Solution:* Dramatically increase proportionate potassium intake in order to displace the calcium retention in soft tissues which in effect *forces the calcium to migrate into bone.*

*Rationale:* Calcium and potassium are positively charged particles and therefore repel each other strenuously. Increase one and you'll hasten the movement or displacement of the other to its respective tissue of dominance or for elimination.

4. *Mass Action/Enzyme Kinetic Loading Effect Principle (MAEK-LEP).* In order to reliably achieve desired rebalancing outcomes, the body's biochemical pathways must be systematically (food) and supplementally loaded (saturated) for a distinct period of time and then the outcome of nutrient retention measured with retests. *Test-to-retest differential comparisons* allow the most thorough interpretation of body response of precisely how well nutrients are being distributed through cells and processed throughout all biochemical pathways. This also provides the necessary insights for further metabolic correction with adjusted (food) and supplement loads.

# Reality Check #8
## A Warning to Us All

Any food or supplement deviation from this approach or what we call a "closed" clinical program will predispose failure. There are simply too many variables as described above that must be taken into account in the quest for therapeutic success. Supplements and foods cannot be randomized or speculated in the process of controlling metabolic response with non-program alternatives. Sadly, when people try to change a personally applied nutrition program in any way, including and especially supplements, they are in essence going against one hundred years of applied clinical scientific research provided by the world's leading medical labs for nutrient/toxic testing and therapeutic results. The whole basis of these programs (and other complementary tests and procedures), is to eliminate all

Note: all problems and solutions are addressed from thelong term perspective.

potential errors and personal guesswork to effectively replace it with solid scientific protocol, in other words, the scientifically proven truth. All else
would be considered non-science or nonsense and therefore is a waste of time
and money. Sadly, non-test-substantiated nutritional guesswork (food and
supplements) is the underlying cause for the U.S. being number one in the
world for nutrient/toxic/metabolic imbalances. Ancient wisdom and standard medicine can only take us so far. This is the real diet secret, there is no
other, only the perfection of this one as history now dictates.

Due to science, the new modern common sense for nutrition is as follows:

1. Measure the nutrients and toxins in your body right now, to know exactly what's inside.
2. Use laboratory medically proven nutrition therapy which is based on the
law of opposites whereby systematically and formulaically the body is fed
more of what nutrients it's deficient in and less of what nutrients are found
to be in excess, until all meet in the middle as confirmed by retests.

The new complementary medicine is personalized nutrition, test-mediated
only, as it will help any body before, after, or during sickness, debilitation,
no matter what their condition or what drugs they are on. As Hippocrates
said, "Thy food is thy remedy." Finally, science has uncovered a proven way
to help Mother Nature to work better for all of us in our time, once and for
all.

# Chapter V

## Target Nutrition Therapy

*To continue learning about yourself*
*you must strive to look at things another way.*
—Robin Williams, *Dead Poets Society*

**What's Wrong With My Body? What Can I Do About It?**
**Going Beyond the Scope of Routine Medicine**
**Tests and Intervention**

The theories of metabolic typing and nutritional individualization from 5,000 years ago to the present have been scientifically reviewed, condensed, tested, and surpassed with a new orthomolecular nutritional technology mega-trend.

In 1956, our orthomolecular Godfather, Dr. Roger Williams, published *Biochemical Individuality.* What was then his theory and is now considered a fact is that each person is biochemically unique in their anatomy and chemical composition. Dr. Williams' research showed wide variations among healthy, normal humans. He related these differences to genetic inheritance and revealed unique needs for particular nutrients due to inherited digestive, absorptive, and enzymatic concentrations and abilities to transport nutrients and to excrete the by-products of metabolism. And as mentioned previously, thousands of years before Dr. Williams, the Chinese, Ayurvedics (described by Deepak Chopra), Greeks (Hippocrates), Egyptians and many more, developed typing systems to uncover individuality. Laboratory science has examined and streamlined **these metabolic typing theories** for any inherent value. Unfortunately, their value is exceedingly limited if not nonexistent because they **give us no direct indication of the actual nutrient retention and functional profiles up to the moment for any individual.** That is they're inherent deficit; this is why they are for the most part useless in today's world.

Old style metabolic typing categorizes certain genetically predetermined constitutional elements into subclasses of physical, psychological and physiological distinction. Blood type, vital statistics, glandular balance, ethnicity, personality, body and face shape, fat distribution pattern and other human distinctions can add up to well beyond the commonly mentioned 37 metabolic/body/blood/constitutional types with corresponding food patterns. This all makes for, at best, interesting reading in comparison of the much more scientific pursuit of discovering our metabolic and biochemical individuality through orthomolecular testing technology. Metabolic typing's dire shortcomings render it virtually useless in light of modern insights. Quite simply, it has nothing to do with what nutritional state the body is in at the very moment of testing, which is all that counts. Only specialized testing beyond the scope of medical routine as featured in the process of personalized nutrition can provide this information fully and precisely.

How much vitamin C, calcium or copper is present in my body? What are my hidden allergies, toxic accumulations and glandular stresses? What aminos and fatty acids are out of balance? Without this up-to-the-moment information derived from direct metabolic chemistry measurement (such as hair, saliva, urine, blood, etc.), you cannot know exactly what nutrition your body needs to be put back into perfect balance. Metabolic profiling (testing) consists of all the tests, which precisely determine every discernable mineral, vitamin, amino acid, fatty acid, toxin, sensitivity, and diet-related hormone pattern present and whether they are in or out of balance relative to all body tissues and functions. These insights allow us to customize diet and supplements exactly to body specifications, eliminating guesswork altogether. One of the important components is that each of us can measure personal wellness success with ongoing retests over time, for comparison, to assess the progress of the personalized nutrition program. Old metabolic typing by itself is a process of grouping genetic subclasses in order to distinguish one's metabolic identity. But without testing direct metabolic need as accomplished in metabolic profiling, we cannot accurately determine our true biochemical individuality.

***Metabolic profiling is where only tests scientifically reveal our innermost uniqueness.*** Clearly light years beyond mere typing theory, 'profiling' eliminates doubts, involves no guesswork, leaves no stone left unturned and ***requires no on-site doctor*** unless requested.

Heart disease and cancer, the two major causes of death in the U.S., are premier nutrition-related diseases which can be anticipated using this metabolic profiling approach, as can the more than 221 other degenerative and germ-instigated diseases. Unfortunately, even most new discoveries in the field of nutrition have been exceedingly slow to be adopted by the medical community. This segment truly operates on a different priority system and has further confounded the integrated connection and holistic application of metabolic typing to the uniqueness of the individual with far too many specialists, specialties, and fragmented tidbits of information organized in a less-than-connected system of body management as it compares to the anti-pharmaceutical or nutritional level. This "put it all together, so it makes more sense on a simplistic level" concept lags even further behind than most people realize.

Good holistic historic examples of this are exemplified by scurvy and beriberi. These are probably two of the best known diet-related diseases, both of which persisted for many years before the British Navy figured out that mere limes arrested scurvy and doctors believed that a B vitamin deficiency, not a bacterium, caused beriberi. Only two decades ago the American medical establishment unequivocally stated that diet had no effect on cancer incidence whereas in August 2005, the American Cancer Society proclaimed that fully 60% of cancers can be prevented by diet and lifestyle changes. They continue to vigorously disseminate information to the public postulating that diet most certainly helps in the prevention and recovery of cancer. Generically multiply this non-health-nutrition connection effect across the board for all disease in conjunction with an inherent lack of concern about each individual's uniqueness and the problem becomes even more evident. Perhaps this is why medical and nutrition tests are so completely different. The substances being examined in medical tests are completely different than those from nutrition tests. A closer comparison between the two is found later in this chapter. For the moment, suffice it to say that medical tests closely examine chemistries of the body, mostly from blood because it is the ideal go-between or sequestering tissue and fluid from which to determine if a life-threatening health crisis from disease or accident is occurring. Medical toxicologists and Barietric physicians sometimes test either toxins or some vitamins as adjunctive tests to standard medical tests but not necessarily with the latest orthomolecular testing/intervention procedures in hand as they have to go outside of their usual medical training in order to learn about them both in diagnosis and therapy.

Orthomolecular tests, designed strictly for personalized nutrition, only examine those chemistries most related to nutrition-related disturbances of any one or number of essential nutrients, non-essential nutrients, toxins, metabolic rate, hidden allergies and certain immunoglobulin, prohormone/hormone profiles and interaction, enzyme function, fatty acids, amino acids, organic acids, parasites, autonomic function, digestive function, toxic elimination, stress, inflammation, drugs, and genetic structure. These particular measurements are predominantly made from non-blood specimens, such as urine, hair, saliva, biopsy, breath, and blood (in some cases where its accuracy is acceptable). Surprisingly, whereas in routine medicine blood is the primary specimen, indication of nutrition levels from blood is not a good representation of the nutritional status of all the body tissues. The following sections will itemize the special nutrition tests which allow us all to go beyond the relatively limited generic approaches to nutrition that we have. Dr. Harry Foster, nutritional researcher and professor of geography from the University of Victoria, describes these tests as providing 25 to 30% more life to our life. In other words, by not testing, you are losing from 25 to 30% of life expectancy and gaining a tendency to become sick, fat, and fatigued by the same amount. These tests have been designed simply to repair the shortcomings of past and present mistakes by amplifying the true power of nutrition.

## The Latest Nutrition Testing and Profiling Procedures

*Minerals:* The smallest particles of matter in the universe are atoms or elements which are interchangeable terms. They are categorized in chemistry and physics books as most of the elements on the Periodic Table. Each of those atoms listed on those tables are the building blocks of all matter and all life in the universe, including our bodies. Their presence in varying degrees and proportions specifies the nature of each life (and non-life) form in all properties and characteristics. The atoms or elements that we are most concerned with are the ones found in soil. Because they are found in soil and can be mined they are referred to as minerals. These 76 minerals are responsible for the structure and function of all life on this planet in combination with oxygen from the air and hydrogen from water. Humans are 4% minerals by weight. The rest of our body weight is matter derived from minerals and/or atoms such as hydrogen, oxygen, and nitrogen—including water, protein, tissue enzymes, hormones, etc. There are the same 76 minerals found in soil, which are identified in humans. They each exert varying electromagnetic force and inertia upon each other (as degrees of attraction, repulsion, and displacement) and their presence relative to one another not only defines "humanoid" within the universe but defines the wellness state of each individual human within itself. They are involved in every process of the body. Their exact proportion to one another, either as synergy or antagonism, affects or defects the efficiency of the entire organism. One's lifespan, state of wellness or sickness, fatness, energy level, and all other factors of one's life process is directly or indirectly related to the presence and proportion (ratio) of one mineral to the next. This, *the body's mineral retention, is the first and most important nutrient factor to test and where scientists always systematically begin the nutrition testing process.* Hair, urine, saliva, and one particular blood test are accurate and reliable indicators of mineral presence and function as deficiency, excess, or imbalance within the body.

*List of Primary Tests:* **1.** TMA (hair analysis) **2.** Metabolic urine analysis **3.** Organic acid analysis (urine) **4.** Saliva **5.** *Blood/mineral profile *Indicates that a blood specimen is required for this particular test.
**Electrolytes are included here. Electrolytes are a group of highly electromagnetic minerals found in blood which can exert a profound effect on other tissues.

*Discussion:* The nutritional role of the trace elements (minerals) revealed in the above tests has only recently become appreciated by clinicians. Diagnostically, doctors mostly look for some metabolic or structural error within the body and try to match a drug to the symptom this error creates. Most other alternative types of clinicians do the same by substituting herbs, generic vitamins and minerals, or homeopathic remedies to the symptom, still passing over diagnosing the root nutritional cause of the problem automatically. The above tests clearly show these mineral (and some directly related vitamin) root disorders. This information is becoming better understood lately by most practitioners and consumers who are more aware of the facts about minerals in relation to illness and wellness. They tend to value this information more so than previously in large measure because the health benefits they've sought are not being realized. Today, it is more widely acknowledged that mineral deficiencies and imbalances affect disorders of the cardiovascular, gastrointestinal, musculo-skeletal, neurological, immune, endocrine, and other body systems and tissues. Still, much confusion persists due to the indigenous nature of mineral's properties and interactions. Minerals are highly interrelated to each other and are directly linked to the metabolism of proteins, carbohydrates, fats, vitamins, proteoglycans and other body constituents. Most clinicians do not comprehend the specificities of these relationships and need to retrain themselves in this perspective. Modern orthomolecular interventional therapies account for these subtleties and institute precise remedies subsequent to the mammoth research efforts of many clinical groups in perfecting this science.

Clinicians and labs favor tissue mineral analysis (TMA) from hair as the frontline entry-level test for our body's overall nutritional and toxic mineral content. In their own research, it turns out to be the most dependable entry level measurement of the body's tissue content of minerals over time (about 6–8 weeks). Other nutritional information derived from urine, blood, and saliva can be compared to this baseline for other functional insights when necessary. Additionally, hair samples are very easy to obtain and is therefore consumer friendly.

Urine measures the component of minerals that are absorbed but excreted. Blood evaluation reveals the component that is absorbed and in circulation temporarily before it is excreted and/or delivered to storage depots. Saliva measurements are taken relative to pH values which help to identify the acid-base balance of the body. In the near future, it is expected that saliva may provide more criteria on minerals which will further help us to reveal one's personal biomineral identity. For now, laboratory science has determined that hair is first and foremost the best for body mineral assessments and especially helpful for screening toxic metal accumulation in the body. Using TMA through advanced mass spectroscopy techniques combined with computer-generated highly precise result interpretation yields vital information for the analytical comprehension of the standing complex mineral relationships within the body and also how to correct these imbalances food by food, mineral by mineral, vitamin by vitamin, phytochemical by phytochemical, amino by amino, etc. The connections of non-mineral nutrients to mineral retention have been demonstrated in side-by-side comparisons of other nutrient tests which has correlated this information. In effect, when the level of a mineral is known, the levels of other nutrients such as vitamins are also known. This is because minerals create the atomic building blocks of virtually everything in the body and therefore are directly or indirectly responsible for the presence and function of those other nutrients.

In other words, if the presence of a given mineral is high or low the other bodily substances that it is a primary ingredient in will be high or low, accordingly. As an example, if calcium is low, bones are weaker because it is a primary ingredient in bone at the tissue level. In a similar comparison, you cannot make your own vitamin D from the exposure to sunshine unless there is an adequate amount of calcium retained by the body. In plants and animals, this relationship is demonstrable as well. These types of atom to atom, molecule to atom, molecule to molecule relationships relative to the structure and function of the body allow us to understand many more relationships besides those just measured in minerals alone, without having to do extra tests on those nutrients. This is a primary reason why mineral testing is so fundamental to all tests with an orthomolecular focus.

Technically, HTMA or hair tissue mineral analysis is a biopsy procedure using hair as biopsy material. Inside the biopsy material are the minerals incorporated during the hair's development. Multiple minerals are tested and their interrelationships are automatically interpolated and displayed accordingly, revealing nutritional status, neuroendocrine activity, metabolic rate, and more, which is all correlated in side-by-side comparisons of varying tests. From the remedial standpoint it's always important to start with a body baseline and then promote an ideal balance using retests in order to examine and better control outcome.

According to Dr. Henry Schroeder, "Minerals are the basic sparkplugs in the chemistry of life, on which the exchange of energy in the combustion of foods and the building of tissues depends." Some of these minerals participate in hundreds of biochemical processes while others participate in the structural support of bone and teeth formation, acid-base balance, nerve conduction, water balance, muscle contraction, enzyme functions, and many other essential processes discussed through out the text. It is accurate to say that minerals have more to do with the structure and function of the body than any other single nutrient substance. Excessive accumulation of minerals, also known as hypermineralosis, can be highly detrimental to health. Hypermineralosis is actually considered to be more dangerous than deficiencies or hypomineralosis due to the disruptive effect on metabolism that mineral excesses cause as they tend to get in the way of, or antagonize, other nutrient functions.

Two excellent examples of what damage even essential mineral toxicities can cause are copper and iron excessively accumulating in body tissue. Hypermineralosis iron causes hemochromatosis and/or hemosiderosis, considered to be dangerous medical conditions which severely disrupt the cardiovascular system. Excessive copper accumulation causes liver degeneration and hepatolenticular degeneration (Wilson's disease) which is a very serious brain disorder. Even the body's concentration of iron relative to copper when out of balance contributes to health problems. Orthomolecular science has demonstrated that the balance of one mineral compared to the next is just as important as their individual levels if not more so. This is why a complete HTMA report must always reveal mineral ratios for maximum understanding and precise therapeutic application. There are some minerals which have very little or no beneficial effects to the body at all and may in fact be very toxic, even fatal at certain levels. These come under the classification of heavy metals which includes aluminum, lead, arsenic, cadmium, mercury, uranium, plutonium, radium, beryllium and others. They collectively are referred to as heavy metals due to their high atomic weight. These high atomic weight metals easily displace and antagonize electromagnetically most of the lighter, more essential elements and are therefore considered highly toxic. This displacement/antagonistic "heavy metal" effect interferes with the function of other essential mineral nutrients which cumulatively adds up to two basic problems:

1.  They reduce the necessary-for-life processes that essential nutrient minerals stimulate, fulfill and/or complete.
2.  Due to their (toxic) sheer presence, they actually interrupt or aggravate the energy flow of the cell, tissue, and even the overall organ and body system. Heavy metals are found in our food and are ever present in the total environment within air, water, and solid substances.

All body minerals, whether essential or toxic, must be nutritionally accountable in order to minimize the potential for all degenerative diseases including cancer. Balancing the body's minerals will also maximize the immune system at large, slow down the aging process, and even to help to stabilize emotions. As mentioned previously, hair analysis is an excellent environmental monitoring tissue for toxic metal exposure in humans and animals. Multiple studies have demonstrated this. A good example of how this works can be seen in one study performed on animals. A test group of animals were given 300 parts per million of cadmium (a very toxic mineral) in their drinking water which added up to an average cadmium intake of 4.5 milligrams over 12 weeks. The liver, kidneys, and hair showed peak levels in 4 weeks. Animals exposed to lesser amounts of cadmium in their drinking water demonstrated peaks at seven weeks in the kidneys, nine weeks in the liver and nine weeks in the hair. The concentration of cadmium in blood remained consistently low despite continuous exposure and did not once correlate with liver and kidney concentrations. On the other hand, the hair-based TMAs did directly correlate with kidney and liver concentrations. This study and many other human studies have drawn the conclusion by researchers that hair can be used as a highly reliable indicator of whole body mineral accumulation and verifies further that blood is not considered as a reliable indicator of tissue accumulation.

An interesting nationwide study performed on children 1–5 years old living near smelters, as compared to those not living near smelters, revealed more interesting data regarding blood/hair relationships. Blood concentrations of heavy metals were not elevated in most of the exposed children while dangerously elevated levels of cadmium and lead were demonstrated in hair. Although not tested in this case, we would expect urine to clearly demonstrate dangerous levels of cadmium and lead temporarily following exposure, as it is a great spontaneous dumping ground for toxic waste and proves highly useful in this regard.

It's worth mentioning another study involving mercury-induced kidney disease. In this research case, hair was found to be the most useful body specimen for demonstrating mercury exposure due to skin lightening creams. The mercury contained in these creams was directly absorbed through the skin resulting in nephrotic syndrome (Michael Jackson, watch out). Similar studies regarding mercury contamination in seafood ingested by humans show the same reliability of this approach.

Historically, TMA from hair is the number one indicator for nutritional status and supplementation in animals. Thousands of studies have precisely correlated the mineral levels in cattle and other animal feeds, to the hair's mineral content. TMA from hair is also used to monitor animals' nutritional status relative to fertility and disease. The same is true for humans, especially in the realm of anti-aging medicine where copper, zinc, manganese (and other powerful minerals) have been linked to certain bodily processes and growth-promoting hormones which, when not at peak levels due to inadequate mineral and vitamin proportions, cause premature age acceleration. In the case of disease tendencies and detection relative to nutrition imbalance before, during and after an identifiable malady, TMA is particularly useful. Cardiovascular disease, cystic fibrosis, PKU (phenylketonuria), diabetes, mental disturbances, cirrhosis, sickle cell disease, acrodermatitis enteropathica, Kashin-Beck and Keshan disease are just a few of the mineral-to-disease connections research has uncovered. The most important minerals to monitor are calcium, magnesium, sodium, potassium, copper, zinc, phosphorous, iron, manganese, chromium, selenium, boron, cobalt, molybdenum, sulfur, germanium, barium, bismuth, rubidium, lithium, nickel, platinum, thallium, iodine, vanadium, strontium, tin, titanium, tungsten, zirconium, antimony, aluminum, uranium, beryllium, cadmium, and lead. Another current use for hair TMAs is to monitor the nutritional status and toxic metal exposure of the unborn fetus through the mother's hair analysis to help ensure a healthy baby (and mom too). Hair can also be used to detect the use of both prescribed and illicit drugs.

Human HTMA lab procedures have been performed for nearly 60 years. Unfortunately, we need to be aware that it is sometimes unjustly criticized or questioned as to its validity in comparison to blood. These misplaced critical references stem from references to data that is over 25 years old when this procedure was not as medically and clinically refined as it is today. HTMA technology has enjoyed quantum leap advances and is comparable to the huge advancements in computer technology. Plus, blood evaluation of minerals has repeatedly proven to be nowhere nearly as useful or accurate. As many millions of these samples have been analyzed over the past few decades, the information explosion and technological refinements relative to HTMA procedures are profound and intensifying. Consequently, we may all (and must) now utilize this extremely convenient and highly economical testing to its fullest potential. Many therapeutic conclusions can be reached when comparing hair TMA to the organic acids found in urine. Organic acids are metabolites of the Krebs cycle and cytochrome enzymatic systems within cells. These enzyme systems produce all energy in the body and rely on the presence of certain key minerals to operate at peak efficiency. The functional capacity of the cell to produce energy (our life force) can be understood in extreme detail using organic acid tests in and of itself and in comparison to the hair TMA. The comparative value of these two tests also help narrow down diet and supplements to extremely precise levels in order to maximize life extension, fat loss, muscular growth, stronger bones and teeth, healthier babies, increased athletic capacities, memory and learning potentials, and on and on.

The organic acid test, a primary component of the metabolic urinalysis process, is considered as a next priority in the mineral profiling process and also begins our understanding of how vitamins, aminos, and fatty acids are being utilized by the Krebs, cytochrome and other related enzyme systems and their precursors. From a symptomatic standpoint this is very much a key test for fatigue or less-than-optimum energy levels much as the TMA is. The enzyme intermediates found in urine most related to mineral function are: alpha-hydroxybutyrate, beta-hydroxybutyrate, succinate, beta-hydroxyisovalerate, HPLA, and orotate. These biochemical markers are further explained in the "Vitamins" section below. At the end, *Your Personal Life* is more about how to take these tests and apply the information given for best results. Taking these nutrition tests is virtually a foolproof process; one only needs to follow the simple directions given for sample collection and submit them along with information sheets, through the mail, to the laboratories. Below is a list of key enzyme intermediates taken from urine, which specifies how minerals are working within the body. This following presentation is to demonstrate just how far our insights currently go in orthomolecular nutritional medicine.

## *Special Enzymatic Markers* (for mineral function):

1.  **Alpha-hydroxybutarate.** Being a ketone body, this chemical reflects dysfunctional carbohydrate metabolism in the liver aggravated by insufficient chromium and vanadium.
2.  **Beta-hydroxybutarate.** Same as above.
3.  **Succinate.** A Krebs cycle intermediate derived from amino acids. Showing a lack of certain amino acids from diet. (See "Amino Acids" Section.) Lowered enzyme function from magnesium and/or other coenzyme inadequacy.
4.  **Beta-hydroxyisovalerate** Although a direct indicator of B10 deficiency, it also signifies inadequate magnesium, along with excesses of lactate, alanine, and odd chain fatty acids.
5.  **p-hydroxyphenyllactate (HPLA).** A metabolite of the amino acid tyrosine and which is classified medically as being carcinogenic. Causing increased fatty oxidation and promotes tumors. Inadequate selenium is associated with this imbalance.
6.  **Orotate.** Seen in enzyme deficiencies and some coenzyme deficiencies where magnesium is considered the key cofactor (coenzyme) of the group.

***Vitamins:*** Also known as "vital minerals" or "vital amines," these are our bodies' molecular minerals. This means that structurally they are slightly larger groups of atoms (molecules = two or more atoms), formally referred to as molecules, made from nonmineral elements and mineral combinations. These 18 highly bioactive biochemicals have less to do with the actual support substance of the body than minerals, like calcium, which gives bone its hardness and strength, or copper, which gives muscle elasticity. However, vitamins are involved with every life process much like minerals. In fact, collectively, vitamins and minerals are the sparkplugs of life. Much as sparkplugs ignite gas in autos, vitamins and minerals provide the spark of life to enzymatically create and process energy from air, water, and food for all aspects of our existence. Their internal presence, properly proportioned, affects wellness from life to death. Vitamins are both synergistic and antagonistic to each other and to minerals as well. ***The nature of this attraction-repulsion pattern renders all A–Z multiple vitamin–mineral supplements functionally useless.*** The exact interrelationships are well understood and direct amounts and proportions within the body must be precisely measured and then synergistically remediated in order to reliably effect perfect balance. Urine, hair, and a blood test reveal all one needs to know for truest accuracy.

***List of Primary Tests:*** **1.** TMA (hair analysis) **2.** metabolic urine analysis **3.** *antioxidant profile (blood) **4.** organic acid analysis (urine)

***Discussion:*** The nutritional role of vitamins, especially antioxidants, seems to have drawn the most consumer and clinician attention lately. On any given day you'll encounter some media focus on antioxidants, multiple vitamins, or some other vitamin-related topic. Even many medical doctors are routinely recommending that their patients take some extra vitamin C, antioxidants, or a "multiple" for added health insurance. It is generally conceded by all that vitamins play an essential part in maintaining the health of the organism at large. They do so primarily by stimulating enzyme action at various levels within the biochemical pathways of metabolism. This stimulation also triggers a glandular response due to the vitamin's other molecular properties in relation to and in conjunction with the surrounding physiochemistry outside of bodily enzyme function of the body. Generally speaking, it is conceded that one can randomly just take whatever vitamins or vitamin-containing food desired and the body simply takes what it wants and excretes the rest. As we have repeatedly stated, nothing could be further from the truth – and this includes vitamin supplements, even the water-soluble ones which are thought of as being harmless in excess amounts. This is because vitamin antagonism and synergism is of vital importance for rebalancing the human body much as in the case of minerals. Furthermore, in similar fashion to minerals, vitamins in deficiency, antagonistic imbalance and excess are closely associated with a myriad of degenerative diseases. Their relationship to each other, to minerals, to aminos, to fatty acids, to all the body's metabolic food processing, to cellular properties and functions, to systemic and organic efficiency, is very critical to good health. But, these interrelationships are not quite as critical as certain minerals. As an example of this, if we removed all the mineral potassium from the body, immediate death would ensue. Conversely, remove all vitamin C from the body which then causes scurvy and eventual death could take numerous weeks and maybe even months to occur. Remove all calcium from the body – death is instant. Remove all B1, thiamine and beriberi follows and will intensify for some time before death occurs. And, as in the entropy of all nutrients, when you remove, increase to excess, or infuse an imbalance of one vitamin, all other nutrients and functional efficiency are affected. This includes all classes of nutrient elements from minerals to fatty acids. We previously referred to this as the see-saw principle.

The first choice in understanding one's personal vitamin profile again is the HTMA already taken for mineral content due to certain mineral-to-vitamin relationships that are revealed. Vitamins, however, are not found in hair as directly as they would be in a blood antioxidant profile. The vitamin measurements of HTMA are considered indirect.

HTMA correlates vitamin retention information from well known relationships of vitamins to minerals in the body. A good example of this relationship can be seen regarding rickets. Rickets is a condition characterized by a disturbance in calcium metabolism causing soft bones. Vitamin D is usually the first clinical recommendation given without ever testing for vitamin D status. If a HTMA reveals a very low calcium level, not only is a greater intake of calcium indicated but almost unequivocally more vitamin D will be necessary as well in order to functionalize both. Similarly, the metabolism of zinc requires adequate B6, while copper relates to vitamin C requirements, and vitamin C aids in iron absorption from the gut. Vitamin A's immune fortification properties are severely impaired during zinc deficiencies. This type of vitamin-to-mineral relationship continues throughout the total spectrum of vitamin mineral synergisms and antagonisms. When a HTMA is taken, a thorough analytical interpretation of results automatically sorts this physiochemical phenomena out for us in food and supplement terms. Metabolic urinalysis further helps to pinpoint vitamin/mineral dependent weaknesses within the system like those which can be found in fat, protein, or sugar metabolism. Organic acid analysis takes this one step further by revealing vitamin utilization directly by the intracellular enzymes found in the Krebs and cytochrome systems. Functional deficiencies and excesses are quickly revealed from this procedure, especially in relation to the B vitamins which are so instrumental to all intracellular energy production. Blood antioxidant panels (profiles) accurately reveal the presence of lipid peroxides (an indicator for free radical buildup), beta-carotene, vitamin A, E and coenzyme Q10 (a vitamin-like factor) while the previous tests mentioned can correlate their functions within the body as compared to their presence. In fact, all of the tests mentioned so far collectively synergize a wealth of scientific information allowing for the most effective food and supplemental customization ever achieved before in history.

A word about enzymes is in order at this time given how it's been lightly referenced throughout this text. As the glossary states, an enzyme is a protein particle within cells which accelerates a chemical reaction of a substance into a different product without being destroyed or altered during the process. Enzymes actually carry out thousands of different chemical reactions between substances that under ordinary circumstances would not react with one another. On a daily basis, our bodies burn about a pound of fuel, mostly carbohydrate as glucose and also fat, all to create body heat and energy (ATP). This chemical process takes place at 98.6 degrees (body temperature). The substances that we ingest: butter, starches, sugar, oils, etc., which initiate enzyme actions are called substrates. These food substances or substrates do not burn at ordinary (room) temperatures and it's difficult to make them burn at much higher temperatures in extreme contrast to a 98.6 degree body temperature where they can burn. A good example of this could be demonstrated by holding a lit match to the edge of a sugar cube. We will find that some sugar will melt but it will never catch fire. This may not seem to make much sense when you consider that the body routinely makes carbohydrates and fat react with oxygen (burn) at average body temperatures. It's the enzymes that make all the difference when reactive temperatures are low. A human body is only able to burn food substances at body temperatures because it has these auxiliary substances, enzymes, which can speed up the burning process without being affected themselves. A good example of this outside of the body can be seen when we place some cigarette ash on the corner of the sugar cube you attempted to burn previously and then put a match to it. We'll find that the sugar catches fire and continues to burn until the sugar cube is completely consumed. The actual burning takes place on the surface of the ash particles which do not change as it catalyzes (speeds up) the combustion of a much larger amount of sugar. The word enzyme is derived from the Greek word for yeast. Yeast contains certain enzymes which accelerate the fermentation process. Fermentation is a chemical process whereby the substrate (starting product) glucose is converted into alcohol after reacting with oxygen. This profitable enzymatic process alone sustains about one-fifth of the U.S. economy as the basis for the liquor, wine, and beer industries.

Enzymes are proteins made of very large molecules containing thousands of atoms (up to 20,000 atoms per molecule). Each enzyme is highly specific to the chemical reactions they catalyze (induce). Some may only speed up a single biochemical reaction while others can effect 100s of other reactions. Our bodies typically contain about 50,000 different kinds of enzymes which are all derived from our genetic blueprints. Folded chains of amino acid residues constitute some pure protein enzymes while others consist of protein with certain additions which are required to give it function as a catalyst. The added parts are referred to as coenzymes or cofactors.

Vitamins and minerals (especially the metallic minerals) serve as coenzymes or cofactors and usually work in combination. As a random example, the enzyme step which oxidizes alcohol to acetate in the liver allowing you to sober up (if you've overindulged at the party last night), is reactively catalyzed by the enzyme alcohol dehydrogenase. Alcohol dehydrogenase contains two atoms of zinc and is derived from vitamin B1 and phosphoric acid. Phosphorus, B1, and zinc have to be sustained by the body from diet in order to replace themselves on enzymes (deficiencies of these coenzymes keeps you drunk noticeably longer due to a much slower deactivation of alcohol's inebriant properties). There are many thousands of examples like this but it is most important to see that it is at this biochemical level (the level of the enzyme) that orthomolecular testing can calculate the most precise vitamin/mineral needs.

This is where the therapeutic action incorporated in personalized nutrition is most critical to efficient enzyme function—whether for those enzymes which directly liberate energy like those found in the Krebs/cytochrome systems or those responsible for building collagen, RNA, immunoglobulins, brain neurotransmitters, or virtually anything in the body. This critical-to-life phenomenon is where much of the sum total of orthomolecular nutritional science is focused. Stimulating life-sustaining enzymes with the proper coenzymes in the right amounts provide the foundation for human life to thrive. Categorically, many enzymes consist of two parts. The pure protein part is known as the apoenzyme whereas the nonprotein part is called the coenzyme. The entire active enzyme including both apoenzyme and coenzyme is termed the holoenzyme. In some gene-related or genetic diseases certain enzymes are missing altogether, as in PKU (phenylketouria) whereby the amino acid phenylalanine, due to a lack of a certain enzyme, cannot be enzymatically metabolized and consequently builds up in the body until death painfully ensues. In the Spielberg movie "Jurassic Park" the lysine contingency was a built-in genetic disorder whereby the faulty enzyme was engineered into the dinosaurs so that they could not turn other amino acids into lysine and would die if not fed lysine directly.

In most cases of genetic disease, the troubled or defective enzyme is present but can only propagate a diminished activity due to a gene-induced abnormal structure of the apoenzyme precluding it from readily combining with its related coenzymes in order to react properly. Perhaps because of this inherent gene defect, only a tiny fraction of the related holoenzyme is present. According to the laws of enzyme kinetics and principles of chemical equilibrium from the Law of Mass Action, a greater amount of the specific coenzyme, proper in quantity and synergistically infused into the body, will automatically increase its concentration in body fluids which will then activate more of the coenzyme resistant apoenzymes, in effect achieving more enzyme output. This enzyme stimulation technique is the basis for megavitamin therapy. A much larger amount of the target coenzyme can stimulate a near normal amount of the given enzymes reactivity resulting in the reinstatement of close to normal enzyme activity and subsequent fulfillment of its related functions.

The disease methylmalonic aciduria is healthfully controlled by this type of holoenzymatic restoration therapy. This fatalistic disease is caused by a holoenzyme deficiency. This target holoenzyme converts methylmalonic acid to succinic acid. Vitamin B12, (cyanocobalamin, made from the mineral cobalt), serves as the apoenzyme's target coenzyme for this reaction. Very large amounts of B12 given to patients causes increased cellular fluid concentrations of B12, stimulating this enzyme-mediated chemical conversion reaction to proceed at a normal rate. Another condition known as schizophrenia favorably responds in much the same way, using niacin and vitamin C to stimulate enzyme output.

Coenzyme deficiencies slow all related enzyme reactions down. Consequently, precisely synergizing coenzyme restoration therapy (ending nutrient deficiencies, excesses, imbalances) speeds up these "make more energy and cell proteins" reactions to optimum wellness levels. Coenzyme excesses can slow enzyme systems down by increasing the antagonisms between coenzymes simply as a function of creating molecular resistance (antagonism) to each other and also due to a crowding effect from too many being present at one time which in turn makes the competition for enzyme and receptor binding sites much greater. The Law of Mass Action is affected negatively by an increase of inert or non-activating particles versus the bioactive ones resulting in less reactive efficiency each time. Less reactions equals less energy and body substance/cell replenishment. Furthermore, coenzyme excesses also burden the excretory mechanisms of the body, leading to many direct and indirect stresses and potential breakdowns in body systems. Too many minerals, for example, can damage kidney membranes over time or a major excess of ascorbic acid (vitamin C) can lower the pH of the body which in turn depletes the buffering systems of the body like those present in the kidney. Kidney-produced bicarbonates become exhausted, which allows more acid buildup, which in turn further leads to kidney stress susceptibility – due merely to an overload of acidic coenzymes – most especially vitamin C in this case. At high levels and/or in significant antagonistic proportions, coenzymes can be very toxic regardless of whether fat or water soluble, contrary to the popular belief that only the fat-soluble, vitamin-based coenzymes A, D, E and K are dangerous in excess.

The overriding goal of Personalized Nutrition is to provide a maximum amount of stimulation to enzyme systems in order to subsequently create a maximum amount of metabolic target products such as energy (ATP) or collagen, muscle fiber or antibodies, stomach acid or neurotransmitters etc. with no stress or backup (slowed metabolism) to the body whatsoever. This equates to providing the body what nutrients exactly it needs up to the moment for fast enzyme-mediated metabolism in accordance with genetic signature and expression. In the case of enzymes, the speed of reaction is always the key factor. As an example of this, consider fatigue, which is directly related to enzyme activity. Fatigue results from the body not having enough energy to meet the demand which is consequential to insufficient ATP production. ATP provides 99% of the body's energy. When the speed of reaction of ATP's formative enzyme systems (Krebs/cytochrome) slows down, less ATP is made no matter how much you eat. Less ATP available to energetically run the body equates with fatigue, and then, resultant degeneration. The body has no choice but to slow down in order to conserve what little energy is available, which causes further feelings of fatigue (especially as your thyroid and adrenal glands can only reduce their outputs in order to play along).

Energy can then only be restored by direct replenishment of the ATP-making enzyme's speed of reaction so that more ATP is available from less food once again. This can be accomplished in six ways.

1. Increase the availability of energy substrate which in this case is pyruvate, which is the chemical end-product made from sugar, fat, and/or protein breakdown to begin the step-by-step formation of ATP. Pyruvate is the only starting product now called a substrate for this ATP-forming, enzymatically catalyzed biochemical reaction. Pyruvate is derived from the specific pathways involving the step by chemical step enzymatic breakdown of carbohydrates (glycolysis), fats (beta-oxidation) and protein (deamination) so that it can next be processed by the Krebs/cytochrome enzyme systems for ATP only. More pyruvate as delivered from more efficient breakdown (or catabolism) of sugar/fat/protein (macronutrients) increases reaction speeds.

2. Fewer products formed, which ends up accumulating at the end steps of ATP production speeds things up. In the subsequent converse case, the buildup of unused enzyme-liberated organic phosphates for ATP production slows reaction speed down, as will the buildup of carbon dioxide, water and ammonia – all end products of this particular chemical reaction. Their buildup literally pushes the reaction backwards instead of forwards because these chemicals aren't moving out of the way fast enough for the reaction to proceed. Enhancing their removal from the cell removes this blocking effect and subsequently increases reaction speeds.

3. Less acidity increases chemical reaction speeds. In the case of ATP formation without oxygen (anaerobic metabolism), lactic acid accumulates in cells which interferes with coenzyme binding sites which in turn slows the reaction down. Keeping the pH as close to neutral (neither too acidic nor alkaline) is "enzyme friendly."

4. Heat increases the speed of reaction by increasing the frequency at which apoenzymes, coenzymes, and substrates align and react with each other and also improves byproduct removal from the cell.

5. A greater cellular concentration of normal apoenzymes allowing for a greater number of reactions also increases the speed of reactions.

6. More available coenzymes within the cell increase reaction speeds and amounts.

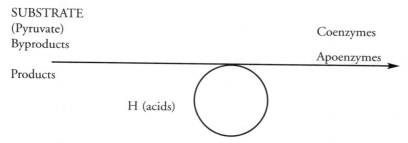

The seesaw of enzyme-mediated biochemical reactions for energy

Greater = gr    Lesser = le

| gr Substrate | = gr | Product | – speed increases |
|---|---|---|---|
| gr Acid | = le | Product | – speed decreases |
| gr Coenzymes | = gr | Product | – speed increases |
| gr Apoenzymes | = gr | Product | – speed increases |
| gr Product | = gr | Substrate | – speed decreases |

| gr Heat | = gr Substrate | – speed increases |
|---|---|---|
| gr Excess antagonistic coenzymes | = le Product | – speed decreases |
| gr Deficiency synergistic coenzymes | = le Product | – speed decreases |
| gr $Co^2$&$H^2O$ | = le Product | – speed decreases |

Another interesting enzyme phenomenon which we can nutritionally manipulate is called "induced enzyme formation." The French biologist Jacques Monod along with Francois Jacob and Andrew Lwoff, won a Nobel Prize in 1965 for investigating this phenomenon. They discovered that the rate of a given enzyme manufacture (remember, more enzymes = greater speed of reaction = desirable for more energy release and anabolic tissue buildup/maintenance) is controlled by a specific gene, which in turn is controlled by another gene called a regulatory gene. This regulatory gene slows down or stops the manufacturing gene from creating more of the enzyme. The regulatory gene turns on the manufacturing gene in response to available substrates from food. This is the exact mechanism which increases athletic performance from glycogen loading for example. Getting more glycogen to accumulate in cells through precise dietary and exercise manipulation starting a few days prior to an athletic event increases both the availability of substrates and enzymes (through gene action in this case) for an increased reaction speed which notably increases energy output for better competitive performance. When glycogen loading isn't applied, the regulating gene simply turns off any extra enzyme stimulation. Lower stored glycogen levels, fewer enzymes and subsequently less ATP is produced due to lower reaction speeds and fewer reactions. To some extent this "use it or lose it" physiological check and balance system is built into the body and works throughout the entire cellular system and all related body systems. Because of this, maximum enzyme utilization with this technique necessitates a personalized nutrition approach in order to optimize all functions and not just glycogen loading.

Another way to stimulate enzyme action is to add certain other substrates, usually amino acids and/or fatty acids, which convert directly into certain enzyme intermediates to feed the enzyme system in targeted spots while skipping other enzyme steps which may be slowed or blocked. Using the previous tests to measure the retention levels of minerals, vitamins and vitamin-like substances allows us to better and more precisely manipulate the enzyme system and related gene function for greater desirable product results, very much as in the case of **creating more energy or ATP from less food**. We accomplish this by accurately calibrating macro (protein-carbs-fat) and micro (coenzymes) nutrient intake to optimum levels and proportions as indicated by the tests. Certain minerals like calcium and vitamins like vitamin E also assist cells in keeping acidic concentrations low which makes for better gene and enzyme function. The proper zones of protein, carbs, and fat, (macronutrients are those nutrients that must be taken in larger than gram amounts daily for survival), ensure a proper balance of substrates-pyruvate, in this case, and apoenzymes. Apoenzymes can be manipulated further from proportioning amino acids and fatty acids as accomplished in the following amino and fatty acid testing sections. The buildup of unwanted byproducts, like carbon dioxide and enzyme intermediates like orotate or succinate can also be reduced by balancing minerals-vitamins-fats-aminos. These all cumulatively improve cell membrane and systemic function so that these metabolic blocks or toxins can be excreted quickly so as not to build up in cells. Intracellular body heat automatically increases enzyme activity but enzyme reactivity should be enhanced further from better blood circulation, more balanced thermoregulation and exercise. Yes, exercise helps all enzyme systems in the body, not just those found in muscle cells to work harder and more efficiently. More exercise speeds up all biochemical reactions much as the other factors do and should never be overlooked in the process of nutrition for this reason.

## *Special Enzymatic Markers* (from urine)

1. **Adipate** – identifies condition known as dicarboxylic aciduria; seen in environmental and viral toxin accumulation and when B2, B5, C, l-carnitine (an amino) and CoQ10 are suboptimal
2. **Suberate** – same as above
3. **Ethyl malonate** – identifies an enzyme (acyl-CoA dehydrogenase) deficiency which suppresses the ability to oxidize fatty acids for energy; considered a genetic disorder which may not cause any noticeable symptoms for many years and varies in severity amongst individuals; B2 and CoQ10 help to activate the enzymes involved
4. **Pyruvate** – is the breakdown product of glucose which builds up unless ample B1, B2, B3, B5, and lipoic acid are present to activate the target enzymes involved so that pyruvate can be quickly processed for energy or converted into useful fatty acids
5. **Lactate** – reveals suboptimal energy metabolism, lactate acidosis and lack of physical activity and suboptimal CoQ10 and B2 levels
6. **Citrate** – shows lack of branched chain aminos which indicates a suboptimal amino acid availability to drive the enzymes involved in energy extraction from food; vitamin C also helps, or can indicate need for more coenzymes and amino substrates including arginine and the B complex vitamins, both directly needed to activate the Krebs cycle enzyme system which is the absolute core metabolic engine of the body for all energy production
7. **Cis-aconitate** – lack of precursors/catalysts such as cysteine, arginine, B complex vitamins, iron
8. **Isocitrate** – lack of arginine, B complex, magnesium and manganese
9. **Alpha ketoglutarate** – reveals need for greater dietary intake of this enzyme intermediate in combination with arginine and glutamine to drive the energy cycle faster, or demonstrates lack of the coenzymes B1, B2, B3, B5, and lipoic acid
10. **Succinate (see Aminos)** – need for more of the precursors: leucine, isoleucine, and valine, or can reflect low levels of magnesium, B2 and CoQ10 to cofactor enzyme function
11. **Fumarate (see Aminos)** – more tyrosine and phenylalanine and their synergists needed
12. **Malate** – more B3 and CoQ10 needed for enzymes
13. **Hydroxymethylglutarate (precursor for cholesterol synthesis)** - more CoQ10 needed or not
14. **Alpha ketoisovalerate** (primary marker for B complex sufficiency)—reveals insufficient B1, B2, B3, B5, and lipoic acid present

15. **Alphaketoisocaproate** – Same as above
16. **Alphaketobetamethylvalerate** – Same as above
17. **Methylmalonate** – can indicate a functional deficiency of B12 if homocysteine is elevated, showing both B12 and B7 to be deficient; homocysteine elevation by itself indicates only B7 and B6 insufficiencies
18. **Betahydroxyisovalerate** – can indicate B7 deficiency by itself and also in combination with increased lactate and/or alanine in urine and excess odd chained fatty acids in blood
19. **p-Hydroxyphenyllactate (HPLA)** – is a carcinogenic metabolite of tyrosine which increases lipid peroxidation in the liver and is related to estrogenolytic (estrogen breakdown) enzyme activities in cells which can increase tumor growth when not in balance; excess HPLA can be reduced by more vitamin C, E, and selenium intake

*Amino Acids:* The smallest constituents of proteins for wellness. They organize 70% of our body's water content into the matter that we see, feel and refer to as "the body." Created from minerals, vitamins, air, water, and sunshine, 40+ amino acids combine to form enzymes, hormones, immunoglobulins, neurotransmitters, cellular, and tissue proteins. Collectively, they provide all body structure and many functions. From the way we're physically built and think intellectually, to the way your body moves and fights disease is directly related to an amino retention pattern. Specific patterns within the body as measured in urine, blood, hair and feces give us dramatic insights into the body's current state of metabolic efficiency (in conjunction with the levels of vitamins and minerals evaluated by the other tests mentioned previously).

*List of Primary Tests:* **1.** Blood plasma **2.** Organic acid analysis **3.** Comprehensive digestive function (stool/urine)

*Discussion:* There are 40 amino acids which can be tested using the profiling procedures listed above. They are utilized within the personalized nutrition process as reactive substrates from whose presence we can troubleshoot metabolic problems and manipulate the key enzyme systems for many chemical processes within the body. Amino Manipulation is accomplished in conjunction with related coenzyme catalysts which will optimize many bodily functions for supreme wellness. Below is a condensed list of the most relevant amino acids and with which bodily function and/or need that they are connected:

1. **Alanine** – can indicate hypoglycemic (low blood sugar) conditions or low cellular energy substrates

2. **Anserine** – connected to proper zinc and/or protein balance or indication of too much poultry intake and/or zinc deficiency

3. **Arginine** – demonstrates low-quality protein intake, reduction of nitric acid levels which in turn causes upsets within the cardiovascular and other systems, or an enzyme block in the urea cycle which interferes with cellular waste disposal; can show manganese imbalance as well

4. **Asparagine** – reflects magnesium imbalance or deficiency, or may indicate problems with purine synthesis

5. **Aspartic Acid** – shows aggravated ammonia detoxification in urea formation process; reflects decreased energy production by cells which results in fatigue, sometimes observed in epilepsy and stroke patients due to low magnesium and zinc levels

6. **Carnosine** – demonstrates deficiency of carnosinase enzyme and/or zinc

7. **Citrulline** – shows enzyme block in urea cycle causing excess ammonia; can indicate low aspartic acid and magnesium levels and/or excess protein intake

8. **Cystathionine** – shows B6 deficiency (pyridoxal 5 phosphate); may also cause low cysteine levels

9. **Cystine** – shows dietary deficiency of methionine and/or cystine; this can reduce taurine levels or high dietary intake and/or dysfunctional cysteine metabolism which causes slowdown of tissue antioxidant mechanisms which can lead to free radical damage and cellular death.

10. **Ethanolamine** – shows slow enzyme conversion to another amino acid phosphoethanolamine which can reduce a primary neurotransmitter (acetylcholine) synthesis adversely affecting brain activity.

11. **GABA (gamma aminobutyric acid)** – demonstrates enzymatic slowdown of conversion to succinate which is directly used by the Krebs cycle to produce energy; this directly causes fatigue; also indicates shortage of B6 and alpha ketoglutarate coenzymes

12. **Glutamic Acid** – reflects buildup of ammonia in blood most particularly in conjunction with excess glutamine; may reflect too high a protein intake and/or B6, alpha ketoglutarate and/or branched chain amino acid deficiencies or enzyme resistance to alpha ketoglutarate conversion in liver which in turn slows down the Krebs cycle causing energy deprivation; functional of niacin and B6 worsen this.

13. **Glutamine** – reflects-long term deficiencies and/or poor absorption of essential amino acids; can also be due to excess catabolism (breakdown) of protein or indication of B6 deficiency; also excess ammonia buildup is suspected if low to low normal glutamic acid is seen; this also increases the need for alpha ketoglutarate which in this case is overutilized to counteract toxic ammonia levels which in turn causes more energy deficits

14. **Glycine** – signifies generalized loss of tissue as glycine, is a vital part of the nitrogen pool and its presence is important to build up glycogen (stored sugar) in cells, or demonstrates a slowdown in metabolism of glycine into pyruvic acid which in turn slows down the Krebs cycle enzyme reactions and glycogen retention by cells, ultimately lowering energy production which leads to fatigue

15. **Histidine** – reflects low-quality protein intake, protein malabsorption and/or lack of other essential amino acids; indicator of rheumatoid arthritis and B12 deficien-

cy or  excessive protein intake; muscle protein breakdown when high levels of 3 methylhistidine are present

16. **Homocysteine** – associated with increased risk of atherosclerosis and other dysfunctions within the ocular, neurological, and musculoskeletal systems; B6, B12, B7 and betaine deficiencies are indicated

17. **Hydroxylysine** – (D) – Not particularly significant – (E) - Indication that connective and osseous (bone) tissue breakdown is present; Iron, alpha ketoglutarate, vitamin C, manganese, and chondroitin sulfate are usually low when this occurs

18. **Hydroxyproline** – In conjunction with low hydroxylysine, an indicator of bone breakdown due to collagen breakdown; the coenzymes mentioned above in number 17 are usually suspect

19. **Isoleucine** – associated with hypoglycemia, other sugar metabolism dysfunction, loss of muscle mass; inability to build new muscle tissue; B2 is low in this case as can be the other branched chain aminos, or when too high an intake of this amino and/or an impaired metabolism of it.  B6 may also be low

20. **Leucine** – indicates potential breakdown of skeletal muscle; low 3 methylhistidine confirms this; B3 and other branched chain aminos are usually low or too high an intake of this amino and/or its incomplete metabolism and/or an ongoing B6 deficiency

21. **Lysine** – low dietary intake or too large an intake of arginine; inhibits collagen synthesis by aggravating transamination of other aminos; may be low carnitine levels or a dysfunctional metabolism of this amino due to coenzyme imbalances involving vitamin C, B2, B6, B5 and iron

22. **Methionine** – shows low-quality protein intake; interferes with sulfur metabolism or if too much methionine-rich protein and/or inefficient metabolism; when other sulfur aminos are low, magnesium and B6 deficiency are also suspect

23. **Ornithine** –reflects  inadequate arginine since ornithine is synthesized from arginine  Ornithine is a source of regulatory polyamines which when low can slow cellular metabolism or reflects metabolic block in the urea cycle which allows ammonia buildup; low glutamic acid/ high glutamine confirms this

24. **Phenylalanine** – reflects thyroid dysfunction and reduction of catecholamines (adrenal hormones) causing symptoms such as depression, mental dysfunction (reduced cognition), accelerated memory loss, fatigue and autonomic nervous dysfunction, excessive protein intake or an inhibition of this amino's conversion into tyrosine; low iron levels can impair the enzyme responsible for this conversion

25. **Phosphoethanolmine**–shows inhibition of choline and acetylcholine synthesis stemming from impaired mythionine metabolism; low B12 , B7, betaine and/or SAM (S-adenosylmethionine) further aggravates this problem

26. **Phosphoserine** – a direct indicator of magnesium deficiency which aggravates this amino's conversion into serine

27. **Proline** – low tissue concentration reveals defective connective tissue synthesis as this amino is a primary component of collagen or reflects the body's lowered utilization of this amino which can be due to low vitamin C and vitamin B3 levels.

28. **Sarcosine** – good indicator of functional B2 deficiency

29. **Serine** – shows distorted methionine metabolism and breakdown in acetylcholine synthesis when threonine is found to be excessive, this means that B6, magnesium,

and manganese are inadequate; when threonine is low in conjunction with this amino, this reflects the loss of protein from cells to be broken down and used as sugar (catabolism) which weakens tissues and causes premature muscle/bone loss; threonine and all branched chain aminos are inadequate when this happens

30. **Taurine** – Increases potential for impaired fat digestion, high blood cholesterol, atherosclerosis, angina pectoris, arrhythmias, seizure disorders and oxidative stress from free radicals; low cysteine levels and reduced B6 function may be present as well; this deficiently occurs much more in women than it does in men or shows improper amino acid supplementation and/or an intensive inflammatory process

31. **Threonine** – shows hypoglycemia most particularly when body levels of glycine and/or serine are low or improper diet and/or impaired metabolism of the amino itself, partly due to low levels of B6 and zinc

32. **Tryptophan** – reflects depression, insomnia and even schizophrenia, or B3/B6/enzyme problem

33. **Tyrosine** – shows in blood pressure disorders, depression, and hypothyroidism (slow thyroid). When phenylalanaine measures on the high side an iron deficiency is probable (a high phenylalanaine can also be as a result of PKU – a very serious condition) or poor utilization from low iron/copper/ iodine/ B6/ascorbates.

34. **Valine** – demonstrates loss of muscle tissue in conjunction with generally low branched chain amino levels; when other essential aminos are low, this indicates poor digestion most probably due to low stomach acid and/or pancreatic enzymes or too high branched chain amino acid intake and/or B6 deficits

35. **1 – Methylhistidine** – reflects inadequate methyl group transfer which in turn suppresses histidine; B12 and B7 levels are inadequate also or dysfunctional; methionine metabolism affected by low intakes of B12, B7, dimethylglycine, and zinc (via inhibition of the enzyme carnosinase)

36. **Methylhistidine** – indicator of muscle protein breakdown related to low antioxidant activity

37. **Alpha Amino n-Butyric Acid** – shows shortage of alpha ketoglutarate and B6 or demonstrates impaired utilization for energy generation and specifies B12 and B10 problems

38. **Alpha Aminoadipic Acid** – signals lysine metabolism aggravation, reduction of amine group transfers in production of other aminos and protein in general and greater need for B6 and K.G.

39. **Beta Alanine** – associated with bowel toxicity from beta alanine production by intestinal bacteria and/or Candida albicans; cause for many food sensitivity and allergic reactions when in conjunction with low taurine levels, high levels of 3 methylhistidine, carnosine and anserine ( from kidney dysfunction)

40. **Beta Aminoisobutyric Acid** – shows lack of an enzyme (transaminase) necessary to process this amino in the presence of alphaketoglutarate

## *Special Enzymatic Markers* (from urine)

1. **Adipate** - Reflects suboptimal fatty acid oxidation and dicarboxylic aciduria which is associated with many metabolic toxins from viral infections; more l-carnitine is needed in combination with certain vitamins (see Vitamins)

2. **Citrate** – shows lack of branched chain aminos and need for more vitamin C or need for more arginine and B complex vitamins.

3. **Cis-aconitate** – reflects lack of precursors/catalysts such as cysteine, arginine, B vitamins and iron

4. **Isocitrate** – shows lack of arginine, B complex, magnesium, and manganese

5. **Alpha-ketoglutarate** – indicates need for greater dietary intake of this compound along with arginine and glutamine to drive the energy cycle faster or a lack of the coenzymes B1, B2, B3, B5 and lipoic acid

6. **Succinate** – shows need for more of the precursors: leucine, isoleucine and valine or low levels of magnesium, B2, and CoQ10 to run enzymes

7. **Fumarate** – indicates when more tyrosine and phenylalanine needed to form enzyme intermediates

8. **Vanilmandelate (VMA)** – associated with low profiles of certain neurotransmitters called catecholamines, (epinephrine and norepinephrine) which require tyrosine to balance especially if low fumarate is present or agreater intake of phenylalanine and tyrosine

9. **Homovanillate (HMA)** – Derived from the neurotransmitter Dopamine which requires phenylalanine (Phe) and tyrosine (Tyr) for its synthesis; (Low Fumarate also signals need for Phe&Tyr)

10. **5-Hydroxyindolacetate (HIA)** – demonstrates low levels of the neurotransmitter, serotonin which is made directly from tryptophan (Tryp); greater Tryp intake improves this condition rapidly

11. **Orotate** – reflects enzyme function impairment of the pyrimidine synthesis and/or the urea cycle; seen in arginine deficiency, when diets contain a high lysine to arginine ratio and when ammonia buildup is present; arginine, aspartic acid and alpha-ketoglutarate are needed in greater quantities to offset

12. **Pyroglutamate** – indicates a glutathione depletion which diminishes the kidney's ability to prevent the loss of amino acids from the body. N-Aceytl-cysteine (NAC), taurine and cysteine help repair

13. **Sulfate** – reflects the liver's diminished capacity to detoxify chemical products produced from drug biotransformation, steroid hormone accumulation, and phenolic substances; a low sulfate to creatinine ratio signifies the need for more sulfur-containing compounds including NAC, taurine and cysteine

14. **Benzoate** – reflects intestinal bacterial metabolism of phenylalanaine left over from protein digestion and/or from high benzoic acid levels in food, and/or an outright glycine deficiency

15. **Hippurate** – Made from benzoate, requires glycine as a cofactor and better digestion is indicated

16. **Tricarballylate** – demonstrates overgrowth of certain intestinal bacteria which may bind magnesium at such a fast rate that it creates magnesium deficiencies; greater glutamine intake will improve.

*Fatty Acids:* Considered by science to be the body's homeostatic equalizers. These special substances provide many functions ranging from nerve and body insulation to immune system fortification to hormonal synergy.

Their combined effect is to provide a template from which other biochemicals can work in harmony. They also provide a slow-release energy source to help fill in, or back up, the body's energy needs. ***Excessive storage of fat on the body is the #1 problem facing the U.S. today over all other nutrition issues.*** Fatty acid imbalances create a large amount of metabolic short circuits which can severely undermine good health and prevent a lean physique. A special blood test reveals which of 47 fatty acids is in or out of balance and why.

***List of Primary Tests:*** **1.** Blood plasma **2.** Organic acid analysis (urine) **3.** Comprehensive digestive function (stool/urine)

***Discussion:*** For the purposes of simplicity fatty acids are divided into the 8 groups as listed below:

**I.    Polyunsaturated Omega-3**
**1.    Alpha Linolenic Acid (ALA or LNA)** – an essential fatty acid (FA) of central importance to the whole enzyme mediated system of fat metabolism and marks dysfunction of nervous, reproductive, cardiovascular, nephrotic (kidneys), and immune systems; upsets in the balance of all other fatty acids and their specific relationships to their respective body systems or imbalance between Omega-3 and 6s
**2.    Eicosapentaenoic Acid (EPA)** – statistically cited as the most prevalent fatty acid abnormality affecting the health status of Western society showing uncorrected inflammatory responses that in turn create arthritis, heart disease, and accelerated aging; can result from delta-6 desaturase (enzyme) impairment from low levels of zinc, magnesium, B3, B6 and/or high levels of saturated, monounsaturated and trans–fatty acids and also cholesterol
**3.    Docosapentanoic Acid (DPA)** – marks impaired growth and development of the nervous system; typical in Attention Deficit Hyperactivity Disorders and visual system disorders; very important in breast milk and can be correlated with nursing mothers' intake of fish oils to ensure baby's health.
**4.    Docosahexanoic Acid (DHA)** – same as DPA (#3) although a low DHA specifically increases one's potential for high blood pressure problems

**II.    Polyunsaturated Omega-6**
**1.    Linoleic Acid (LA)** – an essential FA that is the most of all FAs found in human tissue, demonstrating impairment of cell membrane integrity and eicosanoid synthesis both can severely disrupt many cellular functions or abnormally greater inflammatory responses.
**2.    Gamma Linolenic Acid (GLA)** – when low suppresses dihomogammalinolenic acid (DGLA) formation which is anti-inflammatory in and of itself but is also precursor to the highly inflammatory FA arachidonic acid; when more zinc is present, less arachidonic acid will be made
**3.    Eicosadienoic (EDA)** – represents low levels of other Omega-6 FAs
**4.    Dihomogammalinolenic Acid (DGLA)** – demonstrates poor dietary intake of

essential FAs along with DGLA, causing disruptions of cellular activities and tissue responses. In medical history of tumor formations DGLA must be balanced with ALA for best results.

5. **Arachidonic Acid** – the most principal proinflammatory FA; this FA is what NSAIDS (non steroidal anti-inflammatory drugs) inhibit for pain reduction; increases inflammation throughout all body systems and promotes formation of gallstones

6. **Docosadienoic Acid** – classified as a very long chain FA or VLCFA made from DGLA; usually seen when LA and DGLA are adequate and enzymatic mediated elongation process is efficient; the related enzyme works best with lower insulin levels in the body

7. **Docosatetraenoic Acid** – reflects too much fat and sugar intake; highly prevalent in overweight and obese people

**III. Polyunsaturated Omega-9**
1. **Mead Acid** – Identifies depleted essential FA levels (LA and ALA).

**IV. Monounsaturated**
1. **Myristoleic Acid** – low levels show reduction in cell membrane fluidity; membrane influidity is a consequence of high-saturated-fat diets, so typical of overweight people or can promote tumor growth

2. **Palmitoleic Acid** – Reflects adequate status of essential fats or deficiencies of LA and ALA

3. **Oleic Acid** – makes up 15% of all red blood cell membranes as a fluidity enhancer and shows decrease in red blood cell (RBC) causing RBC abnormalities

4. **Vaccenic Acid** – a mirror image of oleic acid at the molecular level with similar properties showing loss of RBC membrane fluidity

5. **Eicosenoic Acid** – when low can be due to low oleic acid levels

6. **Erucic Acid** – reflects adrenal gland dysfunction most notable in a condition known as adrenal leukodystrophy.

7. **Nervonic Acid** – Particularly affects nerve cell membranes including the myelin sheath and can be caused by high carbohydrate diets and reflects low insulin levels from diets that are too low in carbs.

**V. Saturated (even-numbered amount of carbon atoms)**
1. **Capric Acid** – a medium chain FA (MCFA) not found in meats, indicating inhibition of peroxisomal oxidation which in turn relies on B2, found to be inadequate when this happens.

2. **Lauric Acid** – Same as above

3. **Myristic Acid** – Same as above

4. **Palmitic Acid** – signifies low cholesterol production by liver and overall upset in FA synthesis or when excessive increases blood cholesterol, atherosclerosis, cardiovascular disease, and stroke.

5. **Stearic Acid** – a cancer marker when low in comparison to oleic acid showing too much saturated fat in diet, high triglycerides, and development of atherosclerosis

6. **Arachidic Acid** – shows inhibition of energy availability for cell membrane synthesis and EFA metabolism by inhibiting the delta-6 desaturase enzyme which

then produces less EPA, DGLA, and AA

7. **Behenic Acid** – classified as a VLCFA (very long chain fatty acid); associated with degenerative disease syndromes of the central nervous system and certain enzyme shortages from genetic impairments.
8. **Lignoceric Acid** – same as above
9. **Hexacosanoic Acid** – same as above

   Special note: The average American lifestyle of low physical activity combined with a high-saturated-fat diet induces a metabolic pattern which leads to increasing levels of all VLCFAs in the blood. This VLCFA buildup in plasma and RBC membranes causes dangerous hormonal responses to counteract such events by increasing norepinephrine and insulin output. This problem is further exacerbated by drugs that modulate energy metabolism like trimetazadine for angina pectoris (a form of heart disease).

**VI. Saturated odd chain (odd = actual number of carbon atoms)**
1. **Pentadecanoic Acid** – Signifies low or deficient levels of B12 and/or carnitine and may indicate a high degree of intestinal malfunction known as dysbiosis
2. **Heptadecanoic Acid** – same as above
3. **Nonadecanoic Acid** – same as above
4. **Heneicosanoic Acid** – same as above
5. **Tricosanoic Acid** – Same as above

**VII. Transisomers (From hydrogenated oils) – (Trans Fat)**
1. **Palmitelaidic Acid** – shortest in length, least amount in family of trans fat. See below
2. **C18 Trans Isomers (Elaidic Acid, Petroselaidic, and Trans Vaccenic Acids)** – shows impairment of cell membrane functions, increased cholesterol buildup in blood, inhibited desaturase enzymes from assembling necessary products, presence raises LDLs (low density lipoproteins) and suppresses HDLs

**VIII. Ratios of Fats**
1. **LA** – DGLA when increased demonstrates unhealthy delta-6 desaturase enzyme activity due to deficiencies of magnesium and zinc, high levels of insulin, excess saturated, monoenoic and/or trans fats
2. **EPA** – when DGLA is too high compared to EPA shows upset in the balance of prostanoids, leukotrienes, and 1, 2, 3 series local hormones which consequently impairs a multitude of cellular functions
3. **AA/EPA (or enough Omega-6/Omega-3)** '– when decreased is desirable due to greater amount of anti-inflammatory eicosanoids present whereas increase denotes excess of pro-inflammatory fatty acids
4. **Stearic/Oleic** – when low identifies a medical marker for prostate cancer
5. **Triene/Tetraene** – when increased demonstrates deficiency of the essential fatty acids overall

**Special Enzymatic Markers** (from Metabolic Urinalysis)
1. **Adipate** – can demonstrate a serious health-threatening condition known as dicarboxylic aciduria; signifies a low rate of fatty acid oxidation; this can be seen when B complex, choline, CoQ10, vitamin C, and carnitine levels are suboptimal and/or

when there is toxic presence resulting from certain viral and environmental poison accumulation

2. **Suberate** – Same as above

3. **Ethylmalonate** – Reflects an enzyme (acyl-CoA dehydrogenase) deficiency reducing the ability to oxidize fatty acids for energy; deficiencies of B2 and CoQ10 are present.

*Hidden Nutritional Sensitivities:* These hidden immune system disharmonies act as cumulative killers when left undetected. They can predispose more than 25 major disease states and can make daily living downright miserable due to the intolerable symptomatic responses which are not necessarily classic allergic symptoms. This special class of sensitivities does not cause the typical immediate allergic reaction that we can easily identify. The sensitivity effects are very subdued and therefore hard to detect, which is why they're called hidden or delayed. In fact, the majority of hidden sensitivities, when triggered, cause an immediate release of adrenaline which in turn gives us a lift similar to a couple of sips of coffee. This stimulating adrenal gland mediated response can actually lead to an addiction cycle where we begin to crave foods that we're actually allergic to. Dr. James Braley labeled this the food allergy addiction syndrome and considered it to be a very dangerous problem. A hidden allergy works like this: Within 72 hours of eating an offending food, concentrated vitamin/mineral, sugar or spice, the body becomes deadlocked in a biochemical war that can literally tear up the body with inflammatory responses. According to Braley and others this sensitivity problem has emerged amongst humans from the constant interbreeding of genetically different populations in combination with the increasing rejection of traditional ethnic diets in favor of modern generic diets which have little connection to our individual genetic digestive, absorptive, assimilation and excretory capabilities. This causes a huge array of resulting problems, ranging from heart disease, and headaches, arthritis, fatigue, and premature death. There is a special blood test to identify the offenders and customized food rotations treat the problem naturally.

*List of Primary Tests:* **1.** TMA (hair analysis) **2.** IgG/IgE/IgA sensitivity test and glucose tolerance (blood) **3.** Comprehensive digestive analysis (stool)

*Discussion:* As we examine different types of allergies, it's important to understand that there are several types of allergic responses to specific foods based upon certain antibodies. The two types of allergic responses we are most focused upon are based upon immunoglobulyn "E" (IgE) and immunoglobulyn "G" (IgG) reactions. G and E reactions represent the majority of allergic reactions people suffer from. Ds, As and Ms are also considered to a lesser extent but fall into place after Es and Gs are evaluated. Es account for about 3–5% of food allergies while Gs account for about 85% of those tested. This can vary slightly between individuals. G reactions are hardest to detect symptomatically. E reactions are quite obviously detectable symptomatically, but what are now referred to as "weak" E reactions are not. Both type of sensitivity reactions need to be measured for best wellness results. Both can be controlled and improved upon by proper nutritional intervention. Es are also known as classic allergies which are referred to as immediate onset allergic responses. After eating an offending food or inhaling an irritating airborne particle or touching some allergenic (allergy-promoting) environmental substance (or for some, being stung by a bee), the body has an immediate, sometimes life-threatening, but always an uncomfortable reaction. Strong reactions to allergens range from asthma attacks and instant hives to outright anaphylactic shock which can lead to death. Weak reactions can cause mild to severe headaches, mouth itchiness, itchy skin, mental fogginess, sore joints, heart palpitations, visual disturbances and even stomach discomfort, to mention a few, although IgA immunoglobulins have more to do with the digestive tract. E reactions are very easy to identify since they occur within seconds to minutes of allergen exposure – especially in the case of food or topical exposure. Airborne particles are more difficult to trace unless there is some overwhelming presence like smoke or sprays. Type E reactions illicit histamine secretions by certain immune cells (mast cells) which can be medically counteracted (not cured) by antihistamine drugs (really enzyme inhibitors or cell membrane stabilizers/blockers). These antihistaminic drugs are taken, sometimes indefinitely (chronically), to help control histamine production so that severe reactions do not occur. Chronic use of antihistamines, like any drug, has cumulative side effect consequences of varying range and degree. Fortunately, there is an alternative cure embodied in the personalized nutrition process. It starts by focusing upon food intake instead of drugs. One single exposure to a reactive food can elicit an E reaction or repeated exposures may be necessary for a noticeable reaction to occur. Or, sometimes simply a larger quantity of an offending food is sufficient to set off a reaction. This depends upon the number of reactive antibodies present, which varies by individual for different reasons. Fast metabolisms seem to have a greater susceptibility to histamine allergies than slow metabolisms, especially in the presence of calcium and copper deficiencies, nickel toxicity and sympathetic nervous system dominance. Avoidance of E-reaction foods causes the reactive IgE antibodies to significantly reduce in number within a few weeks. Unfortunately, these same antibodies may reappear when the specific E-reaction food is eaten again, especially when the mineral imbalances and sympathetic stress is not addressed properly. Some of these E-reactive foods may need to be avoided for life, others may be consumable again without problems only if customized food rotations and proper supplementation is instituted in direct combination with any G reactions measured and counteracted.

G reactions are categorically considered as delayed allergies due to their lag time in producing any discernable symptoms. Unfortunately, the majority of symptoms they cause are hidden from obvious sight and sensation and can manifest over time into many serious degenerative diseases if not confronted and corrected. Typically, G's delayed allergic reactions occur in cycles, coming and going in relation to whether offending foods are eaten or avoided. Interestingly, G reactions result from ingesting too much of a certain food too frequently over periods of weeks to months. (This underscores the need for seasonal food rotation and diet variety versus eating the same foods all the time which many Americans do habitually). Some Gs may never be solved as they are genetically incompatible to an individual, while others will be eliminated in time under the right nutrition circumstances. G incompatibilities cause many delayed symptoms including chronic headaches, fatigue, joint pain, muscle soreness, gastrointestinal instability, mood changes, skin discomfort, and many others. Slow metabolisms tend to have a greater number of low histamine and G allergy tendencies.

Because our individual genetic design is not compatible with all foods on this earth, we will inevitably have some G and E problems when profiled. The foods which are not genetically and metabolically compatible from the start will always stimulate some degree of allergenic response no matter how hard we try to correct them, even if you are genetically programmed to be an "eat anything" omnivore. These sensitivities are called fixed allergies. Reactive foods which are genetically compatible by primal design or at least neutral by design are correctable to a very large extent by a systematic process of underindulging. The only reason they may be measured as either or both G or E reactive at the moment of profiling is due to some repairable disorders in body chemistry caused by certain environmental and emotional stresses. These standing disorders are out of synchrony with genetic signature or design. In other words, the genes want metabolism to be one way but due to improper diet and lifestyle has accumulated biochemical imbalances which in essence block the genes from directing metabolism for peak efficiency. Consequently, one's metabolism becomes imbalanced, increasing its susceptibility to misplaced sensitivities. Like a computer on overload, the more of these misplaced G and E responses are allowed to build up, the more new G and E responses will appear. And the more imbalanced the other nutrients become (minerals, vitamins, aminos, fatty acids, etc.) and the more toxic accumulations, the more this cumulative allergy syndrome will persist. This process is further intensified by any dysfunction of the gut lining, referred to as dysbiosis, which allows larger than normal (incompletely digested) food particles to pass into the blood, stimulating reactive antibody responses. Fortunately, the outright majority of misplaced Gs and Es can be effectively alleviated with precise digestive correction and proper food rotations in combination with specific nutrient customization. The fixed responses probably will never completely disappear but may reduce in intensity quite measurably and noticeably. Thankfully, the fixed Gs and Es are usually few in number relative to the misplaced or correctable sensitivities. Like Es, G food avoidance triggers significant antibody reductions within months. E's can take longer sometimes. Once the circulating antibodies drop down, reactivity diminishes to nothing in most cases provided digestive disorders are addressed. These antibodies can return to previous levels if offending foods are eaten again for a prolonged period of weeks to months. A proper food rotation in combination with digestive correction and nutrient/toxin rebalancing ensures minimal genetic and metabolic irritation for life. All that is required is knowing what foods you must confront.

Thanks to orthomolecular medicine advancement beyond standard medical testing, it's easy to itemize hidden allergy test results that relate to specific foods, spices, toxins and even airborne allergenic irritants. There are three phases of allergenic correction in relation to food and spices addressed during formal therapeutic intervention. Specific supplementation is predicated upon other metabolic retention factors and correlations, in combination with G and E test information.

***Hormone Patterns:*** Your personal glandular profile is revealed in saliva and hair and sometimes blood tests. Any imbalances found are most often nutritionally correctable. Hormones are the chemical messengers of the body connecting the brain to each cell as complement to nerve connections. When synchronized properly, life force is maximized.

***List of Primary Tests:*** **1.** Saliva **2.** HTMA (hair analysis) **3.** Blood plasma

***Discussion:*** Hormones represent a category of chemical messengers which help to control cellular functions. These particular compounds are synthesized by a given ductless or endocrine organ directly from nutritional factors and once secreted into the blood act upon specific (targeted) cells and tissues outside of the organ of origin. A good example of a typical endocrine organ is the pancreas, which secretes the hormone insulin which in turn acts upon blood sugar and its effect upon the brain and muscles. There is a type of gland called an exocrine or duct gland, which the pancreas is also. The duct-connecting glands within the pancreas secrete digestive juices–actually, enzymes–such as amylase, which is a key starch digestion enzyme. Although the process of personalized nutrition improves the function of these exocrine glands, it is the endocrine glands that are considered first priority, inasmuch as they have so much to do with controlling exocrine gland function. The tables below provide a simple overview of some of the key relationships we must take into consideration.

## TABLE III:
## PHYSICAL FUNCTIONS OF THE ENDOCRINE GLANDS
### TARGET GLANDS

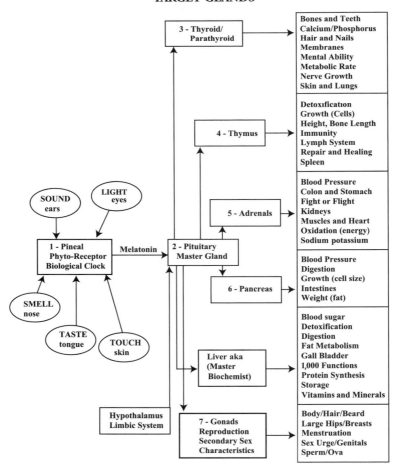

In Table 3, each one of the target gland numbers 3 - 7 put out hormones that affect the organs listed next to them. The pituitary or master gland (2) is controlled by the hypothalamus, which in turn is impacted by the limbic system which is connected to all other parts of the basal system of the brain. The basal system primarily controls a person's emotional behavior. The following represents a list of the key hormones and effects they have on the body which we are now able to better optimize:

### TABLE IV: (Use in conjunction with TABLE 3)

## OVERVIEW OF ENDOCRINE GLANDS, HORMONES, AND FUNCTIONS

| GLANDS | HORMONES | FUNCTIONS |
|---|---|---|
| Hypothalamus | Direct neural stimulation<br><br>TRH, CRH, GHRH, GHIH, LRH, PIH | Blood pressure, pupil dilation, satiety, shivering, hunger, rage, feeding, reflexes, thirst, water conservation, heart rate, temperature regulation, panting, sweating, control of pituitary gland |
| Pituitary | GH, TSH, ACT, TSH, FSH, LH, Prolactin, MSH, ADH, Oxytocin | Control of thyroid, adrenal, parathyroid, pancreas, ovaries, testicles, placenta, some liver functions, some kidney functions, thymus functions |
| Thyroid<br><br>Parathyroid | Thyroxin, Calcitonin, Triiodothyronine<br>Parathormone | Metabolic rate, mental state, nerve growth, bones and teeth, mental ability, etc. |
| Thymus | Thymosin | Immune system, etc. |
| Adrenal | Steroid Hormones:<br>Gluccocorticoids, 17-Ketosteroids, Mineralocorticoids, Estrogens, Androgens, Progestins, Epinephrine, Norepinephrine | Fight or flight, muscle and heart functions, sodium/potassium balance, oxidation amounts, blood pressure, kidney functions, colon and stomach functions, etc. |
| Pancreas | Insulin, Glucagon | Blood sugar levels, etc. |
| Liver | Direct chemical stimulation | 2,000 metabolic functions |
| Ovaries | Estrogens, progesterone | Reproduction, etc. |
| Testicles | Testosterone | Reproduction, etc. |
| Placenta | HCG, estrogens, progesterone, somatomammotropin | Regulate embryonic growth in relation to mother's metabolism |
| Pineal | Melatonin | Direct effect on gonadatropic hormones in time/light cycle |

*The interconnection of the endocrine system and nervous system in controlling human behavior and metabolism is better clarified and controlled when using orthomolecular principals application of nutritional elements.*

There are numerous hormones which affect multitudes of physiochemical actions. As many as 350 single and multiple hormone profiles are available as tests from laboratories, mostly from blood or saliva specimens. The scope of this text is limited to those glands and their respective hormones which are the most directly related to nutrient status and vice versa. The endocrine system is very complex and in much the same way that vitamins and minerals function synergistically and/or antagonistically, the endocrine glands have antagonistic and synergistic influences upon one another. The system of checks and balances between these glands is more technically termed "negative inhibition." Below are key antagonisms: (anterior = front, posterior = back):

1.  Adrenal Medulla – posterior pituitary, pancreas, ovaries
2.  Thyroid – pancreas, parathyroid, ovaries
3.  Adrenal Cortex – pancreas, thymus
4.  Ovaries and other estrogen-producing tissues – adrenal medulla, thyroid, progesterone-producing tissues
5.  Parathyroid – thyroid, adrenal medulla, anterior pituitary, progesterone-producing tissues
6.  Thymus – adrenal cortex
7.  Posterior Pituitary – adrenal medulla
8.  Anterior Pituitary – parathyroid, pancreas, ovaries, and other estrogen-producing tissues
9.  Pancreas – thyroid, adrenal medulla, adrenal cortex, anterior pituitary
10. Progesterone producing tissues – ovaries and other progesterone-producing tissues, parathyroid

***The PMS Story:*** A good example of hormonal antagonism can be seen between estrogen from ovaries (adrenals, liver, and other tissues) and the thyroid gland in consideration of its production of thyroxine. An overactive thyroid gland can suppress estrogen production while too much estrogen can reduce thyroid activity. This condition often manifests in women who take estrogen as hormone replacement therapy (HRT) or oral contraception.  Affected women often develop increased fatigue, weight gain, blood sugar sensitivities, and depression. The extra estrogen from the contraceptive pill slows thyroid activity and subsequent thyroxin production thereby reducing the metabolic rate. As this proceeds during the pre-menstruation phase of the cycle when characteristically estrogen levels normally increase, lethargy, depression, and weight gain intensify to a greater extent than would have been the case without the added hormone. Dr. David Watts, in his book *Trace Elements and Other Essential Nutrients,* describes this phenomenon of PMS as "premenstrual hypothyroidism" due to this phenomenon of estrogenic thyroid suppression. Many symptomatic women taking estrogen-dominant birth control pills experience total relief from this problem when switched over to progesterone-dominant birth control pills. Progesterone is directly antagonistic to estrogen and when increased relative to estrogen subsequently diminishes estrogen's adverse effect upon the thyroid gland. Progesterone is actually synergistic to thyroid function.

The thyroid-estrogen connection also works in reverse whereby an overactive thyroid or one that is being overstimulated by the body or by HRT which is too strong, will adversely affect estrogen status, which in turn will lead to calcium loss and eventually osteoporosis (and other potential problems relative to calcium loss).

The Chinese medical principles of yin and yang are very much applicable to the endocrine glandular system (and minerals as well, especially in relation to weight loss). This system works based on a balance of opposing forces whereby one gland and its dominant hormones work to counteract the next gland and its dominant hormones until perfect balance is achieved throughout the body. Even within each individual gland this opposition phenomenon occurs. This can be seen in the case of ovarian function. Ovaries secrete both estrogen and progesterone which are in opposition to one another. The Yin–Yang phenomenon is a simplified reason as to why any endocrine problem develops alone. When one hormone is out of balance, everything else (in this case the other glands and cells that they exert influence on) try to functionally adjust or compensate, which in turn can lead to more imbalances. In reverse, a lot of hormone imbalances can occur causing intensification of one gland's imbalance in and of itself as it tries to adjust to the added stress. Plus, the two most opposing forces of the nervous system, the parasympathetic and sympathetic components of the autonomic nervous system, exert their influences as they attempt to moderate the cause and effect in this glandular balancing act. Parasympathetic nervous input slows things down (especially glands), while sympathetic input speeds things up. A given gland does not become under-or overactive without affecting another, especially its most opposing gland. This is true for mild disturbances (sub-clinical imbalances) and severe disturbances (clinical imbalances). One need not have a serious glandular pathology such as Cushings, Addison's or Hashimoto's disease to experience a disturbed relationship between the glands and resultant hormone antagonisms which can seriously undermine bodily functions.

It's most simple to understand the nerve-to-gland connection that is based upon whether a given gland or hormone is stimulating or sedating by nature in conjunction to its corresponding parasympathetic or sympathetic nerve component, since the two work together so closely. The following table is based upon the research of Dr. David Watts. Please note that anterior = Front, posterior = back, lateral = side, anabolic = building up, catabolic = breaking down:

| SEDATIVE OR PARASYMPATHETIC GLANDS AND HORMONES | STIMULATING - SYMPATHETIC GLANDS AND HORMONES |
|---|---|
| Posterior Pituitary | Anterior Pituitary |
| Lateral Hypothalamus | Medial Hypothalamus |
| Adrenal Cortex (anabolic hormones) | Adrenal Cortex (catabolic hormones) |
| Parathyroid | Adrenal Medulla |
| Ovaries (estrogen) | Thyroid |
| Pancreas (insulin) | Ovaries (progesterone) |

### *Stress, Stress, Stress*
### *The Biggest Pollutant and Health Problem*

The above glands and hormones counterbalance each other, striving to achieve a healthy balance. But they can still vacillate widely due to changing circumstances such as emotional stress, physical activity levels, eating patterns, sleep cycles, overweight tendencies, certain diseases, toxin accumulation, allergies, age, and nutritional disorders. This is a very dynamic system of checks and balances which can adjust quickly to help the body to maintain a homeostatic (stable) consistency under all terms and conditions of life as a matter of survival. The endocrine hormones have many varied functions within the body but can be divided up into two very basic classes of regulatory function. They regulate metabolic activity by either slowing it down or speeding it up in similar fashion to Yin–Yang. Stimulatory glands and hormones directly oppose the sedating ones and vice versa. This phenomenon can clearly be seen in the regulation of heartbeat and blood pressure. A surprise or anticipated stress causes the heart to speed up and blood pressure to increase as a result of increased neuroendocrine discharge (nerve-to-gland-to-blood discharge). The sympathetic nervous system stimulates tissue-direct (in this case muscles in the heart and blood vessels) and gland-direct (in this case primarily the adrenal and thyroid glands) glands, which in turn secrete stimulating hormones. These stimulating effects add up to a faster heartbeat, increased heart rate and oxidation/metabolic rates, more dopamine (a brain neurotransmitter that wakes you up) and a consequential suppression of all body activity which slows things down (sedates) like an intensification of energy put into the digestive processes instead of other more stimulating functions. Hence, parasympathetic effects are reduced in favor of a more sympathetic dominance in all related body function.

Any stress, good and bad (eustress and distress) in any degree can trigger increased sympathetic responses to help protect/ready itself. Whether weightlifting (a eustress), experiencing an auto accident (a distress), the sympathetics (nerves and glands/hormones) take over. When this occurs a stage of fight or flight takes over as the body becomes extremely awake and full of adrenaline. Some time after lifting weights or experiencing a fender bender the parasympathetics then intervene to calm down the excitatory effects present under sympathetic dominance before they wear down body reserves any further, causing any more damage. Many, other bodily functions are affected as well, with some that are rather obvious and others that are not so obvious. The sympathetics and parasympathetics keep each other in check, vacillating from their more stimulating to their more sedative output as needs arise. Always they strive for a synergistic balance, or homeostasis, so that all needs of the body are met on all levels without sacrificing too much during periods of stress. A gland and its related hormone group can dominate over the others when their particular balance is disturbed, which can ultimately cause one's metabolism to either become overstimulated or too sedated, such as the case in adrenal stress syndromes. This always has nutritional consequences.

***The Nerve-Gland-Stress Nutrition Connection in Action:*** A dominant sympathetic input will over stimulate the body. This in turn causes it to use up, not fully digest or lose from the body (as well as urine, sweat, and feces) essential minerals such as calcium and magnesium while other minerals such as potassium, sodium, and phosphorus build up. This phenomenon occurs from direct changes made to the intestinal absorption rates and the kidney's retention of these elements plus a loss of certain vitamins, mostly the water soluble ones–the B complex. The elevation of stress, which can cause sympathetic overstimulation elevates metabolic rate, which in turn causes an increased utilization of these nutrients and others such as certain amino acids and fatty acids. The sympathetic gland/hormone groups mentioned in the table above can be classified as the front-line stress glands due to the fact that they are most directly activated by perceived stress and as a result, defensively and very quickly turn up the metabolic rate. This reactive phenomenon, fight or flight is easy to experience when someone comes up behind you and scares you. Fight or flight is in place to help protect you from blatantly recognizable harm, like being chased by an angry dog. Through a strong neuroendocrine response, it temporarily and automatically potentiates the body's energy, strength, and clearness of mind for better physical and mental performance so that your survival chances are at a maximum, allowing you to effectively wrestle the angry dog into submission (good luck), as Sylvester Stallone would in a movie, or run away and quickly climb a tree for protection (which is probably what most people would choose to do in real life).

However, an occasional dog scare is not the real stress problem for most of us. More damaging is the chronic elevation of stress levels over the long term. This type of prolonged stress creates cumulative and long-lasting imbalances, which slowly but surely undermine our health. As an example, some high blood pressure syndromes people suffer from as activated by long-term stress result from the body's ongoing and increased retention of sodium with a corresponding loss of magnesium and calcium. When sodium retention is higher, blood pressure automatically becomes higher, whereas the loss of magnesium and calcium exacerbate the small muscles surrounding your blood vessels ability to relax. An increase in sodium concentration causes more water to build up inside of the blood, which in turn increases pressure within vessels. The muscles surrounding the blood vessels and the heart itself then have to contract harder in order to compensate, most especially in light of calcium and magnesium losses, which when in proper balance, tend to relax those same muscles which reduces pressure (sodium is considered the yang in this case while calcium and magnesium the yin). For those individuals who suffer from this type of problem, it's a well known fact that ingesting less sodium as salt and more dietary and supplemental magnesium and calcium help to lower blood pressure.

The metabolic reverse of this sympathetic dominant phenomenon can be seen when instead the parasympathetic dominant gland and hormone group dominate, creating a sedative effect on body functions. A total lack of exercise can cause this. Progressively increasing fatigue levels are experienced when this lack of eustress or exercise stress occurs and in many cases blood pressure that is too low and even depression can develop. The fatigue experienced from parasympathetic dominance results primarily from lowered energy production which in turn is directly correlated with increased retention of calcium and magnesium, which are considered the most sedative of all minerals and are especially antagonistic to the thyroid and adrenal glands in their job to stimulate energy production.

### *Pregnancy Revisited as a Physiological Stress*

All physiological responses affect the neuroendocrine system and therefore the body's nutritional needs. Good examples of this occur during and after pregnancy. Due to the load, or stress, of the fetus on the mother's body, a pregnant mother's need is greater and sometimes very different in nutritional requirements than those before or after pregnancy as the body adjusts itself to better meet the extra and special nutritional needs of the growing fetus. After the baby is born, the mother's body has a new set of nutritional requirements necessary to optimize the nursing process. Infants and children have different nutritional requirements for growth and development than adults who aren't growing. These nutritional need changes occur through each stage of growth, development, and maturity from birth to death. Differing stresses exert their effects on the neuroendocrine system which in turn alters nutritional requirements, as stated before.

Stress is highly multifactored and includes viral, bacterial, and fungal infections, all active disease including degenerative and diet-related syndromes, emotions, toxic metals, chemical exposures, drug-induced side effects, and even athletics. Highly intensive training and competition is stress to an athlete (or fitness buff) which in turn changes nutritional requirements quantitatively and qualitatively. We categorically consider exercise stress as being calculated eustress because of its beneficial physiological effects when not overdone. Exercise helps to tune up the body's physiological efficiency and metabolic capacities. Over-training creates distress because it exceeds the body's ability to adapt favorably. During the early stages of distress the body responds with what researchers call an "alarm reaction." The sympathetic nervous system creates this alarm reaction by increasing its rate and intensity of electrochemical discharge, which in turn alerts the neuroendocrine and immune systems of a stress assault. These nervous discharges stimulate the metabolic rate to increase immediately. This first *alarm reaction stage* is officially known as the previously mentioned fight or flight phenomenon (ffp for short). The ffp alters nutrient need and nutrient utilization in all nutrient categories (minerals, vitamins, vitamin-like substances, aminos, fatty acids, hormones, proteins, and sugars). After the initial ffp kicks in as an overall part of the alarm reaction, two more time-related stages of stress evolve. The ***resistance stage*** occurs next as the body then attempts to recover its lost balance from the initial ffp stage by adjusting itself physiochemically to settle down before any real damage can occur from overstimulation (unless of course you've been bitten by the dog that you mistakenly wrestled and are now in a state of total shock, which could again change nutrient need from the initial ffp levels to completely new levels). Last is the ***recovery stage*** of stress where again nutrient needs differ as part of the body effecting changes necessary to put it back into better balance.

The stages of stress mentioned above are created by different degrees of neurohormonal inputs that adjust the body back to a normal steady state. Each of these degrees of stress has its own set of nutritional requirements which is very similar to other individuals but is still highly unique to one's own biochemical individuality.

Dr. David Watts has measured changing vitamin and mineral needs during the three stages of stress as mentioned above and has compiled a partial list of the key nutrient changes indigenous to each stage:

> ***FFP Alarm Stage:***
> Minerals depleted – calcium, copper, cobalt, sodium, selenium
> Vitamins depleted – B1, B6, B12, C, D, E
> ***Resistance Stage:***
> Mineral depleted – potassium, zinc, iron, magnesium, manganese
> Vitamins depleted – B1, B2, B3, B5, B6, A, C
> ***Recovery Stage:***
> Minerals depleted – calcium, cobalt, copper, magnesium, selenium
> Vitamins depleted – B1, B6, B7, B12, C, D, E

The above three stages of stress are normal body reactions which should progress from one stage to the next in healthy individuals. But in some cases, a given individual may get stuck in one of these stages, unable to progress to the next due to inadequate nutrition research or sustained stress that does not allow the body to calm down normally. Getting stuck in any stage carries with it a certain group of disease-promoting phenomena which can manifest over time into very serious health problems.

A good example of this disease-promotion process occurs as a result of being literally stuck in the alarm stage of stress, unable to progress to the next. This high stress problem consequently results in chronic inflammation tendencies which eventually lead to arthritis, colitis, gastritis, cardiovascular diseases, and many other degenerative conditions. Remaining stuck in the resistance stage creates an across-the-board destruction pattern throughout the body which can result in chronic degenerative diseases including cancer. Movement into the recovery stage is most desirable but full recovery may never be achieved if certain nutrient imbalances persist along with the lack of stress management. In fact, if one's unique nutrient needs are not addressed effectively, he or she can easily move into an exhaustion stage also known as burnout where one's stimulatory glands are dramatically weakened, allowing the sedative glands to totally dominate, shutting everything off and causing collapse. Both target nutrient management and stress management are exceedingly important to prevent this from happening. Some interrelated mineral proportions or relative ratios affected by different endocrine glands with their respective hormones, which Dr. Watts and other researchers have extensively studied are in the following list of glands, hormones and mineral ratios:

Adrenal cortex (anabolic hormones) – Na/K, Na/Mg, Fe/Cu, Ca/Mg, Ca/K, Ca/P, Ca/Na
Adrenal cortex (catabolic hormones) – Fe/Cu, Na/Mg, Na/K, Ca/K, Ca/P, Ca/Mg, Ca/Na
Thyroid – Na/Mg, Fe/Cu, Ca/P, Ca/K
Parathyroid – Ca/P, Ca/Mg, Ca/Na, Ca/K, Cu/Fe, Ca/Fe, Fe/Cu
Pancreas – Ca/P, Ca/Mg, Ca/K, Ca/Fe, Ca/Na, Zn/Cu, Fe/Cu,
Estrogens – Ca/Mg, Ca/P, Ca/K, Ca/Na, Ca/Fe, Na/K, Zn/Cu, Fe/Cu
Progesterone – Zn/Cu, Fe/Cu, Na/K, Ca/K

It's important to keep in mind that stress inputs from the neuroendocrine system can dramatically change these mineral ratios as well as the related levels of vitamins and other nutrients which are ultimately synergistic and/or antagonistic to these particular minerals. In other words, change one ratio and other retention changes follow automatically, whether from what is consumed or from what kind of stress is being processed by the nervous system and glands. An example of this can be seen when the level of calcium goes down in the body due to an overactive thyroid gland which allows phosphorus retention to increase and then displace calcium further. This displacement effect in turn creates a greater need for vitamin D retention automatically, since vitamin D is a primary synergist for calcium retention by the body and its need increases when the ratio of calcium to phosphorus goes down. This effect chain reacts throughout the entire body in regard to related nutrient balances.

Inasmuch as the neuroendocrine system affects nutrition, so does nutrition affect the neuroendocrine system. A good example of this occurs when a magnesium deficiency exists, which in turn stimulates certain adrenal cortex hormones, which, in conjunction with other associated mechanisms, speeds up the rate of muscle tissue breakdown (catabolism) which is a key phenomenon of premature aging. Exactly how this type of information specifically relates to your unique body would be revealed from testing the body directly so that therapeutic intervention can be precisely calculated. For the moment it is important to understand that both glands and nutrients exert biochemical forces upon each other. Less nutrient availability undermines proper glandular function, hormone output, and hormone balance, while more stressors activate the glands to strongly impact upon the body's demand for specific nutrients. In the case of an underactive or hypothyroid, there is a greater demand for and utilization of vitamins C and E while the conversion of beta carotene to vitamin A is enzymatically suppressed. Conversely, a lack of iodine causes the thyroid to slow down and produce less thyroxin. This leads to a slowing or underactive thyroid with its respective patterns of nutrient need and utilization as effected from both directions; stress to gland to nutrient, and from nutrient to gland, which both meet in the metabolic middle somewhere depending on which is the most influential force at that time.

The following is a summation of many classic hormonal effects upon nutrient status as studied and cataloged by Drs., Bralley, Lord, Watts and others.

| Hormones | Body Level | Affected Nutrient | Effect On Nutrient |
|---|---|---|---|
| Thyroid | Higher | C, E, I, Na, Fe, K, P, B1, B3, B5, B6, B10, Mn | Increased utilization |
| Thyroid | Lower | A, Mg, Ca, Cu | Decreased carotene conversion<br>Increased retention of Ca, Mg, Cu |
| Thyroid | Lower | Iodine | Iodine deficiency |
| Testosterone | Lower (Males) | Zinc, Aminos, C | Increased utilization |
| Estrogen | Lower (Females) | Ca, Mg, D | Decreased bone mineralization |
| ACTH (Adrenocorticotropic Hormone) | Higher | Amino Acids | Increased utilization |
| Cortisol | Higher | B Complex, Aminos, many minerals, Fe, C, Fatty Acids | Increased loss<br>Increased utilization<br>Lowered Omega-6 levels |
| DHEA | Higher | E | Increased oxidative stress |
| Growth Hormone | Lower | Fatty Acids, Amino Acids, D | Decreased fat oxidation<br>Increased catabolism |
| Insulin | Higher | Most minerals, aminos, Zinc | Increased losses |
| Insulin | Lower | Glucose | Decreased metabolic utilization/increased urinary losses |

The following is a simplified classification of many nutrient chemical influences on hormones and other related cellular controls as cataloged by Drs. Bralley, Lord and Watts.

| Nutrient Chemical | Control Factors | Effect of Reduced Nutrient Supply On Hormones |
|---|---|---|
| Iodine | Thyroxin | Reduced synthesis |
| Amino Acids | Tryptophan: Serotonin<br>Arginine: Nitric Acid<br>Tyrosine: Thyroxin | Reduced synthesis |

**Continued**

| Nutrient Chemical | Control Factors | Effect of Reduced Nutrient Supply On Hormones |
|---|---|---|
| Essential Fatty Acids | Eicosanoids<br>Thyroxin #4 conversion into Thyroxin #3<br>T3 to T4 conversion) | Reduced synthesis<br>Reduced conversion rate |
| Selenium | T4 | Reduced conversion to T3 |
| Manganese | T1, T2, T3, T4 | Reduced synthesis |
| Calcium, vitamin D, Mg, C, Cu, Zn | Parathormone | Reduced synthesis |
| Zinc | Growth hormone<br>Testosterone<br>Thyroxin<br><br>Corticosteroids | Reduced levels<br>Reduced synthesis<br>Reduced synthesis and conversions<br>Inhibited ACTH action |
| Molybdenum, Boron, D | Estrogen | Reduced levels of converted estrogens, most particularly 2-methyoxyestrone |
| Dietary Fiber | Butyrate | Unregulated colonic membrane growth |
| Soy | Isoflavone derivatives | Modified estrogen activity |

### Which Came First – the Nutrient or the Hormone?

In conclusion to this section on hormones, it's important to note that our personalized nutrition discussion is not complete without answering the question – which came first, the nutrient or the hormone? The unequivocal answer is both at almost the same time. Because nutrient and hormone levels are so interdependent upon one another it may seem confusing. In fact it's always best to start the personalized nutrition process with an evaluation of your body's nutrient and toxin levels first before directly examining hormone levels. Nutrient and toxin presence and balance provides the most fundamental interactive template from which the glands synergize themselves. And in all actuality, each cellular control mechanism, including hormones, is derived from nutrients in the first place. Luckily, it's easier and safer to modify diet first before upsetting delicate hormone/glandular balance. In the majority of cases nutritional rebalancing affects hormonal rebalancing most effectively. Synthetic or bioidentical hormone replacement rebalancing doesn't necessarily impact upon nutrient balance as favorably and can cause more harm than good when other glands are unnaturally suppressed.

Then there's the effect of stress to consider. Stress can easily push the glands into secreting hormones which will always throw nutrient balance off, thus creating strong shifts in nutrient demands. If your nutrient reserves aren't adequate, your own body chemistry will be stressed further, sometimes to the point of complete exhaustion. This in turn opens the door to all disease. So what can we do? Test first nutrients and toxins so you can know what is really going on at the deepest levels of atomic and molecular interaction long before a hormone is ever created. Then, based upon nutrition retesting, determine if special interactive hormone tests are needed to reveal other factors or to accelerate the process of balancing the metabolism so that results can be achieved even faster.

### *Gene Profiling or Clinical Genomics*

Whereas most testing techniques discussed so far measured the internal biochemical environment in order to locate harmful nutritional and toxic inconsistencies, this type of examination involves looking at the DNA directly for genetic defects that can contribute to disease. The so-called defects are called single nucleotide polymorphisms, or SNPs for short. These SNPs incur certain protein and enzyme production in cells, leading to many diseases, especially chronic diseases. This genetic information is directly connected to the way that our body processes food, most especially in light of the role of manufacturing and regulating genes (mentioned previously under "Enzymes") in creating healthy or unhealthy enzymes. The overall genomics project is based on the belief that all human diseases result from the interaction of genetic susceptibility to modifiable internal and external environmental factors. SNPs have been categorically associated with almost all known diseases, but these genetic variations are not considered to cause a given disease itself. Instead, they are considered to influence a person's susceptibility to specific environmental factors that are known to increase disease risk. There are certain SNP sets which can be connected to a given disease or physiological imbalance such as immune dysfunction, detoxification, bone metabolism, or cardiovascular metabolism, to name a few. There is a question as to which SNPs are and which are not clinically useful and the labs involved with testing this have four critical requirements:

*Relevance* - The activity of enzymes and individual proteins can be simultaneously coded by hundreds of SNPs. The ones that are carefully chosen are the ones which have the most direct influence over specific biochemical imbalances, which are known to create disease or symptom clusters.

*Prevalence* - SNPs are common genetic predispositions associated with extremely prevalent conditions.

*Modifiability* - Examinations focus on those genetic variations whose expression is most directly influenced by environmental factors so that interventional options related to dietary, nutritional, lifestyle, and pharmaceutical methods can be better organized and implemented.

*Measurability* - A well-developed clinical test is routinely recommended for follow-up functional laboratory testing* of nutrient balance and metabolic disorders.

*List of Primary Tests:* **1.** CardioGenomics profile, DetoxiGenomics profile (more in the next chapter), ImmunoGenomics profile, OsteoGenomics profile. **2.** HTMA (Hair Analysis ).** **3.** IgG/IgE/IgA sensitivity test** **4.** Organic acid analysis**

*Discussion:* Roger Williams' concept of "the biochemical individuality" as postulated in 1956 explored and explained variability in disease susceptibility, nutrient needs, and drug responsiveness amongst individuals, healthy or not. The part that genomics is supposed to play in this has to do with who is most likely to develop a specific disease and who will respond favorably or react unfavorably to a particular supplemental therapy or drug. Ultimately, its overall goal is to help reveal exactly which nutrients are most optimal for a particular individual's most healthful genetic expression. The inherent limitation is simply that it is not directly a measure of the nutrients present up to the moment in the body and therefore it cannot now or ever take the place of nutrition direct tests and other very necessary considerations but are nonetheless a useful adjunct.

One's heredity is dependent on the genes found within the entire genome. A gene is about 3,000 nucleotides long, can vary considerably in this variable, and only 3% of the entire genome itself is actually used for human physiology. Gregor Mendel is the Austrian botanist credited with discovering genetic characters. There are certain Mendelian Laws of Heredity as summarized on the following page:

*Note—In effect, genetic tests automatically refer us back to what the body is retaining and functionalizing at the moment as determined by orthomolecular personalized nutrition testing in the first place. This is because genetic tests cannot account for exactly what is inside the body without nutrition tests and are therefore not helpful in determining precisely what to eat and in which proportions at the moment.

** The genetic tests should not be taken unless these tests have been performed previously for best comparative efficacy.

- *Each physical characteristic corresponds to a single gene.*
- *Genes come in pairs.*
- *Only one gene of the pair is passed on to the next generation by each parent.*
- *It is equally probable that either gene will be passed on.*
- *Some characteristics are considered dominant, while others are considered recessive.*

## Reality Check #9

Genes do not equal fate as many people believe, inasmuch as they do not have to express themselves as a disease when the environment they are in becomes modified favorably.

The idea here is to plan around a potential risk, if you even have one. It takes both your genes and their environment to trigger disease, so the more you can personalize a nutritional and lifestyle route to avoid risks and maximize your metabolism, the more you will enjoy a healthy life. These tests are really only necessary for people who have conditions that run in their family–notwithstanding that familial and learned habits can contribute to these conditions–the idea being that indisputable data on oneself is the inspiration and starting point to begin changing course toward a much healthier future (or else know that we'll suffer the dire consequences). Just knowing this information can reduce stress about the possibilities when otherwise unknown. There's also a complementary genetic science breakthrough known as epigenetics which further sheds light on the role of one's genes in relation to the environment described in the Biology of Belief and the nature versus nurture paradox as presented brilliantly by Dr. Bruce Lipton.

## Reality Check # 10

After understanding the levels of the biochemicals presented previously (and some others as needed), one can be in a position to consume exactly the right nutrients in the correct proportions according to the law of opposites and its other related principles to provide the body with exactly what it needs to correct its own nutritional problems, without fail.

Our last task of discovery is to uncover other substances within us which are considered, at best, toxic or poisonous. Just as specific nutrients must be targeted for rebalancing, these toxins must be first located in the body, then eliminated from the body as efficiently and healthfully as possible.

# Chapter VI

## Target Toxin Elimination Therapy (TTET)

*There is no darkness but ignorance.*
-William Shakespeare

### Where's the Poison? How Slow Can You Go?

Slow death results from the bodily infusion of heavy metals and other toxic elements such as mercury, cadmium, lead, antimony, uranium, arsenic, chlorine, beryllium and aluminum, anti-corrosives like chromium 6 (as seen in a Julia Roberts movie, "Erin Brockovich") and very strong carcinogens such as formaldehyde (FMA), trimellitic and phthalic anhydrides, isocyanates, TDI, benzene, styrene, acrolein, ethylene oxide, benzopyrenes, methyl parathion, chlorobenzene, anthracene, tetrachlorovinphos, naphthalene, petroleum distillates, and many others.

For the record, these types of toxins are found everywhere in the environment and eventually end up in our bodies no matter how hard we try to avoid them, by eating less fish or taking fewer x-rays or whatever. Subsequently, identifying the sources of each of these toxins should come after we've tested and measured ourselves for their presence within our internal environment. This is even more important in light of the fact that each person accumulates these toxins at different rates based on their biochemical uniqueness. Different people exposed to the same amount of toxin can have completely different retention within their body when tested and then compared. Generally speaking, the more nutritionally balanced we are the less toxins will negatively affect us as much as essential nutrients can to expedite the body's removal of toxic material across the board. One variable is clear – children and older folks are more susceptible to toxic infiltration and retention problems. Excessive buildup of nutritional minerals and vitamins (hypermineralosis and hyper-vitaminosis) free radicals and other easily detectable poisons all can accumulate and combine to seriously deteriorate body functions. Special hair, urine, blood, saliva, and feces tests reveal these chemical killers so that the proper detoxification can be initiated long before serious disease takes hold. We can also consider the presence and residues of parasites, bacteria, fungi, and viruses as toxins within this scope of concern. Their detection and target elimination will contribute to the overall well-being of the body.

***List of Primary Tests:*** **1.** TMA (hair analysis) **2.** Antioxidant profile (blood) **3.** Organic acid analysis (urine) **4.** Toxic challenge (blood/urine) **5.** Saliva evaluation/stool evaluation **6.** Standard blood tests (immune function)

***Discussion:*** Inasmuch as proper enzyme function determines the efficiency of nutrient-driven metabolic and physiological functions, the metabolic basis of life, so does proper enzyme function determine the outcome of toxic accumulation within the body as part of this overall homeostatic or equilibrium process. In effect, nutrient-driven enzyme reactions clear the body of poisons which can be significantly enhanced by personalized nutrition or personalized detoxification or Target Toxin Elimination Therapy (TTET). Aside from immunoglobulins and antibodies to fight germs, there are six enzyme pathways, all genetically induced and concentrated within the liver and to lesser extents other cells, to handle the neutralization and/or elimination of toxic chemicals in/from the body including nutrient excesses and excess hormones. Scientists refer to this process of elimination as clearance of toxins. These detox enzyme systems handle the clearance of three major categories of toxins: xenobiotics (toxins occurring in the environment such as mercury), drugs (prescription, over-the-counter and recreational), and substance buildups from either diet or endogenous (made by the body itself) chemicals. These special detox enzyme mediated clearance systems are all concentrated constituents of the master chemist: the liver. They rely heavily upon proper amino and other essential nutrients to function properly. Clearance involves the chelation and biotransformation of toxins into neutral (or harmless) chemicals. These biotransformation reactions are classified as:

1. glutathione conjugation
2. sulfation
3. peptide conjugation
4. glucuronidation
5. acetylation
6. methylation

There are Phase 1 and Phase 2 reactions which divide up the above six classifications into those which involve special substances known as P-

450 cytochromes and those that don't. Breakdowns can occur in the process of biotransformation which can be pinpointed via proper profiling and then nutritionally corrected. In fact, much of the weaknesses encountered in these chemical detoxification systems were originally thought to be genetically determined and therefore fixed or non-inducible (unchangeable). As of late, research has demonstrated quite the opposite, especially in relation to amino acids in certain phytonutrients. Inducing these detoxification systems to be more efficient, in spite of extremely wide variations from person to person, is just a matter of proper lifestyle and nutritional manipulation. Customizing detox protocols specific to one's unique biochemical specifications will effectively rid the body of the burden of chemical killers (toxins). Following is a biotransformation system-by-system explanation of which toxin is handled by which named detox system:

*Glutathione conjugation* – (xenobiotics) – styrene, acrolein, ethylene oxide, benzo pyrenes, methyl parathion, chlorobenzene, anthracene, tetrachlorovinphos, toxic metals, petroleum distallates, naphthalene; (drugs) – acetaminophen, penicillin, ethacrylic acid, tetracycline; (dietary/endogenous) – bacterial toxins, aflatoxins, lipid peroxides, ethyl alcohol, quercetin, n-acetyl cysteine, prostaglandins, bilirubin, leukotrienes

*Sulfation* – (xenobiotics) – aniline, pentachlorophenol, terpenes, amines, hydroxylamines, phenols; (drugs) – acetaminophen, methyldopa, minoxidil, metaraminol, phenylephrine; (dietary/endogenous) – DHEA or dehydroepiandosterone, quercitin, bile acids, safrole, tyramine, thyroxine, estrogens, testosterone, cortisol, catecholamines, melatonin, 3-hydroxycoumarin, 2,5 hydroxy vitamin D, ethyl alcohol, CCK or cholecystokinase and cerebrosides

*Peptide conjugation from glycine* – (xenobiotics) – benzoic acid, phenylacetic acid, naphthylacetic acid, aliphatic amines, organic acids; (drugs) – salicylates, nicotinic acid from nicotine, chloropheniramines, brompheniramine; (dietary/endogenous) – bile acids, cinnamic acid, PABA or paraminobenzoic acid, plant acids, nicotinic acid from niacin

*Peptide conjugation from taurine* – (dietary/endogenous) – bile acids, caprylic acid, propionic acid, butyric acid, decanoic acid, lauric acid, myristic acid, palmitic acid, stearic acid

*Glucuronidation* – (xenobiotics) – carbamates, phenols, thiophenol, aniline, butsnol, N-hydroxy-2-napthylamine; (drugs) – salicylates, morphine, acetaminophen, benzodiazepines, meprobamate, clofibric acid, naproxen, digoxin, phenylbutazone, valproic acid, steroids, lorazepam, ciramadol, propanol, oxazepam; (diet/endogenous) – bilirubin, estrogens, melatonin, bile acids, vitamins A, E, K, D, steroid hormones.

*Acetylation* – (xenobiotics) – 2-aminofluorine, anilines; (drugs) – clonazepam, dapsone, mescaline, isoniazid, hydralazine, procainamide, benzidine, sulfono-mides, promizole; (dietary/endogenous) – serotonin, PABA, histamine, trypta-mine, caffeine, choline, tyramine, coenzyme A

*Methylation* – (xenobiotics) – paraquat, beta-carbolines, isoquinolines, mercury, lead, arsenic, beryllium, thallium, cadmium, tin, strontium; (drugs) – thiovacil, isothane, rimiterol, dobutamine, butanephrine, eluophid, morphine, levaphanol, nalorphine; (dietary/endogenous) – dopamine, epinephrine, histamine, norepi-nephrine, L-dopa, apomorphine, hydroxyestradiols

One particular detox test clinically favored currently due to popularized research on **free radicals** involving the above enzyme systems, is one which directly evaluates oxidative stress. This test evaluates the body's ability to resist free-radical buildup and subsequent damage in the body. Free radicals are leftover oxidation/reduction (electron transferring) molecular reaction particles which are extremely unstable and therefore overreact. These highly reactive molecules irritate and damage other bio-chemicals, cells and cell membranes, and tissues at large, creating upsets in metabolic and physiological functions, eventually causing a cumulative deterioration of health. Oxidative stress caused by free-radical buildup is a big priority amongst health authorities nowadays and the reason for antioxidant mania in the supplement world. It is the role of antoxidants both to help enzymes to counter antioxidant buildup and by directly absorbing (buffering) these molecular monsters. But, too many antioxi-dants present can actually increase oxidant levels, leading to even more free radicals and/or can deplete essential oxidants, like iron, causing more damage or dysfunction. In excess even antioxidants can become pro-oxi-dants and then turn into oxidants thereafter. This irritating chemical stress phenomenon, simply speaking, occurs as a result of synergistic/antagonistic properties of interreacting nutrients at the atom-ic/molecular level. Consequently, we can precisely employ tests to detect and correct any free radical imbalances by using antioxidant-specific ther-apy (AST) as a component of TTET in order to fully eliminate and not mistakenly add to the problem with indiscriminate nutrient therapy not based upon testing the specifics of the matter. Free-radical buildup is only one piece of the overall toxification puzzle but is one, as all the others are, that can be addressed with the proper testing in the place first. So-called detoxification programs which are a non-tested shotgun approach usual-ly fall surprisingly short of achieving a complete and final detoxification of the body in all matters of potential concern. Simple fasts do not guar-antee that toxic material will be removed, either.

# Reality Check #11
## You Cannot Reliably Clean Out Toxins From the Body That You Cannot Identify First.

**Special Enzymatic Markers** (from Metabolic Urinalysis)

1. **Hydroxy phenyllactate (HPLA)** – "A good sign" when low, as the body is counteracting estrogenic effects on tumor growth; when high it works as a pro-oxidant/carcinogen suppressed by C/E/selenium
2. **Methylhippurate** – demonstrates presence of xylene, a common but very toxic compound
3. **Orotate** – marks hereditary deficiencies of enzymes involving the urea cycle; also caused by L-arginine, aspartic acid and AKG (alpha ketoglutarate) deficiencies
4. **Pyroglutamte** – demonstrates glutathione depletion; glutathione recovers valuable amino acids to prevent their loss in urine which in turn helps maintain a higher nitrogen retention in the body; NAC, taurine and cysteine help suppress nitrogen loss via this process
5. **Sulfate** – reveals weakness in Phase II liver detoxification pathways; the body has a reduced ability to clear drug, steroid, hormone, and phenolic compounds (microorganism residues) from the body; when compared to creatinine (from urine) a ratio can be extrapolated (sulfate/creatinine) which, when low, demonstrates low sulfur reserves (sulfur neutralizes toxins); NAC, taurine, methionine and cysteine help to correct this problem

The next group of enzymatic markers reflects the products of abnormal gut Microorganisms typically classified as intestinal dysbiosis markers but for our purposes are grouped under toxic accumulation.

1. **Benzoate** – IDs highly specific strains of bacterial overgrowth and/or glycine deficiency; a high dietary intake of benzoic acid (a food preservative) can also cause this condition; will rebalance with a greater intake of glycine and better protein digestion in combination with probiotics
2. **Hippurate** – same as above
3. **Phenylacetate** – same as above with an indication for greater dietary fiber and glutamine intake along with berberine, pre and probiotics
4. **Phenylproprionate** – same as above
5. **p-Cresol** – directly from bacteria and protozoa (including amebas) within the gut; p-Cresol is highly toxic; antibiotics such as neomyocin should be avoided; Berberine, pre and probiotics, increase dietary fiber and glutamina are all indicated to correct
6. **p-Hydroxybenzoate** – same as p-Cresol
7. **p-Hydroxyphenylacetate** – same as above, associated with small intestinal diseases like giardia lamblia
8. **Tricarballyat**e – same as above and in addition can create a magnesium deficiency if left uncorrected

9. **Dihydroxyphenylpropionate** – demonstrates Clostridium overgrowth concurrent with multiple food allergies due to "leaky gut" syndromes which are also associated with numbers 7 and 8 and the next three enzymatic markers that follow

10. **Citramalate** – reveals yeast and/or fungi overgrowth which requires bowel detoxification using grapefruit seed extract, undecylenic acid and caprylic acid along with beneficial bacteria (probiotics).

11. **B–Ketoglutarate** – same as above

12. **Tartrate** – same as above

Note: Citramalate, B-ketoglutarate and Tartrate are known as antimetabolites due to their connection to the chemical intermediates of normal energy metabolism within the body. They affect energy pathways of the central nervous system and have been shown to be elevated in children who began displaying autistic traits after multiple broad spectrums of antibiotic treatments.

Below is a brief overview of other specific nutrient-to-toxin target effects indigenous to TTET.

*Heavy Metals* What can be done about heavy metal toxicity that is so common today? The four cardinal rules to heavy metal detoxification are:

1. Avoid exposure – you may be inadvertently adding to the amount of toxic accumulation in your body. You need to identify the specific sources of these toxins by checking sources given in your reports and also the contents of other materials to which you have frequent exposure. Begin by reading labels as much as possible but realize that everyone is exposed to certain levels of heavy metals from food and drink and other environmental sources.

2. Reduce absorption by the gastrointestinal tract – generally speaking, the absorption of ingested heavy metals is low but the rate can vary from one individual to the next to a large degree. One across-the-board food component that is probably the most helpful in reducing the percentage of toxic metals and all toxins absorbed is dietary fiber. A nutritional plan replete with a good variety of fiber is healthfully beneficial. The following foods are particularly useful in reducing the absorption of toxic metals.

- All kinds of beans
- Whole-grain breads
- Most fresh fruits including apples and quinces
- Most cooked vegetables
- Whole-grain cereals, especially oatmeal

There are also special supplements which can bind heavy metals such as bentonite, activated charcoal, and algal extracts.

3. Increase elimination of toxics – there are numerous natural chelation and complexing substances utilized as dietary supplements which will expedite the removal of heavy metals by forming certain soluble complexes which the kidneys can clear. There are also more aggressive chelation therapies available depending on the degree of toxic metal exposures. The following are some key dietary supplements which help clear toxic metals from the body:

- Methionine
- Ascorbic acid
- Lipoic acid

4. Ingest more competitive nutrient elements – another complement to the removal of toxic heavy metals is to supply a generous amount of other nutrient elements that directly compete with and displace the toxic metals. These are considered the primary antagonists of each of the metals listed below:

| METAL | ANTAGONIST |
|-------|-----------|
| Mercury | Selenium, Zinc, Iron, Sulfur |
| Cadmium | Zinc |
| Lead | Calcium, Iron, Sulfur, Magnesium |
| Aluminum | Zinc, Selenium |

Before you can truly proceed with a target detox program, just as you must identify nutrient retention for yourself, you must first answer these questions:

1. Which toxic compounds are in my body?

2. How much of each toxin is in my body according to the test results?

3. What nutritional and/or environmental sources do my tests suggest are contributing to my body's burden of these toxins?

4. What does my report say to do to rid my body of these toxins?

Once toxic presence is known it becomes clearer how to therapeutically utilize this information for yourself. A one-of-each approach is not useful and is actually harmful.

## OTHER SPECIFIC NUTRIENT DETOXIFICATION FUNCTIONS

| SPECIFIC NUTRIENT | TARGET EFFECT |
|---|---|
| Vitamin C (ascorbic acid) | Increases toxin mobilization, reduces toxic metal binding to tissues, and increases antioxidant protection in general |
| Vitamin B Complex | Increases liver enzyme function to detox |
| Lipoic Acid | Protects liver and increases antioxidant regeneration |
| NAC (N-Acetylcysteine) | Increases glutathione formation and its complexation |
| Calcium | Protects against lead accumulation |
| Cysteine | Increases formation of glutathione and sulfates |
| Copper | Regenerates glutathione |
| SAM (S-Adenosylmethionine) | Highly active form of methionine |
| Methionine | Acts as a methyl donor and sulfur supplier |
| Glycine | Stimulates liver to conjugate toxins |
| Selenium | Regenerates glutathione and protects against mercury |
| Sulfate | Stimulates liver to conjugate toxins |
| Free-form aminos | Increase energy production by intracellular mitochondria, act as methyl donors and provide organic sulfur |
| Manganese | Regenerates glutathione |

## WAYS TO FURTHER INCREASE RATE OF DETOXIFICATION

| METHOD | EFFECT |
|---|---|
| DMPS (2, 3–dimercapto– 1-propane –sulfonic acid) given intravenously | Increased mobilization rate from bone and soft tissue |
| EDTA (Ethylenediamine Tetraacetic Acid), Penicillamine | Increased mobilization rate from bone and soft tissue |
| DMSA (2–3 –dimercaptsuccinic acid) given orally | Increased mobilization rate from bone and soft tissue |
| Vigorous exercise, sauna, whirlpool | Increased circulation and sweat flow |
| Cruciferous vegetables | Increased rate of toxin conversion by liver |
| Diuretics, increased fluid intake | Urinary excretion |
| Dietary fiber and cholagogues | Excretion by feces |

### Food Rotation and Detoxification for Allergenic Toxicity

Profiling tests mentioned in Chapter 5 reveal hidden nutrition sensitivities and some toxic accumulation as well. Applying the test findings to a strategic sequence of alternating food consumption and/or toxin elimination in the case of anti-nutritive toxins allows us to clean the body out of this chemical stress so that it can function at peak efficiency. Most hidden allergies can be reduced significantly and in some cases eliminated altogether using the 1-4–7 alternation process. Other non-nutritive toxic accumulations (such as mercury, for example) may require special supplements in addition to modified food intake, depending on their nature. For example, if you were found to have a slight sensitivity to spinach and an abnormal mercury level in your body, then you would avoid all spinach 6 out of 7 days per week for the next 90 days, then you would have spinach once every 4 days for the next 120 days, at which time a retest should reveal a major sensitivity reduction to spinach. Mercury detox requires an increase in sulfur-rich foods like garlic, in conjunction with increased intake of supplemental zinc, selenium, iron, sulfur and the herb derivative, dimercaptosuccinic acid. (A $10 mail order hair analysis can confirm results.) Your specific personalized process of rotation and detox is exceedingly important to extend life, promote healthy DNA, and minimize disease potential.

### The Three Phases of Allergenic Correction

***Food Elimination:*** This begins the most necessary first steps taken to remedy allergies. It involves avoidance of very slight, moderate, and strongly reactive foods for two to three months in varying degrees depending on the strength of the reaction and the number measured. All immunoglobulyn E foods should be avoided until the first retest, at which time the elimination format will be adjusted according to what is found. The following only pertains to IgG foods (and spices), not Es: If 25% or less of those allergens tested react positively, two months is required in this phase. If more than 25% test positive, three months is required. E and G blood tests generally have four classes of reactivity strength: 0 = no reaction, 1= very slight, 2 = slight, 3 = moderate, 4 = very strong. This phase consists of the first two weeks, at which time only 0 foods can be consumed; after the first two weeks, one of the foods can be added in at one day per seven. After 60 to 90 days (depending on reactive percentage), 1s can be eaten once every four days, 2s can be eaten once every seven days. This goes on for another 30 (under 25%) to 60 days (over 25%), at which time 1s and 2s can be eaten once every three days while 3s can be eaten once every seven days for the next 60 (under 25%) to 90 (over 25%) days. After the retest, this format is modified according to how much improvement is demonstrated with the goal of reintroducing more 0, 1, 2, 3, G foods and some weakly reactive Es. 4s and strong Es will probably remain on the lifetime avoidance list forever.

***Food Rotation:*** This begins at the start of the food elimination phase and requires a generalized food rotation in conjunction with a specific food rotation. Generalized food rotation involves alternating consumption of non-reactive foods over a three day period concisely and in conjunction with reactive foods which are eaten once every four days. In generalized food rotation (GFR), variety is the key but the food families corresponding to the specific reactive foods have to be properly seeded in so as not to interfere with the specific food rotation (SFR). Proper food rotation entails leaving one full day of related food family elimination after a specific food elimination that is part of that particular food family, even if the other food family members are not G or E reactive. Proper SFR requires ingesting a specific 1+, 2+ or 3+ food only once every four days. Any related food family foods are deleted the day after, as FFR dictates.

Example: Food #1 is cabbage which is a mustard family food. Food # 2 is turnips which are part of the same family. A #1 food is 1+ reactive while #2 is 0 reactive. #1 is eliminated on Monday and cannot be eaten again for six days. #2 is not eaten on Monday or Tuesday but can be consumed thereafter until cabbage is again eliminated, at which time the cycle begins again.

***Reintroduction:*** Subsequent to avoidance of reactive foods for the specified time periods is the reintroduction of these foods. For best results it is most effective to add foods back as the tests recommend and closely monitor yourself for any noticeable adverse reactions. This works best when you have several helpings of the suspect food in the same day, because symptoms will be easier to detect that day or within two more days. Pay close attention – these symptoms can be hard to spot with a wide range of possibilities. And, of course, you can retest Gs and Es before proceeding beyond 1+ foods for more definitive proof of any remaining sensitivities. Retesting is recommended within a year of initiating an allergenic cleansing and antibody detox program. Reintroduction of specific allergenic foods day by day is included in your test results starting with the 1-in-4 alternation method for food offenders. If symptoms reappear, the offending food should be dropped for 21 days and then tried again. There is one absolute: don't, under any circumstances, reintroduce any quantity of food which tests demonstrate 3+ E or G reactions like asthma attacks, hives, anaphylactic shock, itchy and burning rashes, extreme nausea, etc. A significant percentage of Es and a few Gs contain fixed antibody memories which will cause symptomatic flare-ups always, although reactive intensities may lessen over time.

### The Nerve/Gland/Stress Nutrition Connection Revisited

Too much stress is toxic to the body in ways that are measurable and with proper therapy can hold any potential toxic effects to a minimum. Some people believe that you can literally think yourself sick, and this is true as well. One of the more valuable contributions that personalized nutrition can make for each of us is that it can be used to detect and help the correct physiochemical consequences of distress and negative thinking. Inasmuch as and laughing is good for the soul, it's also good for helping to bring the body chemistry into alignment with a perspective that is good to emphasize throughout life. Which brings us to:

## Reality Check #12

### More Conscious Thinking and More Conscious Choices Enables a More Successful Personalized Nutrition Outcome

# Chapter VII

## Clinical Cases
## Problem – Solution – Plan of Action

*It must happen in us before it can happen to us.*
—Raymond Charles Barker

The attainment and maintenance of good health is simply a nutrient and lifestyle control issue.

Controlling the amount and proportion of nutrients and toxins that are being retained, utilized, and/or excreted by your body (and mind) is the key element of control. This is the essence of what nutrition testing is about. The ongoing hypothesis behind personalized nutrition is that if all of the essential nutrients are put into balance in the body and all of the toxins eliminated, life expectancy will dramatically rise and all disease (especially degenerative disease) will dramatically diminish, perhaps be eliminated altogether, and the overall use of side-effect-promoting pharmaceuticals will dissipate over time. Below find a list of the primary variables we need to account for in this control plan. Get these into order and the other structure and function variables of the body will fall into perfect place:

### List of Essential Nutrients Used in
### Personalized Nutrition

### Minerals

Minerals are those atomic elements found in the earth's crust that are constituents of all life, all human tissue, and human food. Many are considered essential to human life while others are considered harmful to human life. Overall, about 76 elements have been isolated in body tissues. There are two types of minerals: macro (major) and micro (trace) minerals. *Macro or major minerals* are required in 100 mgs. (milligrams) or greater amounts every day. *Micro or trace minerals* are required in less than 100 mg. amounts per day, and out of these, many are required in only mcg. (microgram) amounts daily. Minerals occur within the body as:

- **Components** of certain essential organic molecules such as metalloenzymes (or iron-containing cytochromes), amino acids (the mineral sulfur in cysteine and methionine) and others such as iron in hemoglobin and iodine in thyroid hormones
- **Structural components** of various tissues such as calcium, phosphorus and fluorine in teeth, bones, hair, nails, etc.
- **Free ions** (sodium, calcium, and potassium) in blood and all other body fluids and which assist in acid/base balance, nerve impulse transmission, muscle contraction and as catalysts for enzymatic reactions
- **Toxins** when taken in excessive amounts or in imbalanced ratios

| MAJOR MINERALS | TRACE MINERALS | |
|---|---|---|
| Calcium | Iron | Copper |
| Magnesium | Chromium | Zinc |
| Potassium | Selenium | Vanadium |
| Phosphorus | Manganese | Molybdenum |
| Sulfur | Boron | Cobalt |
| Chlorine | Germanium | Silicon |
| Sodium | Antimony | Beryllium |
| | Bismuth | Gold |
| | Lithium | Nickel |
| | Platinum | Ruthenium |
| | Scandium | Silver |
| | Strontium | Tin |
| | Tungsten | Zirconium |
| | Fluorine | |

| TRACE MINERALS – RARE EARTH | | |
|---|---|---|
| Lanthanum | Cerium | Praseodymium |
| Lutetium | Neodymium | Promethium |
| Samarium | Europium | Gadolinium |
| Terbium | Dysprosium | Holmium |
| Erbium | Thulium | Ytterbium |
| TRACE MINERALS – MISCELLANEOUS | | |
| Curium | Erbium | Gallium |
| Gadolinium | Iridium | Neodymium |
| Neptunium | Niobium | Palladium |
| Rubidium | Tellurium | Thallium |
| Thorium | Titanium | Yttrium |

| TRACE  MINERALS – HIGHLY TOXIC | | |
|---|---|---|
| Arsenic | Beryllium | Mercury |
| Cadmium | Lead | Aluminum |
| Plutonium | Radium | Radon |
| Uranium | | |

| SIGNIFICANT  MINERAL RATIOS | | | |
|---|---|---|---|
| Calcium/Phosphorus | Sodium/Potassium | Zinc/Copper | Calcium /Potassium |
| Sodium/Magnesium | Calcium/Magnesium | Iron/Copper | Calcium/Strontium |
| Copper/Molybdenum | Selenium/Silver | Chromium/Vanadium | Iron/Cobalt |
| Selenium/Tin | Potassium/Lithium | Potassium/Cobalt | Zinc/Tin |
| magnesium/boron | sulfur/copper | | |

| TOXIC MINERAL RATIOS | | |
|---|---|---|
| Calcium /Lead | Selenium/Mercury | Sulfur/Mercury |
| Iron /Lead | Zinc /Cadmium | Sulfur /Cadmium |
| Iron /Mercury | Zinc /Mercury | Sulfur /Lead |

## *Vitamins*

Vitamins are organic compounds:

- **Required** in trace amounts by the body
- **That perform** specific metabolic functions like stimulating enzyme action, also known as coenzymes or cofactors because of this property
- **Not fully synthesized** by the body, are considered "molecular minerals"
- **That do not produce energy** in and of themselves; they require enzymes to work with for energy production
- **That in excess** can be toxic to the body condition known as clinical or sub-clinical hypervitaminosis; are either synergistic or antagonistic to each other and minerals
- **That come in two forms:** fat soluble and water soluble

### *Vitamin Names*

**Vitamin A** - fat soluble in three forms:
>        A1 retinol, A2 dehydroretinol, A3 pro vitamin A (beta carotene)

**Vitamin B Complex** - water soluble in multiple forms:
>        B1 thiamin, B2 vitamin G aka riboflavin

## 150

B3 niacin in two forms:
> nicotinic acid, niacinamide (P.P. factor- pellagra preventing factor)
> aka antipellagra factor

B5 pantothenic acid

B6 group (pyridoxine, pyridoxal, pyridoxamine)

B7 Bc vitamin M (folic acid Bc conjugate)

B10 vitamin H (biotin)

B12 anti-pernicious anemia factor comes in two forms:
> cyanocobalamin (B12), hydroxocobalamin (B12b)

**Vitamin C Complex** - water soluble in two forms:
> C ascorbic acid aka anti-scurvy factor aka anti-scorbutic factor
> bioflavonoid complex - multiple forms:
>> flavones, flavanones, flavanonals, eriocitrin, hesperedin,
>> naringen, naringenin, rutin, tumeric, quercetin

**Vitamin D** - fat soluble in three forms:
> D1 aka D aka calciferol, D2 aka cholecalciferol
> D3 aka ergocalciferol

**Vitamin E Complex** - fat soluble in three forms:
> E1 - d-alpha tocopherol (most active form)
> E2 - d-beta tocopherol, E3 - d-gamma tocopherol

**Vitamin F (essential fatty acids)** - fat soluble in 4 forms:
> Omega-6 cis-linoleic acid (LA), Omega-3 alpha linoleic acid (ALA)
> *GLA gamma linolenic acid, *EPA eicosopentanoic acid

**Vitamin K** - fat soluble in three forms:
> K1 phytonadione, K2 menaquinone, K3 menadione

**Vitamin L** - water soluble in two forms:
> L1 isolated from beef liver extract, L2 isolated from yeast

---

* These two forms of fatty acids (activated fatty acids) can be manufactured by the body, but due to severe metabolic disturbances common amongst Americans we tend to consider them as essential and therefore necessary to derive from exogenous sources (food and supplements) through the TNT (Targeted Nutrition Therapy) profiling process. Proper TNT minimizes the inhibition of these two fatty acids in metabolism by keeping resistance factors like insulin and vitamin deficiencies to a minimum.

## Vitamin-Like Factors

Chlorophyll
Choline
Inositol
Ubiquinone (coenzyme Q10)
Octacosanol
Lipoic Acid
PABA (para-aminobenzoic acid)

Pangamic Acid (vitamin B15)
Pycnogenol
All bioactive non-toxic compounds
  and herbs
Glandular extracts
Colostrum

Enzymes:
> Metabolic (produced in body from amino acids—endogenous)
> Digestive (proteases, amylases, lipases)
> Cellulases - (**endogenous** and **exogenous**)
> Exogenous (naturally occurring enzymes in all foods)

## Phytonutrients

Phytonutrients (phytochemicals) are known and unknown nutritive compounds found in all plant life including but not limited to vitamins, minerals and other preclassified nutrients.

Some phytonutrients are known to prevent certain diseases, such as cancer, or help eliminate excess soft-tissue, calcium-like phytic acid, but their full metabolic implications and functions are still not well understood. There are thousands more to be discovered.

| | | |
|---|---|---|
| Alkaloids | Isoflavones | Ginsenosides |
| Allium | Saponins | Disogenin |
| Allyl Sulfides | Indoles | Schisandrins |
| Caffeic Acid | Isothiocyanates | Salicin |
| Ellagic Acid | Polyphenols | Kavalactones |
| Sulfonamides | Hippuric Acid | Glycosides |
| Sulforaphane | Proanthocyanadins | Chlorogenic Acid |
| Limonene | Parthenolides | Polyphenol catechins |
| Dithiolthiones | Eleutherosides | Genistein |
| Protease Inhibitors | Ligustilides | Daidzein |
| Phytic Acid | Anthocyanosides | |
| Phytosterols | Ginkolides | |

152

*Amino Acids*

These are the smallest component parts of protein and provide the building blocks of the body from which all tissues are synthesized and many metabolic control factors are derived, i.e. hormones, enzymes, neurotransmitters, immunoglobulins, etc.

| I. Neutral Aliphatic | I. Neutral Aliphatic |
|---|---|
| Threonine*<br>Isoleucine (aka branch chain amino)*<br>Leucine (aka branch chain amino)*<br>Valine (aka branch chain amino)* | Glycine<br>Alanine<br>Serine<br>Norleucine |
| **II. Neutral Cyclic<br>aka Aromatic aka Heterocyclic** | **II. Neutral Cyclic aka Aromatic<br>aka Heterocyclic** |
| Phenylalanine*<br>Tryptophan* | Tyrosine, Proline<br>Hydroxyproline (loosely classified) |
| **III. Neutral Sulfur Containing** | **III. Neutral Sulfur Containing** |
| Cysteine<br>Methionine* | Taurine<br>Homocysteine<br>Cystathionine |
| | **IV. Acidic** |
| **V. Basic** | Aspartic Acid, Glutamic Acid, Glutamine, |
| Histidine*<br>Lysine*<br>Arginine | Asparagine, Hydroxyglutamic Acid, GABA<br>(Gamma Amino Butyric Acid) |
| | **VI. Miscellaneous** |
| | Citrulline (from urea cycle)<br>Ammonia (from urea cycle) Phosphoserine<br>Methylhistidine<br>Phosphoethanolamine<br>Methionine Sulfoxide<br>Sarcosine<br>Alpha Amino Adipic Acid<br>Alpha Amino - n – butyric acid<br>Ethanolamine<br>Anserine<br>Carnosine, Carnitine |

*Basic eight essential amino acids.

## *Fatty Acids*
The smallest component of fat.

**Omega-3:**
1. Alpha Linolenic
2. Eicosapentaenoic (EPA)
3. Docosapentaenoic
4. Docosahexaenoic

**Omega-6:**
1. Linoleic
2. Gamma linolenic
3. Eicosadienoic
4. Dihomogamma linolenic (DGLA)
5. Arachidonic
6. Docosadienoic
7. Docosatetraenoic

**Monounsaturated:**
1. Vaccenic
2. Myristoleic
3. Palmitoleic
4. Oleic
5. 11-Eicosenoic
6. Erucic
7. Nervonic

**Saturated:**
1. Capric
2. Lauric
3. Myristic
4. Palmitic
5. Stearic
6. Arachidic
7. Behenic
8. Lignoceric
9. Hexacosanoic

**Odd Chain:**
1. Pentadecanoic
2. Heptadecanoic
3. Nonadecanoic
4. Heneicosanoic
5. Tricosanoic

**Trans Fat:**
1. Palmitelaidic
2. Elaidic

**Ratios:**
1. Polyunsaturated/Saturated
2. Stearic/Oleic
3. Linoleic Acid/DGLA
4. Eicosapentaenoic/DGLA
5. Arachidonic Acid/EPA

All of the above nutrients, vitamins, minerals, amino acids, and fatty acids are accounted for through personalized nutrition procedures as frontline body data and are synergistically proportioned within subsequent individualized nutrition programs according to all biochemical uniqueness found. Allergy, digestive function, toxin, low-grade-fungal/bacterial/parasitic infiltrations, genetic, and interactive hormone tests can be utilized also, although they tend to become more clinically valuable when and if the frontline nutritional therapy reaches a plateau or doesn't respond efficiently. Many of the frontline variables have already been lab-correlated with metabolic efficiency, glandular/hormone function, digestive weaknesses, toxic compounds, and allergies so that across–the–board-relationships are understood and addressed. Initially, these other factors can be considered more as Secondary body data as itemized as follows:

IgE, A, G, M, F, D allergies
Digestive function
Toxins beyond the heavy metals
Genetic profiles

### *Research 101*

As we systematically detect and correct nutritional and toxic disturbances one by one, test by test, you then become your own clinical case with before and after biochemistry snapshots. These then demonstrate progress and stories of detoxification elimination, improved health, and accentuated well-being that go along with these biochemical snapshots and far less body fat in overweight individuals as well. For the sake of discussion, I have included some brief overviews of successful stories in the following sections. Each individual is his or her own personalized nutrition test case whereby the success of the nutrition rebalancing experiment is truly in their hands because everything that they ate, drank, or exposed themselves to was important to the outcome of the experiment and therefore considered as part of the clinical case. Consider the case a scientifically expressed story that has a distinct beginning, middle, and end. The beginning is a given nutrition test or tests, the middle is putting into effect the nutritional recommendations created from the test, and the end is a retest or retests. It is the outcome of knowing exactly how well the recommendations which are deduced from the first test have created a reduction in whatever imbalances are found in that first test as demonstrated by retest(s). This is a simple cause-and-effect scenario.

The other two components of this scientific story involve variables and controls. The variables of a given clinical case are those experimental understandings and influences that have to be defined most succinctly in order for the experiment to be best understood, reliable, and duplicable in other people under the same or similar circumstances. The only problem here is that no two people are alike and therefore each experiment will have a different story, even though the variables may be very similar. This requires an even more panoramic deductive process in determining whether a given personalized nutrition case can be duplicated in the same way on another person. In the real world this is where we have to cut our losses and rely more on the controls of the experiment—controls being those factors of the story which minimize variations from its theme, details, and essence—but still in the hands of the participant outside of experiment administrator control, unless studied under the most environmentally controlled conditions, this can only be accomplished as an inpatient type of study. Realize that the more the variables are controlled, the more researchers value it because the data is usually more reliable, duplicable and understandable.

The following clinical stories are based upon outpatient research, whereby many of the controls are in the hands of the participants themselves, and therefore we have to rely on their honesty about what they did. But as you'll see, the success speaks for itself. The predications for what each person did in each case had previously been developed by medical testing labs based on their research—both in-house and out of house—and the scientific literature at large. I acted as a conduit for this information for these people in order to help them integrate it into a daily plan of action. Furthermore, my job was and is to go by the book and integrate the most appropriate and applicable information, as well as educate each person in how to functionally apply the information into their actual lifestyles. Realize, however, that there are no control groups in these scientific stories for comparison other than the fact that the outright majority of Americans exhibit profound nutritional imbalances when tested.

The following case stories (and many others) when initially tested, exhibited the same problems but then changed, as they followed their personalized nutrition programs closely, as verified by retests and their own reports of symptomatic reduction from the original complaints that went along with their initial presentation. The placebo effect, or that variable in every study whereby an experimentee improves his or her results by positive beliefs alone is least controlled here, because everybody described in the following presentations expected to improve which in my mind as a clinician is still desirable because my goal is to help people to heal mind and body under the actual conditions of real life. Positive beliefs do ensure better outcomes but may cloud the issue of how much positive outcome the actual therapeutic intervention by itself creates. So I'll simply leave it up to your own interpretation. But I will say that each person who was given tests knew that this was the vehicle to reliably detect nutritional problems. The dietary and supplement changes were planned as the solution to the problem to be verified by both retests and their own subjective experiences. Although disease and symptomatic presence diminished in the following clinical cases, these findings were of secondary importance and not the true focus of the study, which again was simply to demonstrate that we could eliminate deficiencies and excesses of nutrients and toxins. All else which occurred after this process as reported and revealed, although extremely important to each suffering individual, is nonetheless considered a side benefit of rebalancing nutritional chemistries which is always our primary goal. The overriding theory or the postulation of orthomolecular medicine is that because all disease is diet-related, when you correct nutritional disturbances, you correct most disease syndrome development, increase effective energy, and improve upon life expectancy automatically. Below is a table of diseases that are considered to be prevented and/or respond to the personalized nutrition approach.

### *Diseases and Dis-eases That Respond to Personalized Nutrition*

| | | |
|---|---|---|
| Achiness | Back Pain | Fatty Liver |
| Acclimatization | Bacterial Infection | Fever |
| Acne (All Types) | Bad Breath (Halitosis) | Fibrocystic Disease |
| Acute Pain | Bed Wetting | Fibromyalgia |
| Addiction (All Types) | Bells Palsy | Food Allergies |
| Adrenergic | Birth Defects | Fractures |
| Hypersensitivity | Bloating | Frozen Shoulder |
| Aging | Blood Clotting | Gall Bladder Disease |
| AIDS | (Abnormal) | Gas |
| Alcoholism | Blood Pressure | Gastric Ulcer |
| Allergies | (High/Low) | Gastritis |
| (Airborne, | Blood Sugar | Gastroenteritis |
| Environmental, | (High/Diabetes) | Genetic Disease |
| Atopic, Nutritional) | (Low/Hypoglycemia) | Glaucoma |
| Alopecia | Body Fat Abnormalities | Gluten Sensitivity |
| Alzheimer's | (High/Low) | Gouty Arthritis |
| Amino Acid Imbalance | Brain Allergies | Hair Loss |
| Amoebic Infestation | Brain Disorders | Hangovers |
| Anaphylaxis | Burkitt's Disease | Hay Fever |
| Anemia | Ear Ringing | Hearing Loss |
| Anger | Eczema | Headaches |
| Angina Pectoris | Edema/Water Retention | Heart Disease |
| Ankylosing Spondylitis | Endocrine Dysfunction | Heartburn |
| Anorexia | (Glandular Enteritis | Hemorrhoids |
| Anxiety | Imbalance) | Hepatitis |
| Arrhythmia | Erythematosus | Herpes |
| Arteriosclerosis | Excessive Skin Dryness | Hiatal Hernia |
| Arthritis | (Scaling) | Hives |
| Asthma | Excessive Thirst | Hormonal Imbalances |
| Atherosclerosis | Eyesight | Hot Flashes |
| Atopic Dermatitis | Dysfunction/Loss | Hyperactivity |
| Autoimmune Disorders | Fatigue | Hyperchlorhydria |

Hypermobile Joints
Hyperpigmentation
Hypertension
Hypervitaminosis
Hypochlorhydria
Hypoglycemia
Hypometabolism
Hypotension
Hypothyroidism
Hypovitaminosis
    Immune System
    Dysfunction
Infections (Chronic)
Infertility
Inflammatory Bowel
    Disease
Influenza
Insomnia
Intestinal Parasites
Irritable Bowel
    Syndrome
Jaundice
Joint Swelling
Juvenile Delinquency
Kidney Failure
Kidney Stones
Lactation
Lactose Intolerance
Leaky Gut Syndrome
Learning Impairment
Leg Cramping
Ligament Laxity
Loss of Concentration
Low Birth Weight
Low Self-Esteem
Lumbalgia
malabsorption
Malnutrition
Manic Depression
Marasmus
Memopause
Memory Loss
Menstrual Disorder
Metabolic Dysfunction
    (Including
    Acidosis/Alkalosis)
Metabolic Rate
    Slowdown
Migraine Headaches
Miscarriage
Mood Swings
Mucus Accumulation

Multiple Sclerosis
Muscle Cramps
Muscle Spasms
Muscular Dystrophies
Myalgia
Myofascitis
Nephritic Syndrome
Nervous Disorders
Neuralgia
Neuritis
Neuropathy
Neuroses
Nutrient Deficiencies
Osteoarthritis
Obesity
Osteoporosis
Otitis Media
Overeating Syndromes
Overweight Syndromes
Pain (All Types)
Pancreatitis
Panic Disorder
Parasites
Parkinson's Disease
Pellagra
Pelvic Inflammatory
    Disease
Periodontal Disease
Personality Disorders
Phenyl Ketonuria
Phlebitis
Phobias
Pleurisy
Pneumonia
Poisoning
Polymyositis
Polyneuritis
Polyneuropathy
Post-Partum
    Depression
Pregnancy Discomfort
Premature Birth
Premenstrual Syndrome
Prenatal Health
Prostanoid Imbalance
Prostatic Hypertrophy
Prostatitis
Pruritus
Psoriasis
Psychosomatic Disorders
Regional Enteritis
Restless Leg Syndrome

Reyes Syndrome
Rheumatoid Arthritis
Rhinitis
Rickets
Schizophrenia
Senility
Sensitivities (Chemical,
    Nutritional)
Silicosis
Sjogren's Syndrome
Smoking Dependence
Spinocerebellar
    Degeneration
Spontaneous Abortive
    Tendencies
Sports Injuries
Steatorrhea
Stiffness
Stress Management
Stretch Marks
Systemic Lupus
Tendonitis
Tension Disorders
Thrush
Thyroid Disorders
Tinnitus (Ear ringing)
TMJ Syndrome
Tooth Decay
Tropical Sprue
Ulcerative Colitis
Ulcerative Cystitis
Ulcers (Gastric,
    Duodenal)
Undereating (Loss of
    Appetite)
Urate Stones
Urticaria
Vascular Disease
Vasospasm
Viral Infection
Weight Loss/Gain
Wheezing
Worms
**Zollinger-Ellison
Syndrome**

Outside of the Malibu Health and Rehabilitation Center, exercise and stress were the least-controlled variables of my patients' routines. In the center, a stress management and exercise regime was always included. The essence of these examples was simply a before and after story of test-demonstrated improvement with little or no attention to the details of stress reduction or exercise participation, which was voluntary in each case.

## First Clinical Case
## Myself

### *The Story*

I became excited about nutrition and exercise at age seven when I started developing into a champion swimmer. At that time, I discovered the principles of cause and effect. I had the idea that if cause and effect were really true, I could ***custom design myself*** to have a one-of-a-kind body for which I was the sole architect and builder. So at an early age, I set out on the course to prove these principles either as true or untrue. This process turned out to be very exciting. My first series of achievements included multiple swimming victories leading to local, county, state, and national rankings and a fifth placing in a pre-Olympic track and field meet. I missed the Olympic team qualifying cutoffs for both sports, but I still felt glorious. Imagine, cause and effect enabled me to excel in two completely different sports, and others as well.

I became very ambitious with my newfound success and decided to establish as my next goal power lifting success – something that is even more opposite than swimming and track are to each other. I began my power lifting campaign by gaining thirty pounds in six weeks, which doubled my initial strength levels overall. I used no drugs or steroids— just diet and supplements. Then...all of a sudden one afternoon I couldn't breathe! I started gasping for air and felt like I was going to suffocate! A friend rushed me to the emergency room. The diagnosis was given as a severe case of asthma of unknown origin. The doctors loaded me up with drugs which helped me breathe a little easier. I still had a hard time climbing up a flight of stairs without having to stop to catch my breath. I fell from what seemed "super health" to "super illness" literally in one afternoon.

The attending medical doctors said that there simply was no cure for this condition – just symptom reduction with drugs. Completely devastated, I began losing my lust for life. Realizing that this illness was my greatest challenge ever, I decided not to accept this fate. I realized that my only recourse was to once again practice cause and effect to save my life. Without the help of any doctors, except for the ideas and practices of Dr. Carlton Fredericks, a nutrition-oriented physician who broadcast a health radio show in New York, I systematically implemented cause and effect using alternative nutritional medicine, and within one and a half years from my original attack, I completely overcame the devastating disease of asthma which the nutritional testing had determined was actually caused by a chlorine allergy. I was ecstatic. Cause and effect really worked – it had saved my life. So with unbridled and renewed enthusiasm (and a freely breathing respiratory system) I applied the principles of cause and effect and attained the master's class level in power lifting and then further excelled in the bodybuilding world by capturing the 1st place title in three Natural Mr. America bodybuilding competitions ("Natural" means without the use of steroids or any other drug). Now with the experience that I really do control the destiny of my body, it was crystal clear to me that these principles of nutrition and exercise were more than just something to read about; they are dynamic forces of life. These same principles have since taken me from my youth through countless athletic achievements and eliminated a terrible disease that literally wouldn't allow me to catch my breath.

The ultimate test of cause and effect was in winning my first Natural Mr. America crown in 1981, five and a half years after I couldn't catch my breath. This event was an exciting competition between 150 men who were in a dogged battle for this great title. While I understood that properly applied nutrition and exercise had gotten me to first place, at the time I wondered if maybe I had just gotten lucky. So I set another goal for myself to see if it would work again and it did. In 1982, I received the Natural Mr. America crown for the second time. I reasoned that if I could do it for the third time, I could prove to myself and thousands of others from all walks of life that nutrition and exercise could be organized for your body only and that there could be undeniable and irrefutable data with which to convince others that they too could have the body they chose. In 1982, during the NBA Mr. America competition, competing against over 160 participants, I was crowned Natural

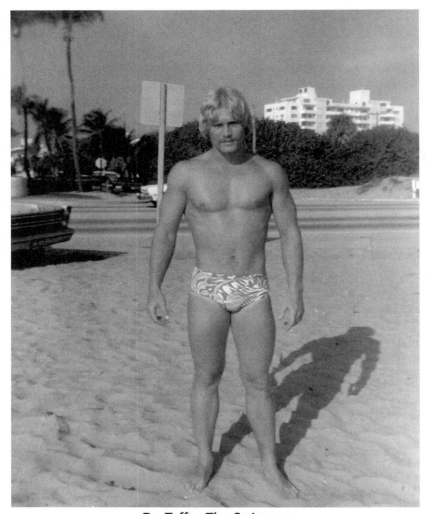

*Dr. Tefft - The Swimmer*

Mr. America for the third time. At six feet tall, my best competitive weight was 216 pounds, which put me in the heavyweight class. It was at this point that I decided to begin a journey to make a difference in other peoples' lives by designing programs for their bodies only, which would provide the basis for a satisfying lifestyle. A better body and good health always makes life more rewarding. I had started on what has since become my life's work.

## Clinical Statistics

The preceding story provides a brief narrative of I developed my directives in life. The real story began when I could not breathe. The medical doctors who examined me in the hospital following my first "unable-to-breathe attack" gave me a shot of epinephrine and officially told me that I had an asthma attack. I had never had an asthma attack before and did

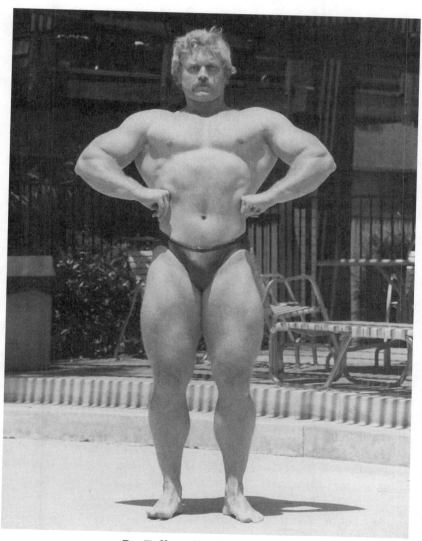

*Dr. Tefft - The Power Lifter*

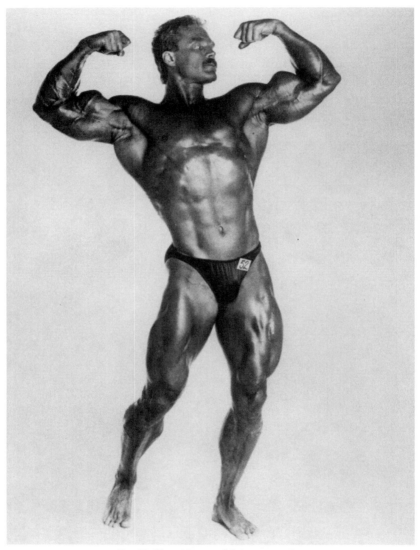

*Dr. Tefft - Natural Mr. America*

not even know what the disease entailed. I was 23 years old. Further examination by *an allergist revealed the following from standard medical and routine allergy testing:*

- All of my regular blood chemistries were normal
- I had allergies to dust, chicken feathers, and cat dander
- Diagnosis: asthma

- Prognosis: poor; incurable disease whose symptoms could be suppressed by medications
- Therapy: corticosteroid pills and two types of inhalers, avoidance of dust, chicken feathers, cat dander and exercise
- Prognosis: with proper detoxification and systematic food rotation, good

After phoning in to a radio show with Dr. Carlton Fredericks, who told me that there were cures for asthma which standard medicine had no clues about, he redirected me to an alternative research clinic that employed orthomolecular nutrition/allergy/toxin tests. These special tests revealed:

- Extremely high chlorine and mercury levels in my body
- Severe mineral deficiencies of calcium and magnesium along with an extreme excess of copper and numerous other mineral imbalances
- (Standard) IgE allergies, determined from blood instead of skin tests, to cat dander, dust, mites, chicken feathers.
- (Nonstandard or non-routine) IgG allergy testing revealed "strong hidden allergies (delayed-onset allergies)" to all dairy products (milk, cheese, yogurt, etc.), string beans, all gluten-containing grains from wheat to rye to oats, egg white, crustaceans like shrimp and lobster, Brazil nuts, spinach, beets, yams/sweet potatoes, pecans, sunflower seeds, chocolate, apples, coffee, strawberries, rhubarb, Concord grapes, parsley, eggplant, Swiss chard, collards, brewers yeast, kelp, and tomatoes
- New diagnosis: chlorine, mercury poisoning, multiple IgG allergies causing status athmaticus
- Prognosis: with proper detoxification in food rotation, good
- Therapy: amino acid/chelation detoxification program for chlorine and mercury including megadoses of L-methionine, L-cysteine, and L-histidine, saturation baths consisting mostly of magnesium salts; lots of carrot juice, special vitamin supplements high in the nutritive factors my body was low in with special foods selected on the same basis; a special food rotation, which was basically devoid of all the allergy foods in the above at first, working them in slowly over time; with slowly increasing low-intensity exercise, adding in an abundance of sunshine and fresh air, drinking only distilled water and special lung-opening massage therapy; plus getting chiropractic adjustments to T4 (the lung spot) and other spinal segments that were related from a reflex standpoint; and at last but not least it was recommended that I remove silver/mercury dental fillings
- Outcome: six-month retests revealed dramatic reduction in chlorine and mercury levels (about 50% and 60% respectively); a reduction of copper excess to within the high end of normal on the hair tissue mineral test; significant

increases in both calcium and magnesium, although both still deficient in retention levels; no more IgG allergies to oats, shrimp and crustaceans, Brazil nuts, spinach, or eggplant, with a reduction in the allergic severity to the other foods except for dairy products, which stayed about the same. IgE tests revealed that I had no more allergies to cats or mites. Also by this time, I was off of all oral corticosteroids; I was barely in need of any inhalers, only having two very minor asthma attacks; was able to exercise with increased intensity; plus my depression was fading fast and I referred to myself as Mr. Happy.

One year later: all nutritional mineral levels were within the reference range, chlorine was non-detectable, IgE allergies to dust was minor with no others present, most IgG allergenic indexes were gone or reduced to very slight sensitivities except for dairy, which remained high in my sensitivity list. Also, I only used one inhaler before high intensity exercise, I did not need the other and did not have one official asthma attack other than from a couple of episodes of shortness of breath after exercise, which seemed to fade quickly when I got into a hot steamy shower after my workouts.

Two years later: no observable mineral deficiencies or excesses, a slight presence of mercury still, slight IgE allergy to dust, IgG allergies to string beans, milk (not cheese or yogurt) and strawberries; absolutely no asthma attacks, no need for inhalers – **cured;** plus, I was breaking every athletic/fitness record I ever set for myself before (which has continued to this day).

Age 35: shortly after adopting a cat, I started to develop allergic symptoms and breathing difficulties; I showed an IgE allergy to cats but all other orthomolecular measurements taken (minerals, vitamins, organic acids, fatty acids) were near normal except for my nagging allergy to string beans and a new IgE allergy to bananas; my wife and I sadly gave our kitty to her mother and father for safekeeping, after which all symptoms went away completely, except for my sensitivity to green beans and bananas.

Age 49: I began to develop an overwhelming itchiness all over my body and began to swell up and break out with pustules and red spots, most notably around my joint areas like wrists, frontal elbow, knees and on my neck; my hair began falling out in bunches; my eyes were red and bloodshot; I suffered extreme fatigue and started becoming depressed; my body odor was horrible and I had a terrible metallic taste in my mouth all the time. I took a routine medical SMAK-25 blood panel with nothing to show except for increased cholesterol levels and ratios – all within range; after taking a hair test (which was slightly overdue) I found my arsenic level was literally off the excess range of the reference chart by almost 20 times— a whopping 1.95 milligram percent, when only up to .01 is considered tolerable; my mercury and aluminum levels were well into the clinically dangerous ranges as my potassium retention skyrocketed and my hard-fought normal retention of magnesium dipped into deficiency status along with copper, zinc, phosphorous, chromium, selenium, cobalt and a host of microtrace minerals—all off dramatically from previous levels tested.

My clinical impression: Arsenic poisoning leading to the intense urticaria and multiple nutritional disturbances.

Medical diagnosis by allergist: Urticaria. Being part of a multimedical clinic run by Dr. Jorge Monastersky, I went to one of our network allergists with my tests for an opinion. I was told he found the arsenic poisoning, as demonstrated in my hair, interesting but wasn't sure that it was causing the urticaria and suggested a cortisone shot and cortisone cream to suppress the itchiness symptoms and skin blemishes.

Prognosis: fair to good with cortisone therapy.

Medical therapy: because my appearance was starting to scare off patients, I took the shot and the cream and within one week the symptoms started to disappear; in two weeks, all trace of the urticaria seemed to be gone.

Nutritional/Chelation Therapy: in 3 1/2 weeks, all the symptoms started to return as the shot wore off, and the cortisone cream seemed less effective, so it was then and there that I decided to focus on the source of the problem, which I believed to be the arsenic and therefore concentrated on a natural detoxification program by doubling the dosage of customized supplements as directed by the HTMA lab and by going on oral amino chelation therapy including 1500 mg of dimercaptosuccinic acid/3000 mg of L- methionine/4500 mg of N- acetylcysteine three days a week with four days off on which I took 750 mg of L- methionine and N- acetylcysteine. within two months, a hair tissue mineral analysis test

revealed that the arsenic had returned to the chart at about .25 mg percent; there were no symptoms of itchiness, exematous patches or fluid-
filled pustules whatsoever; I had stopped using the cortisone cream and
have the same barely used tube to this day as a sentimental keepsake, just
like some of my asthma inhalers. When I told the allergist of this story,
he thought it was interesting but still didn't know what to make of it, but
was glad that I felt better.

New outcome: excellent. After three months of the new therapy, out-of-
range nutrient levels were restored to within-reference-range-values once
again and arsenic levels dropped to such low levels that to this day they
have not been observable for the most part in any retests other than as
only a trace. This includes having the clearest, most comfortable skin I've
ever had. Dr. S., the allergist, still doesn't understand what happened and
to this day refuses to take a nutrition test because he thinks he doesn't
need one.

Additional information: as it turns out, the arsenic originated from a
contaminated insecticide that a builder accidentally used in a clinic
build-out wherein I was a consultant; 13 other people who worked at
this center came down with similar symptoms during this time and their
medical doctors did not know what to make of it other than as urticaria
to be treated with cortisone therapy. They all turned out, when tested, to
have high arsenic retention levels and eventually ended up doing the
exact chelation therapy along with nutrition plans recommended by
their own hair tests as I did to completely remedy the problem. My wife
at that time also exhibited dangerous arsenic levels as she had visited me
on site a few times; although she did not suffer the same intense amount
of urticaria that I did, her hair did start falling out and her eyes were
bloodshot. She followed the same basic chelation therapy in combination with doubling up on the unique recommendations from her own
hair testing, levels of which were entirely different than mine due to different nutritional retention levels found in her measurements.

### *Two Rich and Famous Case Studies from Malibu*

No text regarding the art and science of orthomolecular medicine personalized nutrition would be complete without explicit clinical examples of
this approach on the rich and famous, people who we all imagine can
afford the best of everything. The following two patient studies represent

my actual experience with two of the most common and most interesting clinical problems I've encountered as a professional nutritionist, that illustrate how incorrect generic ideas are and how illness, disease, and discomfort know no boundaries. Naturally, these patients wish to be kept anonymous, but who they are would astonish, lending credibility to the idea that just because you're richer than most, you're not necessarily healthier. For the purposes of simplicity and brevity, and to spare readers many tedious case details which are not the true focus of this particular book, I have condensed my findings into an easy-to-understand discussion format. Let me therefore refer to these patients as Person 1 and Person 2.

### *Person 1*

Person 1 first came into my office at Malibu Health and Rehabilitation looking for a fast way to lose body fat. She had gained almost 50 pounds during a period of depression brought on by a prolonged divorce process. She desperately wished to lose this excess fat poundage immediately; as with most celebrities, she was in a hurry. We began a medical history on her where nothing serious in the way of identifiable organic disease was present according to previous doctors. There was a total absence of nutritional intervention by any previous health professional because as Person 1 stated, "I really didn't need nutritional help before I gained all this weight. Just six months ago I looked and felt great." Consequently she had not sought nutritional help. Now this very well-to-do middle-aged woman wanted to lose weight naturally and without any drugs or surgery if possible. Her existing supplements consisted of a One-a-Day type of vitamin and mineral tablet, an extra capsule of vitamin C (500 mg) and a standard 400 mg calcium supplement with 200 mg of magnesium. This patient had also recently begun exercising three hours per week on the treadmill at a moderate intensity. Person 1 complained of fatigue, restlessness during sleep, more indigestion than normal, occasional constipation, sore feet, aching knees and back, mental haziness, shoulder rashes, no energy, headaches, and suicidal tendencies. She ate whatever was at hand and had a food history that looked like she lived in several countries at the same time, which she actually did. One day it was McDonald's, the next day it was sushi and the next day it was a gallon of ice cream - you name it, it was there - with no cogent rhyme or reason. Just looking at Person 1's routine diet even made my iron stomach queasy. A physical exam revealed slightly elevated blood pressure, a low-back spasm, normal reflexes, and mostly normal conventional findings, although her body fat percentage was much higher (about 30% total body fat) than the statistical average of 24%. We took a **conventional blood and urine sample** which after analysis **revealed very little** other than a high normal concentration of cholesterol and triglycerides in the blood along with a very slight anemia (low blood iron) and a tiny bit of blood in the urine (later determined to be nonpathological). We finished our first consultation and conventional exam sessions with high spirits and future hopes. The third appointment was set and Person 1 cancelled it, having left a message that she was going on vacation for two to three weeks and would resume determining her nutrition program after that time. Three months passed before I saw Person 1 again. She walked into the office at about a 25-pound-lighter body weight. At first I was pleasantly surprised until I studied my patient further. Her face and exposed skin were very pale and saggy, her eye whites had a pinkish tone, allergy spots and kidney reflex points were darkened under the eyes, her tongue was white and pasty and her manner was very sullen, with less energy and expression than on our first visits.

During our consultation, Person 1 proceeded to tell me how she had gone on a pure vegetarian diet (no meats, fish, dairy, poultry, etc.), only vegetables, grains, and fruits. She had joined a network marketing group and took certain herbs and vitamins that they recommended and provided. This group also helped her to stay on a strict vegetarian diet which they consensually felt was healthier than diets containing meat, fish, and dairy products. Person 1 liked the attention and support of her new friends. When Person 1 first converted to vegetarianism and started taking the special network marketing herbs and vitamins, she reported that she felt great. A lot of her former symptoms and especially ongoing constipation seemed to disappear. She began losing weight rapidly. She felt excited about her new lease on life. Then about five weeks into her new program the weight loss slowed, energy levels dropped and the old symptoms came back while some new symptoms arose. Adding to the old list of symptoms, some brand new symptoms appeared during her vegetarian experience including a chronic mild diarrhea problem (as opposed to constipation initially), terrible fatigue (she seemed to want to sleep forever), some touch and go abdominal pain, hair loss and thinning, dizzy spells, bad gas, and building frustration with her new lifestyle. Person 1's only recognizable and consistent symptomatic improvements during this time were: less restlessness at night, no more constipation in favor of mild diarrhea (which she was told was normal and desirable by network marketing friends due to her body "detoxing"), less observable body fat, although she felt untoned and saggy, and a diminished shoulder rash which seemed to have disappeared for the most part. One concern that she expressed regarding her new host of symptoms was a newfound and extreme craving for chocolate and an ongoing unquenchable thirst for fluids. Person 1 also seemed to have a mild cold she just couldn't seem to get rid of replete with sinus and lung congestion. Given these symptomatic changes, I re-examined her and added new but still conventional blood and urine tests to rule out potential thyroid dysfunction and diabetes (fatigue, thirst, sugar cravings, gas, mental confusion, all at age 40, are textbook symptoms for diabetes and thyroid imbalance). Sure enough, her thyroid function had slowed from her last blood test but readings were still within the lower limits of normal. According to the blood tests, she was now suffering from microcytic anemia and had more white blood cells in her blood than the last test, more than normal. The glucose tolerance test given did not reveal full-blown diabetes of any kind so I suspected other problems in this regard that were nutrition-related (hypothetically: deficiencies of chromium, boron, selenium, and vanadium). I then proceeded to organize a new diet for her. Step 1 was to compute calories and qualify those calories with food to develop a theoretical nutrition model for her after considering all reported lifestyle factors, medical history, body fat test results and some simplified genotyping information. Her genotyping information revealed round features, feminine hourglass shape (wide hips, soft skin, etc.) and other categorical physical and psychological factors; blood type (O) and physiological measurements (blood pressure, heart rate, body fat percentage, etc.) scored her as a Pancreatic Dominant Type with a secondary gonadal dominance using the old metabolic/constitutional typing systems mentioned previously, which were in place before nutritional testing was possible. According to this format, hypothetically, her most recessive glands were the liver and pineal gland. Her nerve type was a Type B (endotonic) with a parasympathetic autonomic dominance and low medium oxidation amount and rate **(refer to Tables I, II, III, IV).** Her psychological profile was that of being food oriented and generally happy with a very social and sensual orientation. Given these factors and others, I categorized her using the old metabolic typing systems as a carnivore - vegetarian or carni-vegan in short. Blood type diet categories for blood type O give an indication of what the best food selections would theoretically be appropriate in her case, mostly as red meat and alkaline vegetables.

Based on this postulation, red meat is seemingly necessary for this metabolic type as are the majority of alkaline vegetables and fruits found in nature. A conflict of health interests lay here since she turned to vego-vegetarianism. The next step was to apply nutrition tests. Therefore, I instituted a battery of unconventional laboratory nutrition/toxin tests from various specimens which focused upon where the most metabolic upsets would theoretically be found, given the genotyping information. So we took blood, urine, saliva, feces, and hair samples for the orthomolecular tests that seemed most appropriate. The primary results are summarized below:

- Full-blown deficiencies and ratio imbalances of iron, B12, B6, folic acid, tyrosine (an amino acid), calcium, magnesium, potassium, and phosphorous
- Marginal deficiencies of chromium, selenium, vanadium, boron, copper, zinc, molybdenum, and lipoic acid
- Higher than normal tissue lead levels, boron, tin and free radical stress
- Delayed response allergies (IgG) to milk and milk products, potato, tomato, garlic, citrus fruits, and sesame
- Bowel parasites, leaky gut syndrome, low stomach acid and poor fat digestion
- Depressed DHEA levels (dehydroepiandrosterone) and upset estrogen-to-progesterone ratio and a hair test-correlated Slow metabolism
- Higher than normal creatinine (urinary) level

The metabolic/nutritional evaluation of Person 1 ultimately revealed a complete mismatching of diet and body chemistry. ***This person was genetically not designed to eat only vegetables and fruits.*** Abstinence from eating red meat had created deficiencies of iron, copper, zinc, B12, folic acid and tyrosine which led to thyroid dysfunction, anemia, and fatigue. Having deficiencies of chromium, selenium, and vanadium could well cause chocolate cravings due to their effect on insulin function and the fact that Person 1's genotype is theoretically more prone to diabetic disorders than other types. The increased white blood cell count was a direct indication of her ongoing cold's systemic presence. The deficiencies of zinc and lipoic acid undermine essential fatty acid metabolism in regard to the immune system, thereby increasing recovery rate times from colds and all disease and symptoms. No wonder her current cold was hanging on for so long. Depressed DHEA levels are indicative of accelerated aging, adrenal stress, and endocrine imbalances (along with hypothyroidism). Bowel parasites and free radical stress were due to a depressed intake of immune-related factors and an increased intake of raw and improperly cleaned foods. Parasites also rob the body of essential nutrients and resultantly add to deficiency states as well. Heretofore undetected allergies to foods Person 1 craved and ate regularly (including garlic) only served to further complicate her health status. Delayed food allergies overload the body with even more stress which leads to further imbalances and disease as well. Person 1 required more calcium in the diet in combination with higher amounts of magnesium, proportionately, and less boron (a primary constituent of the legumes that she was subsisting on as a vegetarian) to improve upon these deficiencies. Betaine hydrochloric acid is also helpful in these regards. With all this metabolic and nutritional chaos going on, it's no wonder Person 1 was suffering from chronic diarrhea which only served to further hamper her body's ability to absorb proper nutrients (especially electrolytes and protein) and therefore worsened her condition. Healthy and unhealthy metabolic balance is created by a cause-and-effect chain reaction of metabolic and nutrient factors. Person 1's condition reflects the chain reaction of intensifying poor health and further validates the need to nutritionally test on a highly specific level.

In Step 4 (Diet and Supplement Customization) I culminated all of the above information and laboratory recommendations to design diet and supplements accordingly, based upon the law of opposites and the computer predictions of the laboratory based upon statistical-comparative clinical research on others likePerson 1. At this time (1989-90), this aspect of integrating diet and supplements was less pushbutton than it is by today's laboratory computers. From a disease standpoint, Person 1 was seemingly on the verge of full-blown osteoporosis, heart and circulatory disease, osteo-arthritis, adult onset diabetes, and a host of other diet-related diseases. From a symptomatic standpoint, this person lived in a chronic state of dis-ease, suffering a very uncomfortable day-to-day existence. As she walked out of my office, with her brand new scientifically designed custom diet program and laboratory manufactured custom supplements, my best thoughts and prayers went with her.

Step 4: Upon reevaluation after four months, when I fully retested Person 1, much to my pleasant surprise the majority of all laboratory tests were clear. She had lost another 16 pounds and she looked and felt, as she put it, "better than ever before" and had that special high-energy sparkle in her eyes that I equate with good health. Even though Person 1 had been put on a short-term detoxification and cleansing food rotation regimen to clean out and overcome food sensitivities, she still showed some persistent lead deposition in her hair (to be expected for a while) and some mild allergic responses to tomato, eggplant (night shades), sesame, and milk. All of these sensitivity states were down from the initially moderate and high-sensitivity readings. In effect, Person 1 was gradually becoming less sensitive to these foods. She still had a slight calcium/magnesium deficiency but all other tests were perfectly normal including the parasite profile. Even the back spasms were gone after adjusting her spine and pelvis only three times in conjunction with our house massage therapist conscientiously working on her soft tissues a total of eight times during the prior four-month period. In less than another six months, Person 1 tested negative to all her other deficiencies and imbalances including the occurrence of lead in her system. She also lost another 11 pounds and 6% more body fat to look, as she put it, "like a teenager again." She had fully recovered in less than ten months and reached all desired health and weight loss objectives.

Person 1's story was one of total success. I chose to tell you about it because of its commonality with many other cases I've treated. Here we have a typical person desperate to lose some weight and feel better. Instead of following through with me from our first visit, she falls into the trap of completely changing her diet on the basis of *one-size-fits-all mentalities* as reinforced by the political manipulation of nonqualified nutritionists whose bottom line motive was to sell her their products and to have her sign up more people into their network, all without a true understanding of or honest regard for her health. These networkers further misled Person 1 by reinforcing her pursuit of vegetarianism, telling her only what she really wanted to hear about its benefits and not the downside, which they themselves probably didn't understand. They also lead her to believe that the chronic diarrhea problem was just a normal detoxification response to their herbs when, in fact, it was a warning sign that something more serious was wrong. Along with her new network marketing friends' advice, Person 1 piecemealed assorted supplements from their marketing inventory (multivitamin-minerals, calcium, vitamin C, and others) which did little or nothing to properly nourish her special metabolism. Examining her previously taken supplements, I found them to be of low quality, generally imbalanced—one nutrient level to the next, and very overpriced. When Person 1 first began her new vegetarian diet and network marketing supplements, she only felt better because of the immediate reduction of saturated fat calories in her new vegetarian diet (her body type does not do well with too much dietary fat), the natural cleansing, detoxification and laxative effects of a mostly raw, completely vegetarian food intake, her extreme compulsive excitement about losing weight and artificial placebo-like feelings of wellness due to the highly stimulating effect the network marketing herbs had on her body and mind. After all, they contained MaHuang (ephedra), guarana, caffeine and other feel-good stimulants. But within four to five weeks her newly begun vegetarian-based nutritional program bottomed out as it failed to fully meet her metabolic needs and her body chemistry was unable to make up the difference from its depleted reserve nutrient storage. This was the time when Person 1 really began to feel poorly and therefore reluctantly deduced that something after all was wrong - perhaps even more so than before she actually started her vegetarian diet.

But it took nearly three more months before she contacted me, because her network marketing support group continuously convinced her that everything was okay in spite of her feeling bad, and that her overall response was actually quite normal—to be expected. After all, she had lost some weight, right? Therefore the program must be working. This was their basic analogy: weight loss equals program success. Luckily, Person 1 finally got fed up with feeling progressively worse and overcame the false belief-fostering and brain-washing network support group mentality about her diet and supplement plan and finally contacted me once again.

Unfortunately, Person 1 is like many typical Americans who wait until there's a crisis situation before they take action and then they usually take the wrong action, paying for it later. In this case, Person 1 constantly ignored the way her body really felt because she wanted things to work out socially with her new friends. Consequently she suffered through more physical discomfort than most people would put up with, finally contacting me only when it became truly unbearable. She actually conveyed to me that because her vegetarian-herb program was touted as a form of natural healing, she wanted to give it every benefit of the doubt and therefore hung in there as long as possible. It's all natural so it must be good, is the thinking. At that very moment in our conversation, she had just realized the important fact that her body is so unique that even natural things not right for her body type can cause problems. Just because a product or program is sold or touted as being all natural doesn't mean that it's right or even safe for you (or her) without a test in hand.

Orthomolecular nutritional medicine worked exceedingly well for

174

Person 1 and her true health potential was recovered and accentuated with many positive lessons learned (like no more *one-size-fits-all* and don't believe everything you're told, especially from people in a big hurry to sell you something).

### *Person 2*

Person 2 is an interesting case in point when it comes to demonstrating the inadequate nature of mainstream medicine and sometimes even alternative medicine, and of how novice and even professional non-testing nutritionists can dangerously inhibit a person's attainment of good health instead of promoting it. Person 2 first came to my office after having been to at least 15 other health practitioners within about 3 years. This is a record number of second opinions in my mind. She had contacted various mainstream doctors none of whom could really find any organic disease present after routine examinations. Person 2 brought in literally piles of medical records which contained little evidence of any disorders - at least by conventional testing and exam parameters - other than some slightly elevated liver enzymes (showing liver stress), depressed iron levels, disproportionate ratios between two blood proteins and a slight viral infective process that seemed to have cleared up long ago and which may have caused all of these findings in the first place, except for the low iron levels.

The last three conventional M.D.s fom whom she sought help weren't able to help her significantly so they told her that her 30 or so presenting symptoms were essentially all in her head. This erroneous shortcut-to-thinking analogy was probably made by these physicians because after all, these doctors could not find anything concretely wrong with her using their standard examination and laboratory evaluation procedures. Actually one physician wrote in his notes "Munchausen's Syndrome" which is fancy terminology for hypochondria. Person 2, out of sheer frustration and desperation, fell in with a mail order scheme which guaranteed to fully cure all of her ills with that one magical product. It's the old, obsolete "magic bullet" mentality again - one healthy magical thing that just does it all, which of course, is scientifically impossible. This magic bullet naturally did not help her condition in the least, so she sought help from a nontesting nutritionist who proceeded to give her a canned diet and supplementation program, with no physical exam or lab analysis other than some basic questions. This particular nutritionist's *one-size-fits-all* approach didn't work for her either, except that my new patient liked a special MaHuang/caffeine/gurana/yerba Mate highly stimulating herb mixture supplement she bought from this particular nutritionist. She liked it because this supplement was the only thing that seemed to fully wake her up, other than coffee. Person 2 actually became addicted to the mixture and took it 7–10 times per day, always returning to her nutritionist to buy more when she ran out. The label, by the way, recommended only two servings per day. Without frequent servings of this "health tonic" she stated that she'd have to sleep 24 hours a day. Despite this herbal boost, she was still in bed 14 hours per day on average due to overwhelming fatigue. Out of continued desperation, Person 2 then decided to go to a university medical center where she spied some advertising for a new community nutrition clinic. She visited an M.D. in this facility who put her through more conventional tests which showed nothing remarkable, and then one unconventional metabolic test which yielded three new clinical insights. The treating physician must have just learned about this particular test and didn't fully understand its implications, because his written and verbal recommendations taken from records to this day still don't make much sense to me. Person 2, after some unconventional medical testing, was found to be fructose sensitive, although no organized therapeutic diet was given to help her. Also, there was some disorder in protein metabolism noted by a physician, for which she was given a single, very expensive amino acid to take. I didn't understand why. Then she was referred back to her regular family physician because her blood lipids (fats) were found to be elevated above normal. Person 2 then revisited the family physician with her new reports and tests from the nutrition clinic and he in response told her to eat less fat and that everything should be fine. The family doctor also recommended that she should try the Pritikin diet, but didn't have a copy of it around to give her and told her to buy the book instead. By this time, Person 2 was mad as a hatter and completely abandoned the thought that mainstream medicine could help her with her innocuous problems. She felt she was getting bounced around from doctor to doctor with nothing much accomplished. Consequently, she went to an iridologist who provided a huge written report and told her that she possessed a lymphatic body type. Unfortunately, only about three of the total 50 pages in her iridology report provided any real information that she could use. Most of it was just background information. Person B, however, was given a list of mostly vegetarian foods which according to iridological findings should be good for her, and a list of foods—mostly processed and red meat foods—to avoid, and that was all.

Person 2 was still not really feeling any better at this point and instinctively felt that there was still something missing for what she needed to be well. The iridologist's food list seemed to help her energy a little now and then but Person 2 was still confused about whether this was going to be the end of the therapeutic line for her or whether she should look further for help. Acting on the advice of a friend, she consulted a nutritional allergist (M.D.) who gave her some non-conventional food allergy tests (IgG) and came up with a much more definite list of foods to avoid. Thanks to these new tests, Person 2 felt like she was actually getting somewhere. Unfortunately, just following the "eat this" and "don't eat that" list and taking a multiple vitamin/mineral as given to her from her doctor was still not helping that much, although she did report experiencing some definite mild improvements in her symptoms.

Following an advertisement in a natural healing magazine, my patient then contacted an N.D. (naturopathic doctor) who proceeded to provide a hair analysis for her. More significant information came through from this procedure. Person 2 demonstrated a tissue iron deficiency, a large imbalance in electrolytes (sodium, potassium, etc.), a mineral balance computer correlation with candidiasis (yeast infection), an abnormal amount of aluminum tissue deposition, zinc and chromium imbalances, and a very high tissue calcium concentration. She was then put into one of three body type classifications based on oxidation rates only from the Kelley system (Dr. Kelley was Steve McQueen's doctor). Person 2 was found to be a slow oxidizer/metabolism (Dr. Watts and Kelley and Watson System). At this point, Person 2 thought, "now we're finally getting somewhere." These new findings had been missed by every other practitioner previously. But unfortunately, due to this particular doctor's heavy reliance on just hair analysis alone, only using its nutritional implications, the total personalized nutrition process was still not complete. More was needed to be done since Person 2's full symptomatic relief was not demonstrated during this therapy. Even with the laboratory and naturopathic doctor's prescribed supplements and her new diet recommendations, although she noticed much improvement, many symptoms still prevailed.

Now Person 2 became thoroughly perplexed. Out of pure desperation, once again, she went to a famous "nutritionist to the stars." Her new nutritionist (this person had no presented clinical degrees) had the self-proclaimed distinction of being a celebrity nutritionist - a pioneer in nutrition - because she worked with some celebrities. Person 2 was given an extended (rather egotistical in her opinion) verbal synopsis of this nutritionist's self-proclaimed greatness, which my patient found to be simply disgraceful. Person 2 also didn't like the fact that this nutritionist, much like all of her previous practitioners, didn't have the appearance of being healthy and fit. All of her practitioners, including this one, didn't look particularly healthy or fit and wore overly excessive makeup—all of which was disturbing to her. The celebrity nutritionist was overweight and undertoned and looked older for her age than Person 2 expected. The phenomenon of the "armchair expert syndrome," (do as I say, not as I do) was beginning to take hold in Person 2's consciousness. Looks and extraneous thoughts aside, the celebrity nutritionist briefly reviewed Person 2's medical/nutrition records and told her that she just needed to "touch up" some areas of nutrition for her and then Person 2 would be fine. She charged Person 2 $150 for about 15 minutes of her time and told her to schedule another appointment. On the second visit, Person 2 was given a slightly more detailed diet plan than the previous naturopathic doctor but it was written using only information from her previous hair analysis report. The celebrity nutritionist recommended then that Person 2 take supplements which she personally had "hand selected" in addition to those that Person 2 was already taking, and then come back in one month. Person 2 was charged another $150 for her 15-minute visit and then another $150 for the hand-selected supplements. During the ensuing 30 days, Person 2 faithfully followed this program—gained four pounds and experienced severe headaches. She returned and reported this information to the celebrity nutritionist. The nutritionist reassured her that everything was fine and that the weight gain was normal during her body's metabolic rebalancing process. The celebrity nutritionist then gave Person 2 white willow bark extracts for her headaches, which she promised would go away. The nutritionist also replenished the supplement supply for another 60 days at an overall total cost of $475 including the visit. Symptoms only worsened during the next 60 days to the point where Person 2 finally became truly fed up. Just before 60 days were up she viewed a TV program "CBS This Morning" that I happened to appear on and decided to seek my help. So she came in, quite disgusted, with piles of reports, generic diets, and bags of supplements, all of which she dumped on my desk. She seemed to be blaming me as the closest health care professional available.

Let me tell you what I discovered about Person 2, as amazing as it is. First of all, none of the previous professionals had ever quantified and qualified her calorie levels and actual foods or genotyped her. Not even a fraction of the total evaluative metabolic/nutritional testing instruments that I have at hand were used. Initially, these were her presenting symptoms and my initial impressions:

| | | |
|---|---|---|
| Anger | Indigestion | Itchiness of skin |
| Headaches | Coated tongue | Progressive stress |
| Anxiety | Ear Ringing | syndrome |
| Allergies | Irritability | Intermittent diarrhea |
| Poor muscle tone | Behavior problems | and constipation |
| Depression | PMS | Halitosis |
| Defensive posture | Loss of concentration | Negative emotionality |
| Fatigue | Low self-esteem | Poor memory |
| Gastritis | Suicidal tendencies | Generalized myalgia |
| Candida | Mood swings | Nutrient deficiencies |
| Liver spots | Weak nails and hair | Nutrient imbalances |
| (brown age spots) | Muscle weakness | Toxic accumulation |
| Edema | Premature graying | |

Considering all the professionals she had been treated by previously, this was quite a list of problems Person 2 was still experiencing.

Her only stated objectives were to feel well again, to get her energy back and tone up her body. My body genotyping process by **old standards** revealed her to be a slightly Gonadal Dominant Type followed closely by secondary pituitary dominance and with a strong showing as a tertiary thyroid dominant classification. Her liver, pineal, and lymphatic system were all recessive. Her blood Type O classification designated Person 2 as a carni-vegan type of eater with a special need for dark green leafy vegetables—in theory. (As a matter of interest, Person 2 shied away from leafy greens due to digestive discomforts she experienced and because of her inability to taste them. - Zinc deficiency?) This could all be true, but in order to be scientific we could not assume anything. This patient craved beans and garlic (she reeked of garlic) which were both liberally contained within the celebrity nutritionist's generic diet. In the previous IgG allergy test given by Doctor #13, she was found to be allergic to milk, yeast, pork, concentrated fructose, and dextrose. In Step 3 (laboratory nutrition/toxic assessment), I further allergy tested her and found that she was allergic to garlic and all kinds of beans. This hadn't shown in doctor #13's previous test, which included garlic, so I had to assume that she had developed a garlic sensitivity since the time of that doctor's test (or the possibility that the first test was inaccurate, which is unlikely). Person 2's sensitivity to beans was somewhat unexpected given the fact that she ate many legumes on her celebrity diet. Interesting to note here was Person 2's garlic and bean cravings. Here she shows in specific tests a delayed allergic response to both foods and yet she constantly craves them. Dr. James Braly's "allergy-addiction syndrome" noted in his book *The Food and Nutrition Allergy Revolution* was plain to see in this case (and many others I've seen). These particular foods created an allergy-initiated stimulatory effect in Person 2's body, which actually helped to keep her awake and energetic.

This type of stimulation is much like a person's "wake up" response to a cup of coffee. This wakeup effect was all part of her body's resultant defensive sympathetic response to the allergenic invaders in synergistic combination with the highly stimulating herbal supplements she had become addicted to. In fact, her nervous system was being simultaneously jolted by the IgG 1 & 4 allergen response and the strong herbal stimulants.

Person B also suffered (according to my tests) from a full-blown thiamin (vitamin B1), magnesium, and iron deficiency and from mild to moderate functional deficiencies of all B complex vitamins (as noted through organic acid analysis), magnesium, manganese, lipoic acid, L-Carnitine, CoQ10, chromium, vitamin C complex, L-tryptophan, N-acetyl cysteine, and more. I wondered how this could be happening to this person given all her supplements and special celebrity diet. Could it all be due to being metabolically hyped up on allergens and stimulants in spite of the special nutrition program? Even Person 2's blood amino acid profile showed a huge protein imbalance with some notable deficiencies. Digestive function tests demonstrated huge malfunctions in digestion and absorption and her liver detoxification pathways were completely overloaded. This unfortunate woman also had a marked aluminum deposition in her tissue samples. How could this be in consideration of all the professionals who had treated her? Truly, she was not suffering from Munchausen's (hypochondriac) Syndrome; this patient had many more obvious physical problems. Even the specialized metabolic assessment laboratories were strongly indicating the presence of many more potential health problems and were suggesting that I use other tests to rule them out in their medical reports. One lab, based on certain biomarkers present, even suggested that she may have a serious cancer problem developing.

Person 2's urinary organic acid profile demonstrated a huge outpouring of just about every metabolite and metabolic intermediate from the primary enzymatic pathway that produces energy in the body. There were so many enzymatic upsets present that I could barely count them. With these primary energy pathways dysfunctional—no wonder she needed stimulants to keep her awake—there was hardly enough energy production by her body to keep her awake naturally. Saliva and urine pHs were so low, considering her rather alkaline diet, it all just didn't seem to make much "front-line" sense. It took me a few long restless nights to realize that Person 2 was suffering from a huge mega dosing and allergenic syndrome. She was taking so many of the wrong supplements in such staggering amounts that her body was registering them as toxins and shutting down defensively in an effort to throw them off. I now call this "nutrient-megadose-toxin overload." She must have had the most expensive urine, feces, mucous, and sweat known to man. Person 2 was so completely overloaded with inappropriate supplements that in fact highly valuable nutrients given at these super high dosage levels were actually considered to be poisons by the body. Imagine, too much of a concentrated intake of the same vitamins, minerals, and other nutrients that normally preserve our wellness can end up very seriously damaging our bodies. This is why I always say supplement megadosers and shot gunners beware.

So Person 2 and I quickly dumped all these former diets and supplements (literally into the trash can) and we tested and rebuilt her orthomolecularly from scratch—the right way—with tests and retests guiding us every step of the way. At first my patient went through a special fast and detox/elimination program before she really got into the main part of the customized eating and supplement program which arose from her test batteries. This initial accelerated modified crystallized amino acid (designed from her amino acid and other tests) food fasting/cleansing rotation program" reduced stress on her system by taking away allergens and hard-to-digest materials in conjunction with magnifying the amino acid retention of the body. This also helped the liver and other elimination organs to clean out and regain their functions as the body was given just enough nutrients to sustain itself under these special detoxification/elimination conditions. Even the short-term initial protein-sparing fast we employed for the first week helped Person 2 to feel noticeably better as her body started to come out of its huge vitamin and mineral overload syndrome. Just throwing off the excesses of what we normally construe and value as essential nutrients within our bodies made her feel better. In this case, less vitamins and minerals taken in actually made her feel better, which is the reverse of what you'd expect.

Needless to say, as Person 2 proceeded through the personalized nutrition program she happily experienced gradual yet noticeable improvements although she did have some occasional symptomatic flareups, which are to be expected in any natural healing process. To Person 2's surprise, those green leafy vegetables, that she consistently avoided, became a strong part of her diet that she actually looked forward to once the body's zinc level was in balance and stomach acid was up. In Step 5 (or Test Reevaluation) she showed substantial improvement in all lab tests (minerals, vitamins, amino acids, organic acids and essential fatty acids) and especially those measurements pertaining to the liver and other eliminative systems. The lack of measurable toxic/oxidant stress alone, as seen in the retests, demonstrated that taking away the shotgun, megadose nutrients allowed the liver and body at large to recover very rapidly. This clinical story is proof positive that too many vitamins can damage your liver and body just like alcohol or any recognizable toxin. Mother was right when she said "moderation is the key" and Person 2 knows this much better now than ever before. This same phenomenon has shown up on many governmental studies like the H.A.N.E.S. (Health Nutrition Education Surveys) 1, 2 and 3 studies and as I observed in the many tests that I've administered.

Person 2 was virtually put back into metabolic balance within one year of eating and supplementing specific to her remonitored biochemical uniqueness. She is a case in point when it comes to discussing the dangers of megadosing and shotgunning supplemental nutrients and extreme diets without nutritional/toxic measurements. It should be noted that many other conventional medical tests were recommended to further investigate this patient's problems by the nutrient testing labs. There was so much metabolic chaos present in this person's body that the testing labs felt that this patient should be investigated further for more serious disease patterns. Consequently, generalized mainstream clinical logic, in this case, would be directed towards finding more evidence of serious organic diseases like cancer, autoimmune disorders, chronic fatigue syndrome, digestive inflammation, connective tissue disorders, and others. In effect, Person 2's vitamin/mineral overload syndrome was causing changes within the body, which were being construed as serious disease possibilities by both conventional and unconventional medicine. These disease possibilities all disappeared once metabolic rebalance was nutritionally reestablished.

This case exemplifies the awesome power of individualized nutrition over *one-size-fits-all*, piecemeal and or shotgun diets and supplements and using cover-up symptom relief drugs. If any of Person 2's metabolic symptoms were leading her down the path to any one of the serious diseases suspected by the labs and myself, all clinical concern has now been put to rest, thanks to the reaches of orthomolecular medicine for nipping it in the bud. This approach provides the ultimate system of disease prevention.

Clinical cases really do become a simple scenario when you use the proper nutritional testing and those clinically proven recommendations made by the testing labs themselves in proper order. You simply have a biochemical "before" and "after" and a symptomatic energy and fat loss/muscle gain story to go with what's in between that is reported by the patient. This only happens because the labs are getting so good at proving, with specifically proportioned remedies, what is found to be out of balance. The application of computer correlations has streamlined the therapeutic process light years ahead of where it was just 15 years ago. It becomes a simple case of the practitioner or person concerned just going by the lab book and properly implementing the scientific facts with an actual program of eating and supplementation that is retested periodically until perfection and balance is reached. In truth, the labs are a lot smarter than any individual practitioner, but the trick for the nutritionist is to be up to systematize, integrate and functionalize the test-generated information for the patient or client so that they can put it into action and achieve success. In the most human terms, this approach should remarkably reduce all diet-related disease, fatigue, excess fat accumulation, allergies, toxic compounds, sexual dysfunction, shortened life expectancy, reduced the fitness attainment and maintenance, loss of cognitive or mental functions, and much more. This can all culminate in the healthiest, most productive lifetime ever for each individual. After initiating literally over 100,000 of these tests and following up with each individual, I can safely say that when people follow the laboratory recommendations they always demonstrate improvements in the actual tests and tend to fulfill their objectives to be well and fit. Those that misunderstand or stray from this type of lab-generated practitioner-delivered information generally do not attain the same level of nutritional rebalancing achievements and conditioned/symptom reduction by any stretch of the imagination. This leads to Reality Check number 12:

# Reality Check #12
## Those Who Do Not Follow the Customized Diet and Supplement Recommendations Made by the Labs Following Nutrition Tests Do Not Achieve the Most Desirable Results

One simply cannot think their way through this or make believe that they can deviate from what is known on this level of science. Their best healthy bet is to follow this exceedingly viable information to the point where they are totally in balance—and keep it there with these tests to monitor, just like medical tests are used to monitor disease. It's not the fault of science when these individuals don't succeed because they did not pay attention to what was scientifically determined to be done for whatever reason.

One can literally look at each individual's test and subsequent retests, mineral by mineral, vitamin by vitamin, amino acid by amino acid etc., from one test date to the next, and graphically see the improvements and hear the accompanying success stories. It's that simple. It happens all the time for me and others – laymen and professionals alike who engage this nutritional approach and who I've shared it with. I believe that most people have no idea that this technology exists or that it can improve the human condition because without these tests in hand they don't know it's even occurring. It is not the object of this book to publish a large caseload of studies, but besides my own story and the stories of Person 1 and 2, I've enclosed some brief highlights of a few interesting case studies to illustrate my points, and that of science, further. (In subsequent texts, we will publish more of these types of case studies on a more in-depth basis.) You must also understand that there are up to 1,560 measured/controlled variables within each orthomolecular study due to its multidimensional approach— that is, tracking the before and after time-interval defined snapshots of up to 1,560 (1,400 nutritional/160 medical) body chemistries, body fat percentage changes and symptomatic improvements that are reported, whereas most research studies only deal with a handful of variables. A good example follows.

### *Research 102*

When I was practicing at the Malibu Health and Rehabilitation Center, I was contracted by a marketing group to test the effect of two aromatherapy inhalant products which I had developed in conjunction with inventor Alvin Lemar, and Geoffrey Ward, PhD, from England. You may remember some years back, the National Enquirer featured these special aromatherapeutic food wands that you would sniff to help reduce appetite and therefore lose weight. These particular wands were ineffective versions of the ones that Alvin, Dr. Ward and I developed, which actually worked according to my research study on 37 Malibu patients. The only three tested variables were:

- The use of these inhalant tubes–up to two sniffs–before meals and any time between meals when appetite was increased
- The time interval of the test, which was 16 weeks
- The weight of each patient taken once a week for the 16-week interval

That was it. No nutrition tests, no special foods or supplements, no special exercise program added – nothing. By the way, the average weight loss for those using the nonplacebo tubes was 8.4 pounds in 16 weeks. The eight people in the placebo group lost an average of 2.4 pounds during that same time interval. Now imagine doing the same study, only this time first giving all 1,400 orthomolecular tests and 160 medical tests. Then after this testing of the master list of nutrients (given in a previous section) along with all of the lab-recommended special foods and supplements that went along with each test and total test case and doing an entire analysis of what happened on as many levels as could be scientifically determined – each individual case story could be its own book in size. This is one of the reasons why I believe that it has taken so long to get nutrition testing on humans up and running—it's just so very complicated due to so many connected research variables which cannot be singled out on their own because they're so closely related to all the other ones. The generic and widespread fragmentation, individualization, and oversimplification of research variables to be tested is the reason why most generic research is so weak and also why so many drug studies backfire with such a high degree of side effects. Thankfully, the nutrition-testing medical labs have been putting these trials together and following the cause-and-effect scenarios of their recommendations on millions of people for many years now, so it's becoming a more dependably integrated science than ever. Instead of just looking at one's zinc intake in relation to the development of colds or some other isolated variable, a given lab will look at the relationship of zinc to all minerals and vitamins and other nutritional variables test by test. This in effect is actually a research revolution that the labs have created for us—one that connects the facts rather than separates them out of context.

In the following I have a few typical case studies described in terms of their very condensed orthomolecular highlights (the names have been changed for confidentiality, but some of these same people have given us Web site and book testimonials using their real first names, and some cases—like our pro golfer—their full names).

*Mindy* Age 45, primary complaint, lack of energy, excess fat, yo-yo effect on former diets, depressed, medically diagnosed slight anemia (for which she was on an iron supplement), stomach irritability, and occasional constipation.

*Test #1* (36 minerals only) Slow metabolism type 1 category with dramatically high levels of calcium and magnesium relative to potassium and phosphorous which were being retained in deficiency status; abnormally high sodium to potassium ratio; excess boron; iron deficiency; manganese deficiency; germanium deficiency and many other deficiencies along with a safe level of uranium but enough mercury to antagonize iron; selenium, zinc, and sulfur function noticeably—as reported in the labs statistically proportioned reference ranges; three months of lab-recommended foods and supplements containing fast pattern opposite nutrients (those that are higher in what Mindy was low in and lower in which she tested to be high in).

Without getting into complex and tedious detail, suffice it to say that the foods given were mostly low in sugar, calcium (dairy foods), boron, mustard family, spinach/goosefoot family, most high-fat nuts, purine-rich foods, and saturated fat and high in potassium, phosphorous, methionine, B1 and B6, iron, and all their synergists which were super-synergized and concentrated by the individualized supplements taken.

*Retest #1* Excess calcium retention rate down by 28 percent to dead center of the reference range, excess magnesium retention rate down by 55 percent to dead center of the reference range, potassium up by 66 percent but still considered in a deficiency status, phosphorous up by 8% (in range), sodium dropped by 71 percent, and 8 percent improvement in iron retention. A drop in boron retention of 68 percent and mostly favorable improvements in all of the other minerals except for mercury, which shot up from 0.12 mg percent to 0.52 mg percent—an increase of over 430 percent. At this time we were not sure if the mercury was a new contamination or if the other rebalancing was forcing it out of the body. The patient reported 18 pounds lost, an increase in strength, no stomach sensitivity, a better attitude, deeper sleep and a dramatic increase in energy; her personal trainer reported about a 10 percent reduction in body fat.

Although my description of this case ends here, suffice it to say that this person has lost close to 45 pounds and has referred 30 people to the program out of pure satisfaction.

*Kurt* Age 52, lost his job due to extreme fatigue and discomfort, suspected by doctors through routine medical diagnosis to have everything from cancer to multiple sclerosis to AIDS and went to clinics all over the world, including Europe, Mexico, and the U.S. searching for answers. He thought he was dying.

*Test #1* (Multiple specimen/procedures) Demonstrated extremely high levels of aluminum, mercury, arsenic, cobalt, iron retention five times higher than the top of the excess range on the reference range table, severe deficiency of zinc, severe vitamin A and deficiencies in most B vitamins, depressions of most amino acid neurotransmitters and serotonin precursors and approximately one half of all organic acid, amino acid, fatty acids and allergy (35 out of 80 foods tested positive tests administered were off range). Colonic yeast was detected, so was low stomach acid, glutamine deficiency of the intestines, increased lysosomal intestinal activity (infection), IgA allergies to gluten and dairy and many other orthomolecular abnormalities—probably one of the most extensive array of imbalances I've seen in one set of tests. At this time, this gentleman was suffering deep depression, dramatic psoriasis outbreaks, swollen lymph nodes, and reoccurring herpes outbreaks; sadly, his family medical doctor did not know what to think or do.

*Two years later* After many retests in all body chemistries and after following the test recommendations to the letter, an absolute scarcity of symptoms, save for a very minor and occasional psoriasis outbreak.

Approximately 65 percent of all original nutrition and toxin tests which were out of range are now in range, allergies have diminished to only three as of the last test and he is now a bona fide Fast 1 type metabolism and looks and feels fantastic. It is almost hard to believe it's the same person I first saw at first.

### Two Calcium Overload Cases
One involving weight loss and one involving athletic performance:

*Mandy* This 37-year-old woman was an accomplished power lifter hell-bent on winning a world championship in her class but was overweight and could not seem to get her strength up fast enough.

*Mineral test # 1* 508 mg percent calcium in comparison to a healthy human reference range between 22 to 97 mg percent, 96.4 mg percent magnesium in comparison to a healthy range of between 2.0 and 11 mg percent, 5.83 mg percent of strontium compared to a healthy range of between .03 mg percent and .50 mg percent, 1.44 milligram percent as compared to a healthy range of between .00 and .26 mg percent, severely depressed levels of potassium, phosphorous, manganese, and others.

*Mineral test #2* (three months later) 163 mg percent of calcium, 24.5 mg percent magnesium, 2.45 mg percent of strontium, .67 mg percent of barium, potassium up by 28percent, phosphorous up by 10 percent, and most other minerals closer to desirable ranges. The patient lost six pounds and set her own personal strength records to win the world level power lifting championships during this time.

*Note:* It's worth mentioning here that only minerals were tested and only this one particular lab program was instituted—yet all these results occurred. It's hard to imagine the success potential if we were to take healthy individuals and work them up from all multilab test levels. The good news is that mineral testing has been correlated against other tests with a high degree of correlation so that this procedure is generally agreed upon as being the gateway program of nutrition testing, yielding the most comprehensive picture from a therapeutic standpoint.

*Linda* This 49-year-old woman had started to mysteriously gain weight and develop a very severe fatigue pattern while becoming more constipated, her hair became brittle, skin dried out and began to wrinkle, sex drive went down, frequent urination patterns developed—especially at night, deep sleep was evasive, memory was dysfunctional, spirits were low, and confusion about everything was at an all-time high.

*Test #1* (36 minerals only) 503 mg percent calcium or 5 mg percent less than Mandy, 44.5 mg percent of magnesium or almost double that of Mandy, a severe potassium deficiency of less than 3 mg percent, and fully eight other huge excesses of minerals beside the calcium and magnesium, along with serious deficiencies of nine other minerals besides the potassium. After reviewing this test the patient went into immediate shock. She confessed that she was taking coral calcium at about the time she started to get fat and feel unwell. She wondered if that could be the problem and I told her absolutely; this type of evidence is what inspired the FTC to pull the plug on the coral calcium infomercial in the first place, much to Kevin Trudeau's dismay. Kevin wrote a book called "Natural Cures 'They' Don't Want You to Know About"; if ever there was evidence of overdosing valuable nutrients, this was an excellent example of "if a little is good, a lot more can be dangerous."

*Retest #1* Calcium down 135 mg percent, magnesium down to 12 mg percent, potassium up to 5 mg percent with four previous excesses eliminated and three deficiencies eliminated; 10 pounds was lost during this test-to-test three-month therapeutic interval, constipation relieved and other complaints for the most part fading fast, if not nonexistent.

Then there are Josh, David, Perrine, Bill, Greg, Lindy and so on and so forth, numbering into the many thousands in my caseload alone. Each of these people presents with different problems due to individuality, each of these people have uniquely different test results, and all that succeed have one common denominator – they've undergone nutrition testing and retesting and then follow exactly what foods and supplements the labs and properly trained practitioners recommend they do to correct any abnormalities found.

It's literally a turnkey science project for each and every one of us who want to reinstate the healthiest nutrient imbalances possible in our bodies; the rest will be caseload history. There are five specific steps mentioned above and throughout Chapter VIII, that must be taken in order to refine lab-mediated nutrition testing programs, which in effect will guarantee the most success, as we will discuss in Chapter 8.

# Chapter VIII

## TNT ABCs
## Your Vital Steps for Guaranteed Success

*Nature cannot be fought*
—Ladislav Pataki, PhD

This text so far has been designed to provide a conceptual discussion and a basic framework to illustrate how personalized nutrition works. Clearly, we can see how complex the workings of it are but it is the only way to accurately investigate biochemical uniqueness. No other approach to nutrition employs this proper acknowledgment or is capable of specifying human uniqueness to this degree. Our purpose is to help you understand that *one-size-fits-all* has now been rendered functionally obsolete and is quickly becoming extinct as a nutritional practice.

This final frontier of nutrition provides the only natural weapon against diet-related dis-ease and diseases. It is designed to allow us to synergistically realign with the natural chemistry of our inner universe to that of our outer universe. We can effectively connect to the most nourishing elements from within our external environment in full accordance with how nature has designed us individually. The chemistry of a radiantly healthy life is contained within the chemistry of the land, air, water, and all that thrives upon it. Our ancestors lived in synergistic harmony with the land and its nourishing elements and in time, our bodies became an even closer reflection of those nourishing elements found in our particular areas of origin and from our own interaction with one another.

This phenomena phenotypically compounded us (genetically shaped us) over many thousands of years. Only in more recent times has humankind blatantly defied the rules of nature (and God). Humankind has dramatically rearranged the environment and those nourishing elements derived from it—doing things their way in obstinate defiance of the natural order. Man-made environmental alterations are most apparent within the more civilized nations and in those nations (usually the same) where the indigenous people pay the least attention to their traditional/historical ways of living. It is not possible to rapidly change the natural order of human life which has been established over the last 40,000 plus years without severe consequences—which we inadvertently have, and we are starting to experience as an intensifying epidemic. Our innate genetic constitution simply cannot accommodate radical changes to our environment, our food, our thinking, and our lifestyles in such short order. When referring to diet-related health, this fact is so strikingly evident when you consider the seemingly never-ending modern epidemic of diet-related degenerative disease plaguing our society like never before with no end in sight. Even our ancient ancestors didn't have these kinds of stresses, except for natural disasters.

In sharp contrast, consider modern-day primitives like the Hunzas, Soviet Georgians, Abkhazians, Azerbaijani or Lake Titicacans, who have been shown to double our effective civilized life spans. Also, consider those less civilized and more ritualistic countries, lower on the socioeconomic scale, which far outperform the U.S. in diet-related good health, yet spend a mere pittance on health care by comparison. It should be so dramatically obvious by now to each of us no matter how many drug commercials or newsletters claim that there is some magical genetic technology that will correct everything in one swoop, that the answers to our diet-related disease epidemic cannot be found in some magical drug, pill, potion or lotion, *one-size-fits-all* approach or sophisticated surgery that simply does everything to keep us young. In the clearer understanding of specific nutrients (from minerals and vitamins to amino and fatty acids and phytonutrients), we must learn what each of our bodies needs to precisely consume in order to optimize the way it was designed to function *healthfully.*

Our bodies are designed to last healthfully to 100 years and more, disease-free. They are not designed to be constantly sick or to be dependent on nonnutrient/nonlife-essential drugs for comfort. As humans, we would not have come this far during the thousands of years when there was no such thing as a drug. Our body, however, is and always will be dependent on the natural order of essential-for-life and life-quality nutrients given to us by God and nature. All we need to do to be virtually disease-free is to take what the natural world has given us (our bodies and minds) and synergistically match them back to the environment from which they were spawned. If you take care of the body and mind, they will take care of you.

The three most nurturing factors—diet, exercise, and lifestyle—are the disease-controlling forces of good health that need to be revalued as such and systematically matched back to the environment, because this is where we have strayed away from our roots of origin the most. The process of personalized nutrition shows the way back to what's right for biochemical individuality, which is where the real secrets of wellness lie in the first place. Before you embark on your journey into the final frontier, please consider the following seven mistakes we repeatedly make, which serve only to undermine our quest for radiant health.

### *Our Seven Biggest Wellness Mistakes*

1. Not applying personalized nutrition to diet, exercise and lifestyle; *one-size-fits-all* is dangerous to our health
2. Continuance of the ongoing decimation of our topsoils, processing and genetic modification of our foods through mass production, high-yield quotas and the push-it-to-the-limit-for-profits nature of modern corporate farming/food production philosophies
3. Belief in the magic bullet of good health; you know, that special pill, potion, lotion or devotion that in and of itself does it all and is therefore the final answer to all of our wellness problems and body design needs
4. Self-destructive behavior and lack of self-responsibility; doing what's obviously bad for us and/or just not taking responsibility for ourselves, and taking health for granted, especially the role of nutrition
5. Carelessly polluting our environment; we really don't need any more toxins. Our bodies and our world are already overloaded
6. Perpetuating a "sickness system" of routine medicine rather than a "wellness system"; we're betting on getting sick and then heavily rewarding physicians for our consequential illnesses—it's costing us too many lives and too much money
7. Blindly trusting our government, drug companies, insurance companies, and mainstream doctors when they all have far too many ulterior motives—mostly financial—to be fully trusted in the maintenance of our best interests

Chapter VIII

*Getting Started*

In order to become a full-blooded personalized nutrition aficionado, you first need to modify your attitude and more importantl, your *thinking* about some things. The preceding chapters have given some special, previously unknown secret insights about the full attainment of good health, how our society is inadvertently duplicating instead of eradicating nutrition-related disease, and what can be done about our current degenerative disease health crisis using precisely applied nutrition as our primary restoration methodology. The scope of what we've discussed so far may have been farther reaching with greater implications than you, reader, ever previously imagined, but it needed to be brought to your attention—before it's too late. I hope that this text has really opened your eyes, minds and hearts to a better way of creating wellness. Perhaps it will shake you loose from the bombardment of one-size-fits-all, quick-fix-it brainwashing so overwhelmingly evident in our society. This text's healthful information has been scientifically generated, is continuously being proven time and time again on millions of people, is purely logical and simply creates positive health outcomes. Maybe you are finding yourself relieved about taking the guesswork out of attaining wellness through nutritional programming on the most personal level. To officially begin this process for yourself to achieve the best results, certain reprogramming tasks need to be taken, as follows.

*Task 1*

Truly understand and faithfully believe that your body is designed to be disease and pain-free, full of energy and life, and conducive to all the good that you want to experience and accomplish in your lifetime. You are not meant to be constantly sick, crippled, lethargic, fat, depressed or to settle for only second best in life. Stop betting on getting sick (like our health insurance industry does) and start betting on being well. To be well, you must not take stock in anybody or any medium that tells you that *you* can't be your healthy best (like many doctors do, unfortunately). Never depend only upon your doctors and others for health needs that you can take full control of yourself. And, of course, beware of drug company rhetoric.

In ancient China, the doctor was paid only when the patient was well. He did not receive payment during periods of sickness. The general wellness status of China even today far surpasses the U.S., on only a tiny fraction of the U.S. healthcare budget. In our society, we actually have gone so far as to reward doctors for our sicknesses by paying them huge amounts of money only when we are sick. Why would a doctor really work that hard to get us well when he's paid only when we're sick? Why should he even attempt to convince you that you can be well when he makes more money in repeat visits when you are sick or even when you think you're sick? Why not use quick symptom fixers to temporarily cover up the real problems? This is the way of convenience. Is it any wonder, then, that our $1.4 trillion per year healthcare budget (the largest in the world) is making so very few inroads into resolving the majority of disease processes, especially diet-related diseases, which account for well over 80% of all U.S. diseases? If everyone was able to stay well on their own just by eating and living better, many doctors and the industries that support doctors' drug and surgical therapies would not be necessary. Do you honestly believe that these groups of people would tell us how to be truly healthy even if they really knew? They'd be out of a job. They make more money when we are sick. We're not only paying for their high-profit support with money that can be spent on better things such as wellness promotion, but we're paying them, again and again with our persistent sicknesses. This ultimately decimates the quality of our lives, not to mention breaking all of our financial backs. Reprogramming Task Number 1 is *DON'T BE FOOLED AGAIN.* Don't fall for *one-size-fits-all* rhetoric ever again. Use the personalized nutrition process to control your natural given ability to prevent and reverse disease. From your heart, believe that you can and will be well. This is called the biology of belief as postulated by epigeneticist Dr. Bruce Lipton during an interview on our internet radio show heard at RealPNC.com.

### *Task 2*

Stop believing that your genetics doom you in either life's quality or quantity. First of all, we have no real way to measure what your genetics are all about to the satisfaction of science, other than as afforded through nutrition testing and customized nutritional therapies. So absolutely no one should be all that sure that they are doomed to be fat or die young or learn slowly or whatever "shortcoming," just because some family member with a completely different lifestyle and biochemical identity has suffered. Far too many people mistakenly blame their genetics for their health and weight problems. It used to be believed by researchers that genetics account for about two-thirds of what becomes of you physically (and mentally) over the first forty years of life with one-third physical effect coming from your environment. They commonly believed that there is a genetically determined nutrient reserve that provides a certain measure of metabolic insurance and that in the ten years or so beyond your fortieth birthday, this genetic to environmental ratio reverses to the point where the overwhelming effects of antagonistic environmental exposure catches up with you and either wears you down or kills you off quickly if you haven't taken care of yourself over the previous years. If you have taken adequate care of yourself by eating and living right early on in your life, then these most beneficial environmental effects will guarantee you the greatest life expectancy or longest life span possible. This entire theory has been whittled down to size by advancing science to the point where exactly what is actually happening to you at any given time, healthwise, has much, much less to do with genetics and much more to do with how you're treating yourself than ever thought before. The bottom line here is to utilize the personalized nutrition approach even before birth in order to help you work in harmony with what you possess genetically and where you literally, measure up, to the moment, metabolically, in order to fully optimize and maximize your life from the moment it begins. In this way you will overcome many genetic blocks you may only think that you have. Plus, you will extend and maintain your body's indigenous nutrient reserves at more optimal levels for proper growth and development as well as in crisis situations. The secret again here is simply to have what nature has provided you to work for you.

## *Task 3*

Begin removing the most obvious health barriers from your lifestyle. Some of these barriers may appear generic because there is no doubt to anyone that this is good for everyone. This is illustrated by the obvious notion (small children excepted) that if you put your unprotected hand in the fire you'll get badly burned—so why do it? Unless one wishes to create harm for oneself, why would you defy reason by placing your hand in the fire and suffer burns? I don't believe that anyone really wants to suffer needlessly, wherever they're from.

### Seven Health Obstacles

*These obvious barriers to creating the best health need to be eliminated for one and all:*

1. ***Drinking inadequate amounts of water:*** Every one of us needs to drink pure "toxic-chemical free," highly oxygenated, high energy water for best health results. Distilled, pure spring or adequately filtered water is simply healthier than tap water, although once you're tested we can even be specific about the best purified water to drink. Soft water is good for some people while hard water is better for others—and this can be ascertained scientifically. In general, however, do not rely on non-pure water beverages like tea or soda to account for your pure water intake. Soda pop, juices, tea, and coffee don't count in the least here. A good generic rule of thumb is to drink one ounce of "real" water for each pound of bodyweight divided by three. If your weight is 100 pounds, you should drink at least 33 ounces of water per day. A good clinical tip many of my patients are pleased with is to drink the largest part of your daily water intake at the moment you wake up in the morning. At this time, your body is the most dehydrated that it will be in the 24-hour wake/sleep cycle. Plus, drinking this water upon rising hastens and increases bowel movements. This beneficial megadose of water also helps to dissolve intramembranous waste solids, hastening toxin elimination through the genitourinary and bowel systems.

   ***Rule of thumb***: Always use pure or distilled water to help filter wastes out of your body—***do not*** use your body to filter the wastes out of impure water.

2. ***Smoking (tobacco or anything, really)***: At least six of the 2,000 compounds found in tobacco smoke and nicotine are known to be carcinogens. The nicotine found in smoke is truly addictive and also physiologically stressful. Tobacco smoke and extreme heat literally paralyzes the cilia in your respiratory system, which are only present to push particles which get stuck when breathing out of your trachea. This phenomenon, in turn, allows particulate matter to slide back into the lungs instead of the cilia, literally brushing it back out of the trachea and lung passages. Heart, and lung diseases, cancer, and other conditions have been medically linked to smoking. Each body type has a different capacity to resist the negative consequences of oxygen-robbing tobacco smoke. Some

individuals will tolerate it better than others, with some lucky individuals beating the statistical odds of smoke-related premature death (as far as we can tell by conventional measurement). But I ask you, why play Russian Roulette with something that is proven to be a basic strain on all body types in the first place? Why put your hand in the fire again and again and again with each new cigarette? Your particular body type may be the one that smoke hits the hardest in terms of life-threatening disease. From a nutritional standpoint, tobacco and other types of smoke act as highly potent antivitamin substances which strip your body of many essential nutrients and antioxidants. It also depletes the body of much needed oxygen. When one truly wishes to stop smoking but doesn't know how to, there are numerous options, and personalized nutrition can clearly help in this regard. As an example, it has been postulated by some scientists that nicotine dependence (or any substance or other addiction) is related to nutrient/toxic deficiencies/excesses/imbalances. Although this connection is not fully understood yet nor the exact nutrient factors which are always involved pinpointed in satisfying detail,* the personalized nutrition process will faithfully restore across-the-board, person-specific nutrients that are essential to good health. Because this automatically restores needed essential nutrients to a specific individual and concomitantly balances the metabolism, theoretically any nicotine dependence (and other chemical dependencies and addictions) created from an imbalanced metabolism should dissipate as a result. I have experienced this phenomenon clinically where people's cravings have been reduced when nutrition balance has been restored. I've witnessed cases whereby the person actually quit smoking altogether because their nicotine cravings dissipated over time as their program progressed.

To this day I'm not exactly sure which aspect of the personalized nutrition program was responsible for this turnaround, or to be faithfully scientific, certain that it was not due to some other circumstances. In the case of pica and sugar craving syndromes, deficiencies of chromium, selenium, and manganese have been implicated, and I have observed notable improvement in patients with

*Perhaps this is where tobacco companies should be putting their research money.

these disorders after using TNT (Targeted Nutrition Therapy) on them. I anticipate that someday, thanks to continued orthomolecular research, we will concisely reveal the nutrient–nicotine connection for each body. Perhaps when this happens, smoking as a common habit among humans may disappear altogether (or maybe not, because of man's incessant desire for stimulants). Even amongst high longevity societies and ancient naturally pure societies, there is always something around that people smoke as part of their religious and social rituals or simply as common practice. At this moment in time, it's very difficult to tell if the smoking habit is here to stay and what overall impact TNT will eventually have on it. If you are a smoker, for best health results, make sure that your nutritional program is in order, at least to help protect your health. And if you consequently lose your nicotine craving, all the better.

3. *Long-term drug dependence of any kind to maintain non-pain comfort levels:* In the first place, long-term drug use for pain inhibition of any kind has serious health-deteriorating side effects. In the second place, if you keep experiencing pain and/or discomfort repeatedly, your body is telling you that something is wrong and that the pain/symptom-blocking drug you're taking really has no curative effect because the physical problem returns once the medication wears off, or when you again duplicate the irritation that instigates the pain in the first place.

   *Example:* People chronically take antacids to eliminate stomach pain which could be avoided in the first place with better food combining, appropriate digestive enzymes, slower more relaxed eating and the use of natural curatives like aloe vera or bismuth, d-glycrrhizerated licorice or Nux Vomica (a homeopathic formula). Once you're treated with TNT, our aim is that most if not all pain relief medications should become a thing of the past and no longer will be necessary because the body will heal itself as a result of the personalized nutrition program. Remember that your body is naturally designed to heal itself (homeostasis) and that symptom/pain-relief drugs do not heal anything (no matter what the commercials say) when they, in effect, merely block the soon-to-be conscious symptoms of pain messages your body is constantly sending to the brain. If anything, this pain-blocking effect from the periphery of your body disconnects consciousness from the reality of your body's true health state, which in turn may seriously impair attempts to keep from damaging yourself further at work or play. Natural curatives like herbs, vitamins, minerals, homeopathics, etc., can work in chemical harmony with the body to actually stimulate and reinforce the healing process when properly applied. Sometimes natural curatives do not remove the pain as quickly and may take extra time to turn the condition around—so patience may be required. However, when the pain is gone—under natural healing conditions—it's only because the body has actually healed itself and not because the sensation of pain is artificially blocked off, as in the case of pain-relief drugs. When you're nutritionally/metabolically balanced in the first place, the need for added curatives will diminish. If a person using TNT does require a temporarily applied natural curative for a short period of time, typically the healing process seems to work much faster and more completely than a nutritionally imbalanced person.

4. ***Physical inactivity:*** Regular physical activity is a health-promoting and a very necessary common denominator for all individuals, whether you're from Soviet Georgia or from U.S. Georgia. A full TNT program should match specific physical activities to specific body types. Some individuals simply do better with some forms of exercise than others and this must be taken into account. Some people will require heavy and high-intensity exercise to feel, look, and be their best. Others will do better with slow, methodical stretching and yoga, Tai chi, dance and light aerobics. Those who like vigorous activity sometimes consider light activity to be sissy stuff, believing that you have to lift heavy weights or beat yourself into a pulp to get anywhere in life. Obviously this isn't necessarily true. Other people tend not to be the best weight lifters and tend to shy away from heavy weight training. What is right for you remains to be determined as you participate in your own recovery.

In the meantime, start to move in whatever way that even remotely appeals to you. We were put on this earth to move, and walking regularly is always a good way to get started on your personal war against inactivity. It just so happens that walking, as an exercise, is beneficial to all people—so you can't go wrong. Also, greater amounts of physical activity require an even more nutrient-dense and balanced nutrition program for best results. The higher the intensity of physical activity, the faster your body metabolizes food, vitamins, and minerals. If you already have nutrient deficiencies and/or imbalances to begin with, exercise will only serve to worsen these metabolic inconsistencies. For all of the goodness regular exercise affords the body, there is this downside to consider. It has reached a point where articles are being written to warn people about this problem. For instance, Dr. Joel Wallach, B.S., DVM, N.D., in his dramatically stated article "Exercise Without Supplementation is Suicide," illustrates this point succinctly. TNT should adequately eliminate any concern that you may have about exercise undermining your wellness status, because it precisely accommodates the body's metabolic requirements under all stress conditions including exercise, which is a positive stress, or eustress, as we mentioned previously. A properly nurtured person will obtain only the maximum benefits from their exercise program. I must agree with Dr. Wallach and add that exercise without personalized nutrition is suicide.

5.  *Inadequate sleep, improper relaxation:* A lack of proper rest, recreation, and relaxation over time puts a severe and cumulative stress on the body that will only serve to undermine the quantity and quality of life. Consistent exercise activity will always help in the promotion of better sleep patterns. Research shows that sleep patterns are very individualized. We don't each need the same amount or quality of sleep. Dream and sleep states vary among individuals and are loosely categorized to some personality types. Overall, however, due to the many complexities in our high-pressure lifestyles, it's very difficult to generalize about sleep from person to person. In each individual's case, it is always better to sleep a little more than to sleep a little bit less than we each perceive our actual sleep needs to be. Personalized nutrition, in my clinical experience, has served to lessen both Type 1 and Type 2 insomnias for some patients and has eliminated it altogether for others. The metabolic rebalancing process systematized by personalized nutrition can only help improve sleep's healing functions, unless, of course, too many stimulating nutrients are taken just before bed. Both the presence of consistent sleep patterns and regular relaxation periods are found amongst long-living contemporary primitive societies like the Hunzans, etc. These peoples are without many of the sleep limitations imposed on us by highly structured and work-pressurized modern society. Besides eating and drinking

properly, sleeping properly is probably the next most important health-promoting factor in life, followed closely by regular exercise. The three essential components of eating, sleeping, and exercise represent our most fundamental foundation of life and should never be taken lightly, as they incessantly are these days. A true wellness aficionado should never undermine nor undervalue these three variables or they will surely suffer the painful consequences.

6. ***Don't take responsibility for yourself:*** Blame everyone except yourself for your problems in life; believe that you are always right and everyone else is wrong and when something goes wrong in your life, it's due to a conspiracy against you. This way of looking at life only serves to depreciate your wellness and happiness. Life is about learning. Take control, overcome obstacles and learn from your mistakes. Take 100% responsibility for what happens in your life. Stop being closed-minded or stubborn about this or you will suffer needlessly. Orthomolecular nutritional medicine involves taking steps to learn how to be in living synchrony and harmony with the universe. It offers a new way of thinking about how to think about health. We are using art and science to accomplish this natural state of physical being and are hoping to enhance a person's psychology and spirituality in the process. From an energetic standpoint we want to better align your inner physical and mental energy to the energy of the outside environment that's best for you. Our goal is to help you to help yourself by using the proper foods and lifestyle to align yourself. This alignment process can in turn impact the way you think and enact your spirituality. In fact, the sciences of psychoimmunoneurology, epigenetics and Noetics are constantly endeavoring to translate and outline useful and practical food-body-mind-body-universe connections. These "new" sciences have revealed that the foods we eat have a direct connection to the way we think, which in turn has another direct connection back to our body functions and back again. It all can begin with consciously choosing the foods that we consume as the first basic step in our creating the way we perceive things. This is where personalized nutrition is the most focused. It's no secret that many of our long-living primitive societies and other native societies all have a spiritual conviction to the natural order of the land and a collective commitment to one another to thrive. They see themselves as truly part of the land. This is basic to their healthy secret in being able to live a long productive life. It needs

to be ours as well. Personalizing nutrition, taking full self-responsibility, and thinking of others as part of a connection to yourself
takes us many steps closer to a more natural, healthy, and fulfilling way of life on the smallest molecular/energetic order—food.
*We are what we retain* from what we eat, what we think, and
everything we do. We are part of the total spirit and circle of life.

7. *Obsessiveness and extremism:* My mother always told me, as did
my favorite biology teacher Miss Qualls, that moderation is the
key to life and that too much of one thing or another can do you
harm. Obsessive and extremist behavior is yet another obstacle to
good health that one needs to confront and conquer. Whether you
suffer from fits of anger and rage, all work and no play or the
reverse, eating a lot of one thing and very little else, constant over-
exercising, vicarious thrill-seeking (living through other's actions
as in addictions to spectator sports), a state of all talk and no
action and no listening, excessive complaining, too much or too
little rest, too much suntanning, constant impatience, overt nar-
cissism, unbridled ego, or any other excessive tendencies all need
to be reckoned with for proper balance. We must do our best to
stay in our center for the best life possible. Personalized nutrition
has many implications here in that it monitors one's nutrition-
related health status, which can serve to help us pay detailed attention to and maintain accountability in other areas of our lives.

These *Seven Health Obstacles* must be addressed for our best health.
Your next step is to learn how to better organize your own diet in rough
form and then to further refine it after nutrition testing in your bid to
achieve the greatest genetic balancing possible.

### *Further Defining Personalized Nutrition*

With the above obstacles out of the way or at least being addressed, personalized nutrition then becomes a step-by-step nutrition process which
completes five distinct steps to nutrition success. But before initiating
the steps, it is wise to first put together any pertinent medical history
along with any medically diagnostic test results you know about (such as
high cholesterol and/or an official diagnosis of chronic fatigue). This is
the time to put in writing your health and fitness objectives that you
wish to accomplish:

***Compute and Correct Calories for Quantity and Quality***—This allows us to create a daily food plan. This is not about counting calories; there are food and nutrient zones to take into account for maximum metabolic stimulation which must be addressed.

***Pure Metabolic Typing (Genotyping in Simplified Form)***—In years past this was a lengthy process which led to little information about how to fix the body, and therefore I have simplified it dramatically so as not to confuse anyone or waste time. This essentially serves as a starting point from which to compare phenotypic results (changes in the expression of your genes due to modifications of external environmental input) in the future.

***Laboratory Assessment (Nutrition/Metabolic/Toxin/Genetic tests)***—This aspect provides the heart to the whole system of detection and eventual correction of nutritional and toxic abnormalities.

***Diet and Supplement Customization***—Deducing and correlating from statistical comparisons exactly which foods and supplements are mandated in accordance with the law of opposites, the seesaw effect and the interactive antagonistic nutrient displacement effects mentioned earlier that provide the controls to our laboratory experiment on each person. These foods and customized supplements provide the therapeutic intervention and are modified according to how the body responds over time, until perfect balance is eventually achieved.

***Re-evaluation (retesting)***—Retesting allows us to follow the body's response closely and make nutritional corrections as necessary until complete results are achieved.

All of the above personalized nutrition steps are utilized in order to minimize diet mistakes and ultimately leave little room for human error. Thanks to scientific research and development, these protocols can be put into effect in the privacy of your own home, which removes many doctor errors and costs.

### You Be My Patient For a Moment
### Old School

For some clinical perspective, let's make believe for a moment that you've sought my help and are now in my office to be put on a personalized nutrition program. Maybe you have already been to a fair share of doctors, nutritionists, trainers and the like, who have not fully addressed your symptoms, objectives, and lifestyle needs. This historically is typical for many of my patients. Perhaps nobody has fully integrated or connected the dots of wellness for you and you've still continued to suffer. Perhaps the last medical doctor you visited couldn't find any overtly obvious problems or disease present and therefore told you "it's all in your head." Maybe you believed them or maybe you really didn't and that's why you sought my help. After all, you still have a lot of nagging symptoms plaguing you like fatigue, intermittent digestive stress, nagging headaches, weakness, weight problems, reoccurring rashes, joint pain, high blood pressure, or any of a number of symptoms. You may have already been to an herbologist, acupuncturist, iridologist, kinesiologist, and other assorted healthcare practitioners. You may even have brought your diet plan and a host of other supplements and drugs with you for me to examine along with all of your medical records. Perhaps you've gotten to the point of pure desperation and that's why you're giving the guy down the street (me) a chance. After all, what have you got to lose that you haven't already lost? Maybe you found me likable on a recent local FOX TV segment news broadcast or maybe you liked it when Dr. Bob Torman on "CBS This Morning" referred to me as "quintessential" because this off-the-beaten-path health approach appealed to your instincts to break out of the medical mold and look for nonmedical alternatives. Maybe you simply felt that I knew something that no one else seemed to know and could actually help you. Maybe you simply had nowhere else to turn. These are things patients have told me before. None of this really matters now because here you are in my office ready to be set straight. You are committed to seeing this through. We start off our office visit by having you fill out an extensive medical, nutrition, and exercise history. This allows me to better understand your personal wellness experiences.

Next, we have our initial consultation. We discuss your health history and what has and has not been done for you in the way of fully analyzing and fulfilling your wellness needs. I accomplish all of this by taking a very close look at your diet, supplements, exercise (or non-exercise) patterns, and your lifestyle overall—I look for obvious antagonisms or imbalances. I do this in the hope of identifying certain gray areas in your health history. These gray areas represent the need for investigative procedures that have not been performed on you to date such as personalized nutrition tests and analysis. The more of these gray areas that become apparent, the greater the chance that we can fully restore you to optimal health. Most average people have huge gray areas with regard to clinical-level nutrition intervention. The larger these clinical nutrition gray areas the greater the success potential. My goal as your adviser is to nutritionally (orthomolecularly) rebuild you from the ground up to create a foundation of wellness that you can maintain yourself. Because nutrition is the absolute cornerstone of wellness and in your case you've historically had little, if any, proper intervention (which is typical of most people), we have a lot to work with and can expect many dramatic improvements. I've already noted your ethnicity, family disease patterns, personal disease pattern, you and your family's ages, your weight (on my scale, of course), gender and other background information. After I give you a brief overview on *one-size-fits-all* traps and this concept's complete infectivity in promoting the most optimal health on an individual basis, we then get down to business.

### Step 1
### Calorie Quantification and Qualification

We review your health and fitness objectives. You tell me that you're hoping to eliminate the many variable symptoms that you've included on your health and history forms but first and foremost you simply want to feel younger, more energetic, and not become sick so frequently and easily. Some of the nagging symptoms you've noted include headaches, fatigue, depression, indigestion, rebounding constipation and diarrhea, overt sugar cravings (you're a confirmed "chocoholic"), intermittent skin rashes, joint pain, poor sleep patterns, hair loss, slow-healing wounds, constant scarring, gum sensitivity, halitosis (bad breath), heart palpitations on occasion, muscle cramps (especially in your legs), intermittent blurred vision, inability to concentrate, premature graying hair, a flabby untoned musculature, excessive fat that just won't come off, cellulite, pale complexion, redness in the eyes, extreme mood swings, heavy PMS, chronic sinus congestion and post-nasal drip, anxiety attacks, chronically dry and bad-tasting mouth, constant gas, stomach pain, foul-smelling stools and urine, multitudes of age spots, wrinkling skin, very dry or oily skin (depending on the body area), bad body odor, excessive sweating, craving for stimulants (like coffee), cold-feeling extremities, constant burping, blood in the stool, feelings of stiffness, occasional dizziness, excessive temper, poor memory, inconsistent appetite, and still more. You may find that many of these symptoms are of surprisingly extreme importance to me as your practitioner, whereas prior to our meeting you were told by other health professionals that "it's all in your head" or "it's not that important, stop complaining" or "learn to live with it because there's nothing that can be done anyway." Then when you think about the quality of your life, you realize that these "dis-eases" are making you quite miserable even though the previous doctor said you weren't really sick. I've had people who are on multiple drugs tell me that they're healthy, because the doctor says so. This is scary when you consider that anybody on a drug save for insulin (for diabetes) is not healthy by any stretch of the imagination.

Our first objective here is to naturally eliminate any and all of these symptoms one by one so you can certainly feel better. With that, of course, you want to live a longer life under these conditions with the youthful vitality of earlier days. Your second objective, you tell me, is to drop body fat and tone up, get fit again. Maybe you're one who doesn't exercise at all or maybe your exercise program is just not cutting it or maybe you have an even more pressing need to get into shape again, like post-heart-attack victims. Maybe you're a world class athlete wanting to peak for the next Olympics or prepare for a future body-building competition or a movie star who needs to show some muscle for your next movie which is being filmed in eight weeks. Perhaps you are truly obese and need to drop the fat and get into shape as a matter of an immediate life-or-death scenario. Maybe you need to rehabilitate a nagging injury that just won't go away, or perhaps you are a regular person simply searching for the answers to simply feel and look better.

Now that we know your desired objectives of fat loss and health gain we can begin a general standard physical examination including testing blood pressure; heart rate; listening to your heart and lungs; palpation for abdominal masses examining your body structure and range of movement; measuring limb and trunk size; doing a body fat analysis; looking at your eyes, ears, nose skin, hair and throat under magnification; and perhaps taking a standard blood and urine sample for conventional analysis (if not performed very recently) and maybe even taking an x-ray of an injury site or for some other reason. Once we accomplish this standard examination phase, we can move onto the next phase which is quantifying (or assessing) your actual macronutrient caloric need given your lifestyle and objectives. How many calories does it take to run your body most efficiently? We'll find out directly. By the way, the majority of patients I've worked with nutritionally have been to other so-called nutritionists (mostly novice nutritionists) who have never quantified their diet for them. Instead of assessing caloric need scientifically for each client, these novice nutritionists simply guess about this procedure, or in some cases are not even aware that it exists in the first place due to their lack of training and expertise in its application.

Many of my patients have walked into the office with what I term "standard form diets" taken from a generic source with no real direct connection to them as the patient. As an example of this, one of my patients handed me a Pritikin Diet plan. Apparently, this patient had walked into a nutritionist's office, plopped down $150, talked to the novice nutritionist for about fifteen minutes with no formal exam or medical history taken, and then was handed this generic Pritikin Diet, which of course had no connection to the actual measurable needs of this patient at all. And, there was that same pile of partly used supplements sitting on my desk which my patient had barely taken because they made her feel even worse after she took them than she already felt. What folly. My distaste for this previous treatment of my new patient further intensified when I found out that the particular novice nutritionist in question is a (somewhat) famous nutritionist to the stars but in fact has no actual accredited academic or clinical qualifications. This is in fact a case of the blind leading the blind which we must all be aware of. This is not an isolated case—this type of fraudulent scenario occurs every day to thousands of unsuspecting consumers.

### The Calorie Quantifying Process

In the interest of science, our first task now is to assess your **Basal Metabolic Rate (BMR)**. The BMR, expressed as calories, is the daily rate at which your body consumes calories in a resting state to sustain life. This rate represents an amount of calories that your body needs if you were to lie in bed all day (24 hours). If you were to match this exact rate (BMR) to the exact amount of calories from foods you take in (properly proportioned), your body would not gain or lose any weight whatsoever. You would not gain so much as an ounce of fat, muscle, bone, organ, tissue, or water. The total BMR represents a culmination of the differing rates at which each cell, tissue, and organ uses energy. It is an ideal calorie amount and it is unique to you only. Your BMR is a sustained calorie level that changes throughout your lifespan as you grow and mature and is related to the nutrient balance found in your body.

Better balance equals a higher metabolic rate; in other words, your body makes more energy from less food. The calorie consumption or BMR can also be altered by disease onset, stress, and exercise modifications in your life. Direct and indirect *calorimetry* studies have measured these levels in humans and there are some mathematically derived standard norms I can employ to decipher your particular BMR. Your BMR is then computed based on age, gender, height, weight, and other factors (all of which are mathematically corrected for). In effect, I am estimating your BMR levels without having to utilize expensive, sophisticated, complex, in-lab calorimetric assessment, although a lab can be contacted to do this if you wish.

### The Energy Usage of Physical Activity

Once we have computed a mathematically derived BMR for you (or tested you on a BMR tester) then we add in the caloric energy needs of your body as a result of getting out of bed, moving around, and exercising. We call this the **Energy Level of Physical Activity,** also known as **Daily Physical Activity Need (DPAN)** and it requires an individualized computation of calories. Whether you sit in an office all day, are a blue collar laborer, a professional athlete, exercise intermittently or consistently—all have a direct effect on how many calories your body requires daily over and above your BMR levels. As my make-believe patient, we will look at what you are physically doing literally every hour of your day and night. When you exercise, I will assess both the type of your exercises and the intensity at which you perform them. Whether you are a heavy, medium, or light laborer all has a bearing on this process of determining the exact amount of calories your body requires. I will assess the rate at which you burn calories throughout the day during different activities using mathematical norms based upon calorimetry studies conducted on exercising and sedentary humans. When you sit down you'll burn so many calories, when you lift heavy objects you'll burn so many calories, and so on. If you'd like to have this more directly assessed, there is new lab technology which allows us to more precisely monitor your caloric consumption during your daily routine, which again can be arranged for, if truly required. Once we've determined the specific calorie needs for your individual pattern of activity, then we can add this amount to your BMR. In your hypothetical case, as my patient, let's say we determined your BMR to be 1,500 calories per day. Your Daily Physical Activity Need was found to be another 600 calories per day, so the combined figure is 2,100 calories per day. In other words, your body requires 2,100 calories per day to sustain itself without any net weight gain or loss in and out of bed. But we're not finished with the quantification process yet.

### *Specific Dynamic Activity*

***Specific Dynamic Activity (SDA)*** represents the caloric energy required for the processes of digestion and reflexive brown fat thermogenesis after eating. Thermogenesis is a term referring to heat production by the body. Our body is actually a "heat factory" with about 75 percent of the caloric energy that we consume as food going into heat production. About 25 percent of what's left goes into energy production or in effect is made into ATP or organic phosphorus used to drive muscular movement, thinking, and all other bodily processes, except for the 6 percent to 10 percent that the SDA consumes for its needs. A certain amount of energy usually expressed as a percentage of overall body energy is consumed by digestion and brown fat metabolism automatically. After eating, that warm feeling you experience is a reflexive response to the increased calorie consumption of brown adipose tissue, which gives off extra heat for better digestion. This brown adipose tissue is a primary thermoregulator (heat regulator) of the body and is specifically designed to create heat to stabilize body temperatures. By the way, white (or yellow) adipose is designed strictly for fat storage and body part insulation. There are many thermogenic supplements designed to stimulate brown fat metabolism to increase calorie usage by the body. MaHuang (ephedra) is one of those herbal supplements used for this purpose—but is it helpful or perhaps dangerous for you? So far, we've been able to compute your SDA as a 6% fixed percentage of your BMR and **DPAN**, also known as the **Energy Level of Physical Activity** combined figure.

Next, we will add all three figures together:

|  |  |  |
|---|---|---|
| BMR...................... | 1,500 calories | (Lying in bed all day) |
| DPAN...................... | + 600 calories | (Exercise, job, lifestyle) |
| SDA...................... | + 126 calories | (6% of 2,100 - digestion) |
| TCND.................... | 2,226 calories | |

This all adds up to 2,226 calories which equals your ***Total Calorie Need per Day (TCND)*** that your body theoretically requires to maintain itself at its constant weight after taking all lifestyle factors into consideration.

### *Dangerous Territory*

Dangerous Territory can be found above or below the TCND figure. If you're consuming more calories than the 2,226 TCND level, you will progressively gain weight, primarily as fat. Most people in our country, over time, tend to exceed their TCNDs. This has lead to the U.S. becoming the most overweight country in the world. Over time, our metabolisms tend to slow down as we age, eat improperly, suffer more stress, and exercise less and less. During the aging process we tend to eat more and more of the "wrong" foods due to stress, enjoy less free time and pay little attention—if any—to our precise nutritional needs. This problem is compounded further by the fact that most of the foods we consume typically available in supermarkets contain low-nutrient density with a greater proportion of empty sugar and fat calories, which increasingly satisfies our appetites less while serving to increase our overall appetites more, so that our bodies reflexively seek more nourishment. It is a vicious cycle. Subsequently, we eat more to make up the difference for low-nutrient densities and end up accumulating more fat from empty calories.

Aging in combination with a lack of exercise allows our valuable calorie-burning muscles to shrink away from nonuse, while noncalorie consuming storage fat (white or yellow fat) greedily accumulates in its place. It has been postulated by physiologists that between the ages of 30 and 60, the average American woman or man loses 30 percent of their strength and the muscle that creates it as they gain approximately 30 percent more fat on their bodies. In our hypothetical treatment of you (as my client), your stated objective is to lose ten pounds in the next ten weeks and thereafter keep fat accumulation controlled for the rest of your life for both health and cosmetic reasons. Excess fat accumulation is a generic health risk and is also considered by most to be unsightly. Once we get you going on a program, we're hoping that your worries about fat gain will dissipate once and for all, which serves as a stress in itself, making things worse.

If, hypothetically, your actual daily calorie consumption level is below the TCND level of 2,226, say at 1,600, you are still in dark territory if you are chronically underweight. At this level, you would be consuming 626 fewer calories than your body actually requires to maintain itself, which in turn would cause it to have to burn whatever fat or muscle available to it to make up the calorie difference. Being chronically underweight carries its own set of health risks ranging from deficiency states to immunodeprivation, growth, and maturation impairments. In this hypothetical case, you would need to actually gain "good weight" to be optimally healthy. By "good weight" I mean muscle, bone, and teeth density, better hydration (water weight) and maybe even a little reserve fat. In order to accomplish steady weight increases, you would have to consume more calories than your recommended TCND level and then back your calories down to the TCND level once your ideal weight has been achieved in order to maintain yourself at this ideal level.

As a typical American nutrition patient, you've already expressed the need to lose some body fat (10 pounds in 10 weeks). Let's say that my evaluation of your eating  habits reveals that your **Actual Daily Calorie Consumption (ADCC)**  is in reality 2,700 calories per day, 474 calories over your calculated theoretical need per day of 2,226 calories. It is quite clear that you are consuming more food than your body actually requires. No wonder you've accumulated some fat and are overweight.  Simply:

> ADCC.............................2,700 calories
> TCND..........................- 2,226 calories (Total Calorie Need per Day)
> 474 calories

So you're in the red by 474 calories. This means that you are taking in almost 500 calories per day more than your body actually requires to sustain itself given your daily average lifestyle. This happens all the time to people without them having the foggiest idea that it's a problem. What happens to this extra 474 calories? Yes, there it is—and that is the extra fat layer on your body. These are the calories that your body can't use for energy and heat so it stores them as fat.

The only way to subtract this fat from your body is to subtract some calories from your current daily intake and increase metabolism. This cannot be done in a haphazard fashion if it is to be permanent. There is a method you've probably heard about before:  Given that 1 pound of fat = 3,500 calories, we will quantify your customized diet so that fat will progressively and naturally come off of your body at a rate that's healthy and safe until you reach your ideal weight and fat percentage. This is accomplished by subtracting calories from your TCND and ADCC and commensurately increasing metabolism which we will be doing as we move along. Under slight starvation terms, your body will be slightly deprived of calories and therefore have to burn fat in order to compensate. At the future time that your ideal weight is reached, your diet will again be adjusted so that calories are added in to bring you up to your TCND caloric level, which also should be higher from target nutrient therapy, in order to maintain that ideal fat percentage and weight level for the long term. Otherwise, you would continue to lose too much weight. This new TCND level may have to be adjusted surprisingly higher than your current 2,226 TCND level because your metabolism and caloric consumption rate have so favorably increased since we first started. Of course, a faster metabolism is highly desirable because now your body uses more calories to create more energy in less time. This means that you can eat more without gaining fat. For the moment, we'll subtract 750 calories from your current ADCC level of 2,700 calories or approximately 250 from your TCND 2,226 calorie level for a *new target level* of 2,000 calories per day. Organizing your nutritional plan at 2,000 calories per day as your caloric target will force your body to take 250 calories per day out of fat storage from under the skin, between your muscles and from around your internal organs to make up the difference. This is called a *calorie deficit* or *negative calorie balance.*

250 calories of fat melting off your body every day over a seven-day period equals 1,750 (7 X 250) calories of fat per week lost from your body, or about 1/2 pound of fat (1/2 of 3,500 calories) lost each and every week that you stay on the 2,000 calorie per day target level. So in 10 weeks, you'll theoretically lose five pounds. Because we're going to redesign your daily exercise program so that you will burn off an extra 250 calories per day with physical activity that your body isn't replacing with diet, the calorie deficit will grow to 500 (250 calories from diet + 250 calories from exercise = 500) calories per day less than your body needs to sustain your current weight. In effect, you'll be in a 500-calorie-per-day negative calorie balance (or deficit). Now you'll be losing fat at a rate of approximately one pound per week (3,500 caloric deficit per week) for a total loss of 10 pounds in 10 weeks, which is exactly what your stated objective is. This all sounds simple to some but confusing to most, but when strategizing diet, most people and novice nutritionists blow it from the start because they don't think of computing caloric needs scientifically. This happens due to either ignorance or nutrition imprecision but always ends up undermining potential fat loss results.

Now, with your new 2,000 calorie per day target calorie level you may think that you're all set to go, but you're not even close. Now I'm going to take you to the next phase in Step 1—Qualification.

### *The Qualifying Process*

Now that we (theoretically) know how many daily calories your body needs to healthfully lose 10 pounds in the next 10 weeks, we need to divide this number up into the proper proportion of macronutrients and their correct caloric amount to fulfill our 2,000 calorie-per-day target. *Macronutrients* are the basic nutrients which we need to consume on a daily basis in larger than gram amounts for survival. These macronutrients are protein, fats, carbohydrates, air* and water. They each have their own calorie value and metabolic value.

According to the Atwater Coefficients:

| | | | |
|---|---|---|---|
| 1 gram of protein | = | 4.35 | Kcal = Calorie |
| 1 gram of carbohydrates | = | 4.1 | Kcal = Calorie |
| 1 gram of fat | = | 9 | Kcal = Calorie |
| 1 gram of water | = | 0 | Kcal = Calorie |
| 1 gram of ethanol (alcohol) | = | 7 | Kcal = Calorie |

(alcohol is not a true macronutrient because we do not require it for survival)

The metabolic value of macronutrients (besides as calories) simply put is:

*Proteins:* Provide the building blocks of the body (amino acids) for all cells, tissues, organs, hormones, neuropeptides, etc; protein tends to speed up metabolism and stimulate the Central Nervous System (CNS); it has diuretic qualities; it cannot be stored significantly as usable protein and therefore must be replenished daily; can be turned into fat and uric acid when taken in excess

*Carbohydrates:* Provide the primary high-intensity, short term-energy source all body cells and tissues require, especially nerve and muscle cells; excess carbohydrates tend to slow metabolism down and hold water in the body in larger than ideal amounts; carbs can be easily stored as glycogen and then fat if not used for energy purposes

*Fats:* Provide the primary low intensity, long-term energy source most body cells and tissues require and are involved in a multitude of metabolic processes ranging from immune function to fat digestion, forming body linings and nerve insulation for prostaglandin formation and more; fat

---

*I classify oxygen as a macronutrient because we need so much of it, although most scientific texts do not because it is not considered a weight measure. The fact is that the atmosphere weighs 14.7 lbs. per square inch, so air does in fact have weight.

tends to slow metabolism down but not to the same degree as excess carbohydrates; in excess, fat is easily stored as body fat.

The inter-proportion of one macronutrient to the next has a profound effect on body metabolism, either leading to increased or decreased metabolic rates, proper balance or serious nutrient and metabolic imbalances and disease states, and a longer life or premature aging. The proper proportioning of proteins, carbohydrates, and fats in certain specified zones within the nutritional plan is very important in terms of overall health impact. At this stage within the five step personalized nutrition plan, we are still only at the initial theoretical levels that have not been fully adjusted to unique body specifications yet; this comes later. For the moment, in your case as a hypothetical patient, we are only mathematically estimating your macronutrient needs. Before we apportion the macronutrients into your 2,000-calorie-per-diet-day formula, we need to take a closer look at these macronutrients.

### Protein – Carb – Fat Connections

#### Protein:
There are virtually all types of proteins in nature that have different properties within our own body's metabolism. Foods rich in proteins consist of eggs, milk, fish, poultry, beef, pork, soy, lamb, legumes, nuts, seeds, grains, etc. They each have different body and tissue-building characteristics, various digestive implications, and allergy factor potentials specific to your biochemical uniqueness. Proteins require the presence of fats and carbohydrates for the most efficient metabolism. Their carbon skeletons can be denitrogenized and transformed into sugar (deaminization) which in turn can convert into adipose tissue (fat) but all at a very expensive metabolic and health-denigrating cost. To rely on protein in substitution for carbohydrate and fat needs is completely erroneous and risky. Excessively high protein diets can kill, as demonstrated by the recorded deaths of some people on high-protein diets. Proteins need to be in proper balance with carbs and fats specific to your body chemistry in order to be maximized properly.

#### Carbohydrates:
There are 4 basic categories of carbohydrates (carbs):

1) Complex—calorie dense (starches with high calorie-to-fiber ratio)

2) Complex—calorie dilute (vegetables with high fiber and low calories)
3.) Natural simple sugars (fruits, high-sugar vegetables, and honey)
4.) Man-made refined simple sugars

Each one of these carbohydrate types have different effects on the body, some desirable and some not so desirable in terms of digestion, hormonal and neuropeptide responses, blood sugar levels and insulin response, acidity and alkalinity, short- and long-term energy production, and overall health. Those vegetables and fruits which contain concentrated carbohydrates have a variety of properties including different acidity and alkalinity levels before and after entering the body, varying glycemic index factors, and differing phytonutrient and vitamin/mineral contents. To achieve optimum metabolism requires that these different types of carbohydrates be properly proportioned within the diet relative to each other and in relation to protein and fat, as well as being very specific to your test profiles. Excessive carbohydrate intake, especially in regard to refined carbohydrates, will always slow metabolism. Excess carbs also tend to increase retained body water, strain organs like the heart and other body systems, damage teeth and the digestive system and most definitely cause fat accumulation in as much as carbohydrate quite readily converts to fat.

*Fats*:
There are 3 most basic types of fat from varying food sources:

*MUFA— (Monounsaturated Fatty Acids)*—Found in a variety of foods from all
     macronutrient categories
*PUFA— (Polyunsaturated Fatty Acids)*—Mostly from plant sources,
     particularly grains, seeds, and vegetables; also from fish and poultry
*SAFA — (Saturated Fatty Acids)*—Predominantly from animal sources

The dietary apportionment of each of these types of fat in relation to one another and in relation to proteins and carbohydrates is critical to a balanced, healthy metabolism and is very individually specific to your measured metabolic type. Sometimes people indiscriminately cut fat from their diets and tend to unknowingly remove good fats as well as bad fats, which in turn creates health problems and metabolic dysfunction. The PUFAs are categorized by three primary essential good fatty acids: alpha linolenic, cis-linoleic, and gamma linolenic acids which are absolutely critical to the immune system and metabolism at large. Many people are deficient or imbalanced in these essential fats and their derivatives due to indiscriminate diet practices, enzyme inhibition (delta-6 desaturase for one, as popularized by *The Zone* by Dr. Barry Sears), and cofactor deficiencies (cofactors are vitamins, minerals, and hormones). Probably the most significant consequence of this fat dilemma is immune system dysfunction. All in all, these fat factors need to be balanced in relation to each other, to carbs and proteins, and in relation to your testing specificities for healthiest results. As you probably know by now, excesses of saturated fats and trans fats from frying (most particularly) increase fat accumulation on the body, can be toxic, cause higher blood cholesterol and triglyceride levels and also put a pronounced unhealthful strain on your body's frame and metabolism at large.

We next need to proportion protein, carb, and fat origin foods into a theoretical interproportion category I call Zone I, of 40/30/30, as *The Zone* suggested, or some other rough ratio to build from as we move through the testing process. Within each category of nutrient, I will be able to build a list of food selections with the proper intraproportion category. For example, your theoretical rough diet will consist of:

*Theoretical   Zone I*
50% of its calories from carbohydrates
30% of its calories from protein
20% of its calories from fat

50/30/20 = INTERPROPORTION of the three food categories

*Theoretical   Zone II*
25% of its total protein calories from fish sources
25% of its protein calories from vegetable sources
25% of its protein calories from eggs and dairy sources
25% of its protein calories from red meat sources

25/25/25/25 = INTRAPROPORTION of each protein type

*Theoretical   Zone III*
40% of its total carbohydrate calories from complex, calorie-
    dilute, high-fiber vegetables
25% of its total complex carbohydrate from dense, starchy vegetables
25% of total carbohydrate calories from natural simple sugars in fruit
10% of total carbohydrate calories from the man-made natural simple sugar
    category of sweets

40/25/25/10 = INTRAPROPORTION of each carbohydrate type

*Theoretical     Zone IV*

<u>40%</u> of its total fat calories from PUFAs
<u>35%</u> of its total fat calories from MUFAs
<u>25%</u> of its total fat calories from SAFAs

<u>40/35/25</u> = INTRAPROPORTION of each <u>fat type</u>

The following steps will enable us to understand exactly what specific foods will be eliminated or retained based on what is found, along with a recalibration of your zones from the theoretical breakdown above. The last component of the qualification process is to check the proportion of micronutrients to one another. Right now, most people depend on the Recommended Dietary Allowances for this but sadly, they are very imprecise when it comes to your actual body's needs and therefore really don't apply. This process of micronutrient input from food and supplements and the final refinements made upon the qualification process is reserved for Step 3 and beyond, when all of the other criteria for your biochemical identity is compiled from testing. At that time, after engaging a ruling-in and ruling-out process, we will have a completely customized nutrition program meal by meal, food by food, zone by zone, and essential nutrient by nutrient that's just right *for your body only.*

### Step 2
### *Pure Metabolic Typing or Genotyping*

Just for the sake of "old school" to "new school" comparison, I have enclosed a highly condensed example of the old and now obsolete Metabolic Health and Rehabilitation metabolic typing program which is instituted in my practice there. Please realize that this step has been completely streamlined in view of more recent scientific and technological advancements and therefore is considered obsolete compared to the way we do things now.

Back to our workup. Being my hypothetical patient in a real on-site office interface, by now you've visited me twice: once for the initial evaluation and once to go over the quantification/qualification calorie computation process. Now it's your third visit and we are going to metabolically type you using nonspecimen-related laboratory data, with the exception of noting your specific blood type. This is the part of your typing process that's going to allow me to place you into your basic tribal ancestral line or phenotype and to theoretically deduce other categorical conclusions about how your body functions so that I can place you into the proper diet category for your type of body. It is in this step that we will determine if you potentially are an **omnivore, carni-vegan** (a type of meat-eater) or a **vegetarian** combination or blend. We will at least develop a working idea of what exact foods are best for you hypothetically, what foods are worst for you, and what you're likely to be allergic to. We will be able to better postulate what the best inter- and intra- proportions of macronutrient and individual foods are right for you (Zones I - IV). Do you need a 50/35/15 (inter) and 40/30/20/10, 25/25/25/25, 33/33/33 (intra) or some other inter- and intra- combination of proportions to be in the so-called zone for you without a "slop factor" (gray area)? Only metabolic typing can tell at least theoretically, without the use of tests. Your particular micronutrient ratios will also become more evident as will the proportion of raw to cooked food you'll require The majority of the food we match to your biochemical uniqueness in the proper proportions should automatically yield the right vitamin/mineral/phytonutrient/amino acid composition, but thanks to the nutrient depletion of food in modern times, we will have to precisely customize and synergize your supplements as nutrient insurance, accountability and augmentation so that your diet plan doesn't fail you in the slightest. It is best that we take no chances with your health and well-being.

### Metabolic Typing Procedures

At this point in old school metabolic typing, I would take you through a series of typing worksheets which will allow me to score your body type characteristics and group them into discernible categories of metabolism.

I begin to type you by scoring you on the basis of your blood type (ABO), height, weight range, body fat percentage, pulse rate, hair characteristics (curly, profuse, balding pattern), skin factors (smooth, soft, rashy, thick, bumpy, eruptive, sensitive), bone and muscle descriptions (small, thick, highly toned, soft, medium, long, large), overall shape (long, thin, compact, symmetrical, curvaceous, broad shouldered, angular, round, large forehead), skin color (black, white, brown, yellow, red, albino), dream states (PSI transmitter, PSI receiver), personality factors (nervous, highstrung, meticulous, aware, sensitive, receiver, physically oriented, flirtatious, sensual, food oriented, jolly, charismatic, love oriented), intelligence characteristics (creative, leader, survivor, social, flexible, practical, intuitive, technical). The net result of this process is to fit you into an endocrine gland category based on glandular dominance and to identify the recessive glands and their proportions of balance in relation to one another. Blood type and endocrine type are closely correlated. Blood typing will help in categorizing foods as theoretically right and wrong for you while endocrine typing helps delineate micronutrient needs and proportions. Let's say that in your case you have a "B" type blood and your height is medium (5'5" female). Your weight range is usually pretty stable and medium (except for the 10 pounds you just put on), your pulse rate is 66 beats per minute, your blood pressure is 120/80 mmHg., your hair is curly, your skin is thick, your muscles are toned and thick, your bones are pretty thick and dense, your overall shape is compact, your head and face shape is rather square, you dream a lot and you're very practical when it comes to the physical and you're mildly athletic. In this case, skin can be any color (although a good proportion of African descent people fall into this category). After rating you from the above criteria, it becomes obvious based on typing art and science that you turned out to be a characteristically pure adrenal type (*as presented in Table III in chapter V*). From these charts (hypothetically) your adrenal gland is considered to be the most dominant and the remainder of your other glands are proportionately recessive, although your thyroid is probably one of the weakest glands in your body.

For the purposes of this book, a full explanation of any or all the known metabolic types is outside its scope. Metabolic Typing is a very complex, very "soft" theoretical science which the science of orthomolecular testing has completely replaced. It tends to be too expansive for a complete discussion in *Your Personal Life* and is really not that clinically useful other than for interesting side notes and to let you know that it does exist. For now, for comparison's sake see Chapter 3, refer to **Table I & Table II**; see Chapter V, refer to **Table III & Table IV**. If more details are desired, please refer to Appendix D or contact the publisher (book@Angelmind.net) for special reports and additional information.

For the moment we hypothesize that you are a:

**Sympathetic dominant type with** a weak parasympathetic response. Continuous stress resultantly causes: migraine headaches, nausea, chest pains, diarrhea, rapid pulse, low blood pressure, physical weakness, adrenal crisis, and ultimately suffocation, cardiac arrest and death with a high **oxidation pattern,** making much energy, but need to conserve oxygen, (by taking greater amounts of antioxidant nutrients).

We've now (hypothetically) determined that you are a Blood Type B negative adrenal dominant type. We'll end this visit by explaining more about the implications of being an Adrenal Type in terms of the way your body metabolically functions and in what nutrients it supposedly (that is before testing) requires. Your metabolic characteristics are:

**Physicality:** Adrenal Types generally have: toned muscles that are strong and prominent with large and/or dense bones and large features; hair is usually coarse and curly; skin is dry, warm and thick; neck and fingers are usually short and thicker than average with generally large and round jaws and teeth.

**Personality:** tend to be fairly easygoing and possess great energy and endurance levels. They are strong and physically oriented, like and in most cases love exercise and prefer physically oriented careers. Professional sports, the police force, the military, business (very competitive) and skilled trades are attractive to Adrenals. They tend not to live in fear or suffer much anxiety but do tend to be less sensitive and creative than some of the other types, preferring concrete things over abstract things. Anger is slow to build but can lead to violence when aroused. Generally, Adrenals are more competitive and aggressive than average.

**Metabolic and Dietary Factors:** Possess a large amount of oxidation at a medium rate, which has much to do with their great energy and endurance properties. Along with these properties, they have excellent muscle control and are dependent on vigorous exercise for optimum metabolic function; possess good digestion and are rarely ill by nature; have a full range of digestive enzymes which ensures sufficient digestive function in the consumption of foods and are therefore classified as "omnivorous"; thrive on a high-protein diet to maintain musculature and also require a high protein to carbohydrate proportion with medium fat amounts within their personal zone; autonomic nervous system is considered sympathetic-parasympathetic balanced or slightly sympathetic dominant; typically don't suffer from confusion much nor are overtly lazy and mentally out of it. Milk digestibility is a function of other dependent variables like race and upbringing and of course existing nutritional status, which will be investigated further. The intake of dense starches is limited to exercise output. The thyroid gland tends to be weaker by comparison while primary toxin elimination is primarily handled well by the bowels and kidneys. The greatest lifestyle problem we have is tending to abuse the body sometimes through improper food choices, inconsistent exercise, and inadequate rest, all due to an inherent attitude of invincibility; characteristically think of self as physically tough and almost able to withstand anything. Because of this "invincibility" attitude, tends to suffer from heart and circulatory problems if left unchecked.

**The Diet Connection:** As a "B" blood type, adrenal dominant your best over-all *protein sources* should be by old standards and would <u>theoretically</u> include:

| | | |
|---|---|---|
| Red meats | Yeast | Fish |
| Sea plants | Chinese cabbage | Cucumbers |
| Poultry | Sprouts | Parsley |
| Beans | Milk (conditional) | Eggs |

Your best overall *fat sources* should include:

| | | |
|---|---|---|
| Avocado | Egg yolk | Butter |
| Raw nuts/seeds | Olive oil | Cream |

Your best overall *carbohydrate sources* should include:

| | | |
|---|---|---|
| Whole Grains (limited) | Bananas | Yams |
| Peaches | Plums | Potatoes |
| Grapes | Cherries | Melon |
| Citrus Fruits | Leafy greens | Squashes |
| Broccoli | Cruciferous vegetables | Celery |

### Chart 1:
### Theoretical Omnivore Type Diet Adjusted For Adrenal Patterns

| FOOD TYPES | HEALTHY FOODS | LEAST HEALTHY FOODS |
|---|---|---|
| Dairy Products | European descent: butter, yogurt, cottage cheese, kefir, NO milk | Oriental and other descent: no milk products at all |
| Eggs, Fats | Lightly cooked eggs, unprocessed seed oils, avocado | Margarine, sesame |
| Meats, Poultry, Fish | Most meats: beef, lamb, liver, organ meats, all fowl, some fish (light-colored, deep cold-water fish) | Certain fish: trout, tuna (dark), opal eye fish, salmon, salmon caviar, all caviar, turtle, snake, some shellfish |
| Vegetables | Leafy green vegetables: lettuce, spinach, swiss chard, cabbage, seaweeds, kelp, spirulina, snow peas, celery, bamboo shoots, water chestnuts, alkaline vegetables:, squash, cucumber, starchy vegetables: potatoes, sweet potatoes, yams, beets, carrots, cruciferous vegetables: broccoli, cauliflower, brussel sprouts, asparagus, other: tomato, pepper, eggplant | Unusual mushrooms, artichokes, corn, pumpkin, avocados, radishes |
| Grains | All grains: wheat, oats, rye, rice, millet, barley | All bleached and highly processed grains |

| FOOD TYPES | HEALTHY FOODS | LEAST HEALTHY FOODS |
|---|---|---|
| Nuts, Seeds | Most seeds and nuts: almonds, brazil, filberts, pecans, sunflower | Peanuts, sesame seeds, cashews, pumpkin seeds, pignolias |
| Fruit | All fruits: apple, apricot, citrus, dates, papaya, grapes, plums, figs, melon, pear, berries, pineapple, nectarine | Pomegranates, persimmons, rhubarb, coconuts |
| Beverages | Herb tea, vegetable and fruit juices, pure water, vegetable broth | Carbonated soft drinks, coffee, black tea, hard liquor, cocoa |
| Miscellaneous | Carob, raw honey, maple syrup, malt, onions, herbs, sweet spices | Chocolate, sugar, salt, junk foods, hot spices, pepper, corn syrup |

<u>Adrenal Type Supplementation:</u> The best and worst food groups and supplements are baseline categories to be further refined through Steps 3, 4, and 5 as we approach total nutritional customization.

***Best vitamins and their relative daily intake range:***
(This represents the rough daily intake range most adrenal types will fit into optimally. Typing Steps 3 and 4 will narrow these levels to individual specific amounts.)

> A: 20—30,000 IU as both fish oil and beta carotene
> D3: 400—800 IU
> E: (d-alpha tocopherol) 400—800 IU
> F: (alpha linolenic, cis-linoleic, gamma linolenic acids) 500 - 1000 mg.
> B Complex: 75 – 150 mg.
> C Complex: 500 – 1500 mg.

***Best minerals and their total intake range:***

> Calcium: 400—600 mg.
> Magnesium: 250—400 mg.
> Phosphorus: 10—24 grains from, lecithin origin
> Chromium: 25—50 mcg.
> Vanadium: 5—10 mcg.
> Selenium: 25—50 mcg.
> Copper: 6—10 mg.
> Zinc: 25—50 mg.
> Manganese: 15—20 mg.
> Iodine: 25—50 mcg.

*Best other Vitamin-like substances*:
(Their presence in the diet is of primary necessity but ranges have not been
determined by research as of yet.)

| | |
|---|---|
| Thyroid and adrenal | Melatonin |
| Glandular extracts | Yohimbe bark |
| Bee pollen | Shitake and reishi mushrooms |
| Spirulina | Proanthocyanadins |
| Alfalfa | |
| L-tyrosine | |
| CoQ10 | |
| Chlorophyll | |
| Bromelain | |
| Lecithin | |

## *Putting it Together*

We have developed a strictly theoretical database of information about
you (my hypothetical patient) in terms of your body's metabolic
strengths and weaknesses and created an outline of what food and supplements in their respective proportions should work optimally for you.
Because you are not a pure tribal phenotype descendant like a Hunzan
or Georgian, there has been some genetic interaction between other tribal lines which has modified you in some ways. If you were a pure Lake
Titicacan, I would put you on this society's average tribal diet but with
some other typing specifications unique to your profiled biochemistry
that is different from other tribal members. I would determine those differences in Step 3 (Laboratory Nutrient/Toxin Assessment). In your case
of impure tribal lineage, I still have the majority of categorical and correlational metabolic and nutrient data needed in order to have a thorough understanding of what is generally right for you allowing for small
race-specific and ethnicity adjustments. Adrenal types are found in all
races but with some recognizable race specific differences I have already
noted in your special case.

The information I have collected about you so far is still in a rough theoretical form in this step. This metabolic typing data affords interesting
insights into exactly how to plan and compare against Step 3's reality
checkup laboratory-testing portion of your overall personalized nutrition
procedures. By the completion of Step 3, I will have a very thorough

understanding of your current metabolic status—measured directly—in extreme detail. With that information in hand, we will then be able to fully customize your eating and supplement program specific to your needs and desired objectives.

### Step 3
*Testing aka Laboratory Nutrient/Toxin Assessment*

Up to this point, we should consider all the typing that we have accomplished so far as a fact finding research project on you, as my hypothetical patient. The process of typing works much like a PhD thesis when it's completed. We begin with the hypothesis that we can determine your biochemical uniqueness using the art and science of "typing" as a given. It's then up to us to prove that we can do this, beginning with assumptions about quantification and qualification and then proceeding through more stringent laboratory testing and retesting procedures to progressively narrow down the variables regarding your biochemical nature to a minimum. As an example of this, consider that as an adrenal type, sesame seeds are one of your worst foods. In Step 3, we can take a blood specimen and test the IgG4 immunoglobulin allergic response to sesame seeds, either proving or disproving our worst food assumption. If it comes up positive, the theory is then validated. But most of the time it doesn't match, which in effect demonstrates that our pure "typing" is highly imprecise in relation to this particular criteria because of the most important variable of the moment—the nutrient retention pattern itself. Step 3 allows us to further separate fact from fiction as the specifics of uniqueness are further revealed up to the moment and to the last accountable denominator. This is where the true value of laboratory assessment lies. Ultimately, a synergistically customized diet with supplements will reflect everything we've learned about your body, and if you're allergic to sesame or if it does not contain the right nutrients in the right balance for your body at the moment, you can be assured that it will not be part of your customized nutrition program. If your testing reveals that you need more magnesium in proportion to calcium, it's in there. If your urine is too acidic, you can be assured that you'll find alkalinizing foods and supplements in your program, and so on.

### *The Four Factors of Metabolism*

In this Step 3, our special orthomolecular laboratory tests are most directed towards evaluating the four components or factors of nutrient metabolism. The designated laboratory tests will reveal your uniqueness in each of these: ***digestion, absorption, assimilation, and elimination*** submetabolic processes. This information provides some important pieces in the overall metabolic puzzle that we could only guess about prior to recent advancements in laboratory technology

### *The Four Metabolic Factors Under the Microscope*

### *Factor One: Digestion*

How can we best determine just how well foods are being digested? Upsets in regularity, symptoms of heartburn, nausea, gas, stomach and abdominal pain, diarrhea and constipation are all signs of poor and/or incomplete digestion. Even so, we still need to take a closer look at this process to fully comprehend your nutritional status and customize nutrition accordingly. Are proteins, fats, or carbohydrates individually or all together difficult for your body to digest? Is it one type of protein or fat that's causing the problem? Is your digestion being adversely affected by low stomach acid or some digestive enzyme deficiencies or due to intestinal damage or perhaps from some hidden disease, irritation or parasite infiltration? These and other questions can be easily answered with the appropriate digestive function studies or correlated nutrition tests. The specific laboratory tests (used to examine all four metabolic factors) are not typically considered conventional although at some time in the future (probably within the next ten years or so) they may become standard practice to some degree, inside and outside of the doctor's office once we get beyond our drug-taking epidemic.

The appropriate metabolic factors of digestion can be found in saliva, stool, urine, breath, and blood specimens and correlated by mineral testing to some degree.

In our hypothetical case as an omnivorous Adrenal Type, digestion theoretically should be good across the board. But we really can't be sure about this without the proper laboratory evaluation in this step. Specialized orthomolecular assessment enhances our understanding of your digestive uniqueness up to the moment and in relation to any processes of digestive deterioration we need to know about. Any part of your digestive process not functioning properly, for whatever reason that we don't detect and correct in your nutrition workup program, can upset metabolism and health forever, no matter how good your diet and supplements may appear to be. So it's critical that we get it right from the start and don't miss any details.

Without getting into great detail about all of the possible test procedures that we can apply to your case, I will simplify *the key procedures we examine*:

- digestive markers or the digestive efficiency of food components such as triglycerides (fat), chymotrypsin (an enzyme), pH (acidity/alkalinity) and immunoglobulin presence
- metabolic markers such as your specific short-chain fatty acid fingerprint, L-glutamine and lysosomal levels
- the presence of bacteria both harmful and beneficial to the digestive process such as salmonella (harmful), lactobacillus (beneficial) and the balance of your intestinal microbial flora overall; also yeast and other parasitic infiltration
- stool color, mass, and blood content
- laboratory measurement relationships, so that a dysbiosis index is given representing the relative functional efficiency of the gut lining in terms of bringing the good stuff into the body and keeping the bad stuff out of the general circulation to be solubilized and/or excreted directly; the presence of a "leaky gut syndrome" is something which shows up even more clearly in the toxin profile of metabolic factor four—elimination

When considering the digestive process and aside from poor nutrient absorption and glandular insufficiencies which lead to deficiencies, one of our biggest health enemies is the body's absorption of incomplete or partially digested foods which can ultimately lead to allergic reactions – some easily detectable, others hidden. Hidden allergic reactions are difficult for detection because your body's response is very subdued at this point in the digestive/absorptive process, unless the IgA immunoglobulin reacts, causing some kind of digestive symptom. Realize that at this point most people just pop an antacid or "purple pill" instead of paying attention to this irritation as a defense mechanism. Subdued allergic reaction or a delayed food sensitivity response is an allergic phenomenon that is considered directly responsible for much of the development of degenerative disease people suffer from, since conventional medicine usually doesn't detect or focus upon this less obvious problem. When this sensitivity is properly detected and corrected, symptoms and metabolic degeneration disappear. Proper digestion is so very critical that I suggest ways to maximize the efficiency of this life-dependent process in every way possible. Slow down when you eat, chew your food well, eat according to your nutrition test results, take the digestive enhancement supplements customized for you and don't drink excessive fluids, especially coffee, with your meals. This is good advice for one and all.

### Factor Two: Absorption

When complete and efficient digestion take place, nutrient absorption should proceed smoothly. Leaving nothing to chance in our quest for true biochemical individuality, we must closely examine this process. Blood, urine, saliva, hair, and stool evaluation all come into play here as we look for:

- normal and/or abnormal amounts of long-chain fats, cholesterol, all other fats, and metabolites such as indican (a byproduct of tryptophan, the amino acid, from its own metabolism within the gut)
- the presence of most vitamins, minerals and other vitamin-like substances in blood, hair, and urine, which indicate that at least they are present (or not); this is known as "static status." We can't be sure of their functional status within the body until metabolic factor three, assimilation, with its differential comparisons is examined
- the occurrence of toxic factors such as heavy metals, free radicals, and enzyme inhibitors (alcohol, tobacco, barbiturates, sulfonamides, isoniazid, xenobiotics, formaldehyde, benzene rings, trimellitic anhydride, etc.)

### Factor Three: Assimilation

This physiological process needs to be carefully checked in order to ensure that the nutrients you consume are actually being properly utilized by the body and not just simply passing through, creating systemic stress, concentrated feces, and unnecessarily expensive urine. All laboratory specimens are utilized here as we reveal:

- the presence of vitamin/mineral, fatty acid, and protein (amino acid) deficiencies
- the proportion of macro-and micronutrient ratios
- the presence of vitamin/mineral overload
- certain enzyme activity in the processing of nutrients
- the status of some of our body's detoxification pathways (chemical reaction pathways which convert harmful substances into harmless substances ready to excrete)
- pertinent hormone and immunological activities

### Factor Four: Elimination (Excretion)

This particular metabolic end process is just as critical as the first three metabolic factors and therefore warrants close examination. What goes in bears little resemblance to what goes out, unless your body is a living sieve. Eliminative efficiency is a "sticking point" for the three previous metabolic factors. If it backs up or slows down, a reverse metabolic overload results. Your body then becomes a dumping/collection site for waste materials, the toxicity of which slowly consumes your health, undermining the previous three metabolic factor functions, creating high physiochemical stresses and resultant energy deprivation. You quickly begin to deteriorate. Improper elimination creates resistance to the very energy of life and is therefore exceedingly dangerous. In this regard, the majority of body specimens are utilized to reveal:

- allergic reactions you may be having to foods; the good news is that many of these food sensitivities can successfully be overcome with the right rotational approach
- your individual detoxification pathways and their efficiency, since biochemical uniqueness includes your own characteristic detoxification pattern
- the presence or nonpresence of certain key detox elements or precursors made by the body or lacking in the diet

You can probably see by now that there's a lot more to being an old school "Adrenal Type" (or any type for that matter) than you'd imagine. Through the appropriate assessment of your unique-to-you metabolic factors of digestion, absorption, assimilation and elimination in combination with the other aspects of your personalized nutrition workup we can create a very clear picture of what your metabolic/biochemical individuality really is all about, even replete with disease tendencies due to cross-correlated laboratory studies. We now have all the data necessary to proceed to Step 4 of the process, which entails fully customizing your diet and supplementation specific to what we've already learned about your human uniqueness from the preceding steps.

### Step 4
### Diet and Supplementation Customization

#### Part 1
In old-school terms, I would need to go back through the calorie computation/quantification and qualification of your diet and then compare the criteria revealed by Step 2, Metabolic Typing, and Step 3, Laboratory Nutrition/Toxin Assessment. In effect, I would have to correct and refine your custom diet to the necessary specifications called for by Steps 1, 2, and 3 and according to your specific personal objectives, which are a 10-pound weight loss and an optimum health and fitness gain. To accomplish this, I'd go through a lengthy multistep ruling-in and ruling-out procedure. The ruling in procedure consists of retaining the foods best suited to your

metabolic and biochemical uniqueness according to the sum total of all of our previous personalized nutrition in Steps 1 through 3. The ruling-out process consists of deleting foods that you are proven to be directly allergic to or that we reveal are not right for you due to other testing factors such as your body's mineral/vitamin content, pH levels, enzyme intermediates (organic acids), amino and fatty acid balance, and glycemic index. At this point in the program all other generically obvious land mines are removed as well. These land mines to be eliminated from the diet consist of all the known generic man-made food additives/irritants and carcinogens such as bleached flour and sugar, nitrates, nitrites and erythrobates (additives found in cured meats like bacon); any other food preservatives which are unnatural; and all unnatural additives, binders, fillers, extenders, etc. Suffice it to say that your personalized nutrition program will only recommend the healthiest, most wholesome, properly synergized organic food selection with options for variety and calculated rotations for favorable metabolic stimulation. The intra- and inter- macronutrient proportions will be adjusted to your testing specifications and equal the daily target calorie level (2,000 calories) when added together mathematically. The inter- micronutrient proportions are present in the diet, but we still need to supplement precisely per test results in order to compensate for nutrient density variations (beyond our control) in whole foods, accelerate results, and provide more nutrient input control.

### Part 2

We can proceed to have your supplements customized through laboratories that specialize in customizing supplements in accordance with your specific needs as we've measured them. They must be designed to account for nutrient synergy and antagonism (previously referred to as law of opposites, seesaw effect, IAND, etc.). To go along with Part 1 of our customization process, we may further need to build in certain short-term detoxification procedures of diet and supplements to help your body clean out certain elimination systems and any highly upsetting toxins present. Detoxification procedures should never be taken lightly. According to Dr. Udo Erasmus, "Most healers agree that degeneration can only have two causes: malnutrition and/or internal pollution (poisoning, toxicity)." Nutrition must address the problems of internal pollution and malnutrition with equal vigor.

By now, as my make-believe patient, you've probably been overwhelmed by the complexity of what we've done so far to correct your nutritional program so that it's precisely matched to your actual needs. It seems complicated, at least in old-school terms, but down deep you know that this is what's truly necessary to get you back on the right track for life. In fact, from our workup so far, you've probably learned so much about yourself that you're really becoming your own self-responsible/self-directed nutritionist, replete with a scientifically designed plan of action at your fingertips. You are independent now of useless advice or dependence on others who don't know any better. There's now only one step left to take in about two to four months down the line.

### Step 5
### *The Final Step – Re-Evaluation & Retests*

The next nutritional step consists of double-checking your body's response to the customized nutrition program designed for you. After all, we have to assess and double-check your progress in order to make sure that the program is working on the deepest biochemical levels, aside from the fact that you've probably most effortlessly lost the ten pounds you wanted to lose and you already feel so much better overall that you can hardly believe it. We must always analyze the effectiveness of the program and your personal compliance level. Your test results should demonstrate across-the-board improvements in everything we've evaluated, from your former vitamin/mineral deficiencies to your toxic accumulation factors to the overall metabolic stress indicators regarding digestion, absorption, assimilation, and elimination. If testing demonstrates that there are more program adjustments necessary, they will be made automatically in order to promote even more concise and/or faster results. Future retests must be used to double-check progress again to keep things on track. At this time we must face any compliance issues which may have possibly inhibited optimum benefits or have not been discussed previously. We will adjust the program as needed. Now you are fully immersed in personalized nutrition and your results are magnificent so far and will continue forever. Congratulations and welcome to the best in health.

### *Old School*
### *Typing Process Overview*

### *Step 1: Calorie Quantification and Qualification*
Create a calorie and food-adjusted hypothetical rough diet. This step is based on standard generic scientific assumptions and predictions utilizing the science of

calorimetry and conventional nutritional philosophies. The information from this step is fully refined in accordance with biochemical individuality as revealed from the following steps.

### Step 2: Pure Metabolic Typing or Genotyping
Categorize body types by measuring and grouping physical and psychological characteristics with no specimen evaluation performed (other than blood type). Identify metabolic strengths and weaknesses to strategize the appropriate procedures for Step 3.

### Step 3: Testing aka Laboratory Nutrient/Toxin Assessment
Testing further refines our understanding of body type to its smallest denominator, nutrient retention, in the fulfillment of discerning biochemical uniqueness up to the moment. Nutrient deficiencies and overloads are revealed and a plan of nutrition action designed.

### Step 4: Diet and Supplementation Customization
We correct the rough diet from Step 1 and customize this diet specific to the information revealed from primarily Step 3 and secondarily Step 2. This ruling in/out process will help to fully individualize diet and supplementation in direct accordance with biochemical individuality and therefore manifest as a precise nutrition program replete with short- and long-term detoxification procedures.

### Step 5: Re-Evaluation
Re-measure all previous data to analyze the effectiveness of the program, the body's response and compliance level. This step primarily focuses upon the outcome of all the laboratory retests given in order to pinpoint exactly what metabolic improvements have or have not been made to help us further refine the program if necessary. In this step any compliance issues still remaining need to be remediated effectively.

After going through the steps presented in the Malibu Quick Check Appendix plus highlighting the proper foods and supplements, a fully customized diet and supplement program may end up looking like this for one day out of the week:

### Diet for Tuesday

| | Grams of Protein | Grams of Carbs | Grams of Fat | Calories or Kcals |
|---|---|---|---|---|
| **Meal #1** | | | | |
| 1 large soft-boiled egg | 7 | 5 | 4 | 82 |
| 2 large boiled egg whites | 8 | 0 | 0 | 17 |
| 8 ounces skim milk | 1 | 12 | 0 | 80 |
| 1 cup bran flakes | 1 | 30 | 0 | 70 |
| 1 slice whole grain toast | 1 | 15 | 1 | 70 |
| 1/3 cup grapefruit | 0 | 10 | 0 | 40 |
| 2 teaspoons butter | 0 | 0 | 5 | 45 |
| *TOTALS* | *18* | *72* | *10* | *404* |

**Meal #2**

| | | | | |
|---|---|---|---|---|
| 3 1/2 oz. tuna in water | 24.5 | 0 | 2 | 105 |
| 1 squirt lemon juice | - | - | - | - |
| 2 teaspoons light mayo | 0 | 0 | 5 | 45 |
| 2 slices pumpernickel bread | 2 | 30 | 2 | 140 |
| 1 cup raw celery | 0 | 6 | 0 | 25 |
| 1 cup raw carrots | 0 | 12 | 0 | 50 |
| 1 small apple | 0 | 10 | 0 | 40 |
| 12 oz. ice tea | - | - | - | - |
| *TOTALS* | *26.5* | *58* | *9* | *405* |

**Meal #3**

| | | | | |
|---|---|---|---|---|
| 3 1/2 ounce skinless chicken breast | 24.5 | 0 | 2 | 105 |
| 1 large baked potato w/skin | 2 | 30 | 2 | 140 |
| 2 tablespoons sour cream | 0 | 0 | 5 | 45 |
| 1 medium salad: | | | | |
| 2 cups lettuce | 1 | 6 | 0 | 25 |
| 1 large tomato | 2 | 12 | 0 | 50 |
| 1/2 cup cucumber | 1 | 6 | 0 | 25 |
| 1/2 cup broccoli | 1 | 6 | 0 | 25 |
| 1 tsp. safflower oil | 0 | 0 | 5 | 45 |
| 6 tsp. red wine vinegar | 0 | 5 | trace | 20 |
| 2/3 cup pineapple juice with 2/3 cup water | 0 | 20 | 0 | 80 |
| *TOTALS* | *31.5* | *85* | *14* | *560* |
| *DAILY TOTALS* | *76* | *215* | *33* | *1,369* |
| *ORIGINAL TARGET* | *71* | *214* | *32* | *1,424* |

***Special Note:*** There is roughly a 10% protein loss (1 gram out of each 10 grams ingested) due to a protein quality factor in foods. As a result, the daily protein total seems a little larger than it actually is. Subtract 8 grams (10% of 83) from this figure for a more realistic factor and add 8 grams to the daily carbohydrate total which reflects this protein's use as sugar by the body. A few extra grams of protein for extra exercise insurance is desirable. Calories don't change.

| | Grams of Protein | Grams of Carbs | Grams of Fat | Calories or Kcals |
|---|---|---|---|---|
| *NEW TOTALS* | *75* | *219* | *33* | *1,369* |

Lab/customized supplements:
ParaPak–two capsules with each meal three times a day
Adrenal Complex–one capsule with each meal three times a day
Min Plex B–two capsules with breakfast and lunch, one with dinner
HCL-Plus– one capsule per meal three times a day
Omega-3 Plus–1 capsule per meal three times a day
Vitamin C-Plus–one capsule taken with lunch
Crystalline–Customized aminos

*Welcome to the New School*

The above sample diet looks simple enough, but the reality of its accuracy and the complex task of achieving it was very extensive. Old-school personalized nutrition in-office for actors and athletes as reported on FOX news was a long, drawn-out, expensive, and complicated process. For purposes of discussion, I presented a very condensed picture in the above of what the Malibu Program was about and Malibu Quick Check Appendix contains many more details for your review and information. I processed many patients at Malibu using this approach in combination with a Blitzkrieg of all the metabolic typing worksheets and nutrition tests available at the time. The actual diets and reports made up small books of information unto themselves for each patient. It was not something that was generally conceded as affordable, convenient or efficient for the average person outside of Malibu, as was echoed on "CBS This Morning" by Dr. Bob Torman 15 years ago. But this is how it was.

Now, thanks to quantum advancements in computer and lab technology, it is most convenient and efficient, as you will see in Chapter 9, as you can start to take full control over your own nutritional destiny—something anyone and everyone can now do most economically and efficiently.

*A new scientific truth does not triumph by*
*convincing its opponents and making them see the light,*
*but rather because its opponents eventually die and*
*a new generation grows up that is familiar with it*
—Max Planck

# Chapter IX

## Determining Your Own Nutritional Prognosis— Taking Full Control

*One man's food is another man's poison*
—Lucretius

Old school is out and new school is now in session thanks to the latest generation of computer-correlated nutrition/metabolic/toxic/genetic testing along with its statistically matched, mathematically generated, personalizing, therapeutic, algorithmic protocols. The need to attempt to classify oneself as an omnivore, carni-vegan, or vegetarian with a certain blood type, sympathetic or parasympathetic dominance, neuroendocrine dominance (such as in the adrenal type/blood type B/sympathetic dominant metabolic type of last chapter's descriptions), sensory type, constitutional type, energy type, organ type, etc. is no longer necessary. In the face of orthomolecular medical research, this type of information is actually obsolete when it comes to the actual quality and quantity of nutrition your body truly needs at the moment. **Much of what follows is done simply, and automatically for you in the new school of nutritional analysis by both the lab and certified professionals, but needs to be quickly summarized for a more complete understanding of what is entailed.**

Please realize that in the new face of testing, I clinically have experienced people who have been from old school, fully metabolically typed not using tests and still, after testing, are found to have so many nutritional/toxic abnormalities it's surprising and somewhat alarming, even to me.

As examples of this, I've tested yogi and martial arts masters who thought they could self-apply Ayurvedic/Chinese medicine and spiritually "will" themselves healthy, who after testing turn out to have more nutritional inconsistencies than most of their followers. Other than the Laughing Yogi, Ramesh Pandey (who expected to be out of balance and even showed his first nutrition test on a TV show with me in order to warn his followers about the need for testing in modern times), the other yogis were extremely surprised, as were Ayurvedic/Seyervedic practitioners, martial artists, Chinese herbalists, iridologists, homeopathic doctors, nutritionists, dietitians, muscle testers, holistic health practitioners, chiropractors, medical doctors, personal trainers, and other healthcare practitioners. Athletes and fitness practitioners who all of their lives believed that their self-styled nutrition programs were so effective that they would never have nutrition test results that would be less than perfect, were all quickly enlightened when they found out the sometimes shocking truth—that they were out of balance more than they ever imagined! Vanity, ignorance, and arrogance have absolutely no place in science. A mind that opens to the truth always prospers.

Now it's our turn to stop taking these things for granted and effectively take nutritional control back to the full reality of the moment, and tightly control our own destiny—more precisely than ever.

In new school, no presumptions are ever made, as the true beginning of truth-seeking begins with a nutrition test, as compared to old school where a huge amount of data was compiled without tests and metabolic typing worksheets came first with testing coming later, if at all. In new school, testing always comes first where all else is secondary. Many old school practitioners tend to put more weight on geno/metabolic theory instead of testing first, until they learn about this incongruous pitfall.

After nearly 23 years of clinical experience from old school to new school, providing well over 100,000 types of nutrition tests in conjunction with the scientific literature, continuing educational seminars, and conferences, I must say that mineral testing from hair, or HTMA (hair tissue mineral analysis), has emerged as first and foremost on the priority list of tests necessary to perfect a personal nutrition plan. The high priority of HTMA is due to its focus on the absolutely most fundamental nutrients, minerals, its across-the-board metabolic scope, and correlated relationships to all the other nutrition/toxic tests. HTMA should be conducted in combination with a pH testing survey from urine and saliva (in order to ascertain severe alkaline or acidic states). Although blood type has very little connection to your nutritional needs at the moment, it always pays to know your blood type, no matter what. A highly simplified and condensed genotyping compilation of this frontline physical data as shown below should be undertaken for future comparative purposes:

## Geno/Metabolic Typing Information, pH, Blood Type, and Medical History + Initial Test

NAME_____ETHNIC ORIGIN_____(Caucasian/
Hispanic/Black-African American/Asian/Persian/Arabian/Indian/Other)
AGE_____ MEDICATIONS_____ *COMPLAINTS_____
*CLINICAL DIAGNOSES AND/OR SYMPTOMS_____
*you can refer to the list of diet-related diseases in Chapter 7 in order to help you to compile this information.
PREGNANCY STATUS_____
PHYSICAL DATA: Blood Type_____Height_____Weight Range_____
Pulse Rate (rest)_____Blood Pressure_____ Hair_____ Skin_____
Muscles_____ Bones___Body Shape___Head/Face Shape___
Childhood Dream States**_____Personality___Intelligence___Miscellaneous__
Fill out the following information *as best as you can.* Use the choices from the legend below for extra guidelines.

**NOTE: Vivid dreams – dreams in minute detail, easily remembered, start in childhood, can fade as one matures; intuitive dreams—dreams of future events that often come true; dreams where the thoughts of others are received; transmitive dreams – dreams where the individual takes control and creates a world that s/he wants.

### Legend for Choices

| | |
|---|---|
| **Blood Type:** | A, B, O, A B, Rh-, Rh+ |
| **Height:** | _____feet _____inches |
| **Weight Range:** | example: 110 – 120 lbs._____ |
| **Pulse Rate (rest):** | heart beats per minute at rest _____ |
| **Blood Pressure:** | systolic _____ mmHg diastolic_____mmHg Example: 120/80 |
| **Hair:** | profuse, silky and straight, coarse and wavy, male pattern baldness, slow balding over time, balding from front to back of head, |
| **Skin:** | eruptive, sensitive, dry/thick/warm, soft with rash tendencies, fatty/thick |
| **Muscles:** | small, prominent/toned, medium, soft-medium-sized, fatty/soft/large, long/lanky |
| **Bones:** | small, thick/dense/hard, medium, long |
| **Body Shape:** | thin/delicate features, compact/strong-looking, medium, females–curvy, males–large upper torso |

| | |
|---|---|
| | and/or barrel chest, round/chubby, long |
| **Head/Face Shape:** | delicate/small, square (especially jaw), very symmetrical, females—curvy, males—bald & angular, round/chubby, long, large prominent forehead |
| **Childhood Dream States:** | vivid dreams, intuitive dreams, transmitive dreams |
| **Personality:** | high-strung, nervous, sensitive/aware, very physical, affable/adaptable, sensual/sexual, jolly, emotionally sensitive, charismatic |
| **Intelligence:** | good technical ability, highly intuitive, practical, flexible, social, survival-oriented, creative, leadership tendency |
| **Miscellaneous:** | quick movements, psychic intuition, larger features, no overpowering physical/mental characteristics, Females—large hips and/or breasts, Males—large shoulders, chubby features, large rib cage, love an audience |

## Take pH for Acidity/Alkalinity—Directions for pH Test

1. Please use Precision Lab #114 strips if possible and perform 3-trials over a 3 day-in-a-row period.
2. A trial consists of touching one clean pH paper to saliva and one clean pH paper to urine, both for approximately 2 seconds. After 2 seconds, match the pH stick colors to the pH chart colors as closely as possible.
3. FOR BEST RESULTS, both pH and urine trial should be performed when first getting out of bed in the morning before eating or drinking.
4. Other Tips:
   Saliva Collection – pH paper can be placed under the tongue after working up a little spittle or spit into a very small clean glass and then dip the pH stick into the glass. (Precision pH paper is non-toxic yet we recommend gargling with salt water after testing for antiseptic reasons.)
   Urine Collection – In a small clean glass or Dixie cup collect about 1 to 2 ounces of midstream urine. (Midstream urine is that which is collected after a count of 2 following the initiation of the urine stream.) Dip pH paper into glass or cup for about 2 seconds, shake excess off and then match colors to chart as closely as possible.
5. Place the number that matches best from the pH charts (1–14) for the saliva and the urine stick below and put it on the charts supplied

TRIAL 1/2/3   URINE __/__/__/   DATE __/__/__/   SALIVA __/__/__/

**Blood Type Test:** If you or your doctor does not have your blood type on hand there are home and over-the-counter kits containing special Eldon Cards to collect a few droplets of blood, which are easily elicited from a fingertip by self-sprung automatic high-tech lancets that are included in these kits.

**First Test —Hair Tissue Mineral Test:** I clinically prefer the world's leading human hair testing medical lab which can now be obtained through mail order. After receiving this test report, you will understand your metabolism and know the following (in parts):

**PART I:** *MINERAL MEASUREMENTS and HTMA EXPLANATION*— Graphs on the first two pages provide measurements of: Mineral excesses, deficiencies, significant ratio imbalances, and toxicities in your body at this time. (The ultimate health goal is to be within the whitest areas or reference range on all graphs.)

**PART II:** *METABOLIC TYPE and NUTRIENT MINERAL LEVELS*— Contains your personal rate of metabolism as slow 1, 2, 3, 4, or fast 1, 2, 3, 4. The goal in this part is to understand how effectively your body utilizes nutrients in terms of glands, diet, digestion, infections, and other significant symptoms experienced. It also contains a discussion of nutritional mineral levels which reveal significant deviations from normal, whereby the goal is to understand which of the nutrient levels demonstrated are adversely affecting your health the most.

**PART III:** *NUTRIENT & TOXIC RATIOS and TOXIC METAL LEVELS*— Contains:
1. An explanation of how metabolic dysfunction occurs due to abnormal balances of minerals and related vitamins.
2. Symptoms of mineral imbalances, and common sources of toxic metals found.

**PART IV:** *DIETARY SUGGESTIONS*—Contains:
1. General dietary suggestions to correct your metabolic rate and number classification.
2. Explanation of food sensitivities (not included for those reports with low-allergy profiles exhibited).
3. Specific foods to avoid to improve metabolic balance and rate.
4. Specific foods to eat every day to improve upon metabolic rate and balance.

**PART V:** *CONCLUSION*—Contains objectives of the program and further explanations about excessive nutrient and toxic minerals.

**PART VI:** *SUPPLEMENT RECOMMENDATIONS*—Contains a list of completely customized and synergized laboratory-manufactured supplements which have been clinically proven to rebalance nutritional chemistries in cases most statistically similar to your own.

*TENDENCY REPORT SUPPLEMENT:* This very important section of the report contains a ***statistical correlation of disease tendencies.*** This is simply an indicator of illness or disease that has developed in cases based on other similar measurements.

*STUDY QUESTIONS* These points will help your overall understanding of your issues!

1.  Which minerals do I have in excess? Are there any vitamins associated with these excesses? Which ones and why?
2.  Which minerals do I have deficiencies of? Are there any vitamins associated with these excesses? Which ones and why?
3.  Which mineral ratios are too high? Are there any symptoms, metabolic rate effects, or gland/hormone/nerve antagonisms associated?
4.  Which mineral ratios are too low? Are there any symptoms, metabolic rate effects, or gland/hormone/nerve antagonisms associated?
5.  What is my metabolic type?
6.  Which toxic minerals are most clinically significant at this time?
7.  What are their common sources?
8.  What total caloric percentage of protein should I eat each day?
9.  What total caloric percentage of carbohydrates should I eat each day?
10. What total caloric percentage of fat should I eat each day?
11. Which foods should I avoid? Which foods should I eat more of?
12. Which supplements, by name, should I take? When and in what amount?
    BREAKFAST
    LUNCH
    DINNER
13. When should I take my follow-up tissue mineral analysis test (see special supplemental report). 2, 3, 4, or more months? (Mark the retest date on your calendar.)

From the above test information, a daily meal plan can be strategized very easily once you have the actual foods necessary to eat more of and those to avoid. There are also expanded food groups, which increase food choices, such as the following condensed list of food families:

*The Best and Worst Foods for Balancing Your Metabolism
as Expanded from Report Findings*

*TEST DATE: 1/01/06: #111111, Slow I Metabolism*

| FOOD FAMILIES | | FOODS |
|---|---|---|
| Plum | B | Plum, cherry, peach, apricot, nectarine, almond, wild cherry, prune |
| Papaw | B | Papaw, papaya, papain |
| Blueberry | N | Blueberry, huckleberry, cranberry, wintergreen |
| Mustard | W | Mustard, turnip, radish, horseradish, watercress, cabbage, kraut, Chinese cabbage, broccoli, cauliflower, brussels sprouts, collards, kale, kohlrabi, rutabaga |
| Laurel | W | Avocado, cinnamon, bay leaf, sassafras, cassia buds or bark |
| Sweet Potato or Yam | B | Wheat, corn, rice, oats, barley, rye, wild rice, cane, millet, sorghum, bamboo sprouts, yams, sweet potato, amaranth |
| Grass | B | Parsley, aster, corn, tomato |
| Orchid | N | Vanilla allspice, cloves, pincato, guava |
| Protea | N | Macadamia nut |
| Birch | W | Filberts, hazelnuts |
| Conifer | N | Pine nut |
| Fungus | N | Mushrooms and yeast (Brewer's yeast, etc.), aspergillus, penicillin |
| Bovid | B | Milk products—butter, cheese, yogurt—whey, lamb, beef, goat, venison, bison |
| Tea | N | Sassafras, papaya leaf, mate, lemon verbena, comfrey, fennel, Kaffir, alfalfa, fenugreek |
| Oil | W | Corn oil, butter, fats from any bird on this list, soybean, peanut, cottonseed, safflower |
| Sweetener | W | Cane sugar, sorghum, molasses, corn syrup, glucose, dextrose, date sugar, orange honey, beet sugar, carob syrup, clover honey, buckwheat honey, safflower honey, sage honey |
| Citrus | B | Lemon, orange, grapefruit, lime, tangerine, kumquat, citron |
| Banana | N | Banana, plantain, arrowroot (Musa) |

| FOOD FAMILIES | | FOODS |
|---|---|---|
| Palm | N | Coconut, date, date sugar |
| Parsley | B | Carrots, parsnips, celery, celery seed, celeriac, anise, dill, fennel, cumin, parsley, coriander, caraway |
| Spinach, Goosefoot | W | Beets, spinach, swiss chard, lamb's quarters (greens) |
| Pepper | N | Black and white pepper, peppercorn |
| Herbs | N | Nutmeg, mace |
| Cashew | W | Cashew, pistachio, mango |
| Bird | B | All fowl and game birds including chicken, turkey, duck, goose, guinea, pigeon, quail, pheasant, eggs |
| Grape | W | All varieties of grapes and raisins |

| FOOD FAMILIES | | FOODS |
|---|---|---|
| Pineapple | N | Juice packed, water packed, fresh |
| Rose | B | Strawberry, raspberry, blackberry, dewberry, loganberry, youngberry, boysenberry, rosehips |
| Melon (gourd) | B | Watermelon, cucumber, cantaloupe, pumpkin, squash, other melons, zucchini, acorn, pumpkin or squash seeds |
| Pea (legume) | B | Pea, black-eyed pea, dry beans, green beans, garbanzos, lentils, licorice, alfalfa, peanut, carob, soybeans |
| Mallow | N | Okra, cottonseed |
| Subucaya | B | Brazil nuts |
| Flaxseed | B | Flaxseed |
| Swine | N | Pork, ham, bacon |
| Mollusks | N | Abalone, snail, squid, clam, mussel, oyster, scallop, conch |
| Crustaceans | B | Crab, crayfish, lobster, prawn, shrimp |
| Apple | B | Apple, pear, quince, medlar, loquat |
| Mulberry | N | Mulberry, figs, breadfruit, hop |
| Olive | B | Black, green |
| Gooseberry | B | Currant, gooseberry |
| Buckwheat | B | Buckwheat |
| Aster/Daisy | B | Lettuce, chicory, endive, escarole, artichoke, dandelion, sunflower seeds, tarragon |
| Potato/Nightshade | N | Potato, tomato, eggplant, peppers (red & green), chili pepper, paprika, cayenne, ground cherries |
| Lily (onion) | B | Onion, garlic, asparagus, chives, leeks, shallot |

| FOOD FAMILIES | | FOODS |
|---|---|---|
| Spurge | N | Tapioca |
| Herb | N | Basil, savory, sage, oregano, horehound, catnip, thyme, spearmint, peppermint, marjoram, lemon balm, cilantro |
| Walnut | W | English walnut, black walnut, pecan, hickory nut, butternut |
| Pedalium | W | Sesame |
| Beech | W | Chestnut |
| Saltwater Fish | B | Sea herring, anchovy, cod, sea bass, sea trout, mackerel, tuna, swordfish, flounder, sole, snapper, roughy |
| Freshwater Fish | B | Sturgeon, herring, salmon, whitefish, bass, perch, trout, pike catfish |

*B* = *BEST* "B" placed next to specific family in order to notate that you must take selections mostly from these food groups.

*W* = *WORST* "W" placed next to specific family in order to avoid eating from these food groups.

*N* = *NEUTRAL* "N" placed next to food groups that don't particularly hurt or help in rebalancing metabolism. Ns are generally limited to two times per week.

* *An asterisk (to be filled in after testing) can be used to itemize miscellaneous foods that can be eaten up to 2X per week.*

** *(to be filled in after testing) is reserved for worst individual foods which may be part of a food family that contains other best foods, which can happen on occasion.*

Before you can line up foods in proper amounts and Zoned proportions, we need to understand the difference between fast and slow metabolisms a little more clearly.

## Slow Metabolism

### Definition
Slow utilization of nutrients by the cells
Low efficiency of nutrient utilization by cells

### Reason For
Slowdown of nerve and glandular (hormone) systems which reduce cellular metabolism
Specific disturbances in the nutrient status of the body which undermines all cells (including nerve and gland cells)

### Identification
Telltale signs of nutrient relationships measured in the body (generally, more sedative minerals present than stimulatory ones)

### Heat Production
Low, gets cold easily, especially in hands and feet

### Energy Levels
Very low, tires easily, tending to be more pessimistic and depressed from lack of energy

### Body shape (when overweight)
Pear, usually gains fat in hips and thighs

### Fatigue Factor
High

### Incidence of Obesity
Very high

### Blood Sugar Pattern
When blood sugar is higher, falls asleep easily; when lower, more awake

### Premature Aging Factor
Increases as metabolism slows down due to lack of intracellular renewal from low energy reserves, causing degeneration

### Sleep Profile
Can suffer from Type II insomnia: falls asleep easily, restless sleep, wakes up feeling tired, suffers from sleep-related fatigue syndromes

### Personality
Performs as the perfectionists fast types would like to be, great ability to follow a complicated project through to completion, may face major hurdles to expressing their deeper emotions, low self-esteem and feelings of inferiority, good team players, can have much patience, don't live only for the job, more reserved than fasts

### Personal Goal on Nutrition Program
Turn a slow metabolism into a faster, fat-burning, more efficient one

### Fast Metabolism

### Definition
Fast utilization of nutrients by cells
High efficiency of nutrient utilization by cells

*Reason For*
Very active nerve and glandular tissues which accelerate or maintain strong cellular metabolism
Specific balance of body nutrients which promote all cellular functions (including nerve and gland cells)

*Identification*
Telltale signs of nutrient relationships measured in the body (generally more sedative minerals present than stimulatory ones)

*Heat Production*
High; feels warm and perspires easily

*Energy Levels*
Very high, tend to be more positive, optimistic and self-assured from constant energy

*Body shape (when overweight)*
Apple, usually gains fat in abdomen

*Fatigue Factor*
Low

*Incidence of Obesity*
Low

*Blood Sugar Pattern*
When blood sugar is high, becomes euphoric; when lower, very stressed and irritable

*Premature Aging Factor*
Decreased, unless metabolism becomes too fast, causing cellular burnout which in turn degenerates cells quickly

*Sleep Profile*
Can suffer from Type I Insomnia: difficulty falling asleep, sensitive to noises, may suffer night cramps or tremors

*Personality*
Intellectually cerebral, likes perfectionism, jumps from subject to subject-without completion, difficulty relaxing (hyped up), easily agitated, "stress-aholics," big egos, want to be center of attention, self-important, often late for work, difficulty delegating duties to others, live to work, talks too much so others can't speak, addictive, impatient

*Personal Goal on Nutrition Program*
Bring nutritionally disturbed, over-fast metabolisms into perfect balance

### *What is Your Metabolic Rate? (You Really Need To Know)*

Because we are each so unique, our nutrient requirements vary dramatically from others, even family members, due to the efficiency (speed and completeness) of how we each process every nutrient and toxin in our food and supplements. Some nutrients get rejected, others are processed quickly and effectively, while others are retained by the body in excess. As a result, *we each demonstrate distinctly different nutritional holding patterns* that our primary mineral test interprets and then nutritionally corrects with customized diet and quantum-factored supplements.

After measuring the exact nutrient balance of thousands of foods interspersed through the 50 major food families, we know precisely which foods and supplements are necessary to accelerate or rebalance metabolism back to its genetic best. We retest your metabolic rate to monitor this process for guaranteed success—and, if you follow the personally designed and recommended program, your metabolism will change and become faster, or slow down if its too fast from irritation.

The personalized nutrition medically approved, clinically proven, scientifically engineered, completely customized food and supplement programs utilized will effect a faster, more "maximum metabolism" (burning) of fat and accelerated energy production than any other approach to metabolic maintenance there is. In other words, a faster metabolism creates more energy, less fat and waste, less toxic accumulation, and an overall healthier body.

### *8 BASIC METABOLIC TYPES*
### *As Classified by Rate of Metabolism_*

### *SLOW METABOLISMS Types I-IV*
Approximately 80% of the American population today is categorized as slow metabolizers, more than any other country in the world! The U.S. is also #1 in the world for diet-related disease. This reflects our epidemic state of slow metabolisms characterized by more obesity and overweight syndromes, chronic fatigue syndrome, more osteoporosis, wide-

spread diabetes, rampant heart disease, legal and illegal drug dependencies, unrelenting Alzheimer's, allergies, cancer, and many other degenerative diseases. The U.S. has more of these illnesses and diseases than any other country in the world. We are all born as fast metabolizers, but thanks to personally mismatched and generally unhealthful eating and supplement habits, combined with poor-quality lifestyle habits starting in childhood, we manage to turn them into dangerously (disease promoting, fat-fostering, genetically antagonistic), slow metabolisms. NO EXCUSES APPLY as research shows statistically, unhealthful states and premature aging are not your genes fault, as many would like to think. You have more control over your own metabolism (and genes) than you think, if you only take the time to understand them, and then do what's scientifically recommended to correct them!

### *What's Your Rate?*
### *Slow Metabolism*

### *SLOW METABOLISM TYPE I–IV Characteristics*
(Reminder: Manifestations of the emotional and physical characteristics of both fast and slow metabolizers depend on a number of factors including degree or severity of mineral/trace element imbalances including vitamins and amino acids, endocrine [hormone] activity and the length of time imbalances have been present.)

Parasympathetic Dominant in I–IV- = Energy-slowing nervous system = a sluggish and diminished energy production (less energy to use, more fat stored)

Thyroid gland activity = slow/decreased from ideal levels (low energy)in I & II and increased in III & IV

Parathyroid gland activity = fast or increased in I–IV which increases calcium loss from bone and results in low energy

Adrenal gland activity = decreased in I, & III (causing low energy), and increased in II & IV

Stomach acid = insufficient digestion in I & II which diminishes energy varies in III & IV

Pancreatic activity = decreased enzyme production with increased sugar hormone production in I, II, IV, varies in III, all resulting in lowered energy production

Body shape consideration = usually pear-shaped, sometimes banana (long & tall) when lean, more apple-shaped in III & IV

Energy profile = constant fatigue in Is while IIs, IIIs, & IVs fluctuate

high to low, with periods of extreme fatigue
Disease susceptibility I–IV highly variable relative to other variables but fundamentally degenerative in nature
Toxic retention rate I–IV = very high leading to low energy
Stress/Index = Is–constant low to high degrees equals long-term energy drain, IIs – acute stress; IIIs–prolonged emotional stress with large mood swings; IVs–very acute stress reaction.

### *Fast Metabolism*

### *FAST METABOLISMS TYPE I–IV*
There are a few factors which cause a person to become a fast metabolizer. The majority of children inherit their respective mineral retention patterns from their parents both genetically and environmentally. With few exceptions, almost every child is born with a fast metabolic rate. A fast metabolism is nature's way of ensuring that every child has the metabolic resources for a quick and constant growth rate.

From an environmental standpoint, a family's eating habits can either reinforce a fast rate or slow it down considerably. In effect, a family's eating habits can lock in their offspring's biochemistry as fast or slow, on a highly permanent basis. A faster metabolism is generally better to possess for fat and health control. This is good when balanced, but an unsynchronized over-fast metabolism can be very dangerous, especially when exposed to prolonged stress.

Unfortunately, even though slow metabolisms invite many diseases, imbalanced fast metabolisms are especially prone to cardiovascular disease, peptic ulcers, histamine-related allergies, some types of arthritis and diabetes. Fast metabolic types can usually eat more and gain less than Slows, but they can still pack on excess fat, mostly around the abdominal region, if they constantly overeat. In time they usually end up with an apple-shaped physique when they persist in imbalanced eating practices.

### *FAST METABOLISM TYPE I–IV Characteristics*
Sympathetic Dominant in I–IV = a high-energy utilizing, highly reactive autonomic nervous system
Thyroid gland activity = increased in Is & IIIs; decreased in IIs & IVs
Parathyroid gland activity = decreased in Is & IIIs; decreased in IIs & IVs

Adrenal gland activity = increased in Is & IIs; decreased in IIIs & IVs

Stomach acid = high to moderate in I–IIIs, variable in IVs

Pancreatic activity = enzymes decreased in Is and IVs, variable in IIs & IVs; hormones generally increased in I–IV.

Body shape consideration = lean muscular to apple; when body fat is low

Fast I–IVs usually retain more muscle tone (than slow types) with "squarer" builds, although IIs & IVs seem to fatten into apples easier

Energy profile = very high—with stress-induced and/or hypoglycemic mood swings—to very low at times

Disease susceptibility–highly variable, more relative to less degenerative in Is, more reactive immune response in IIs, IIIs, and IVs

Toxic retention rate = high or low depending upon other variables

Stress Index = usually constant from high to low; IIs are acute, IIIs are very high, IVs are at stress burnout levels

NOTE: According to Dr. David Watts, no matter which type you are determined to be, it's most beneficial to bring all minerals and their ratios into balance over time. When this occurs you will end up either as a fast slow I or a balanced fast I, which are classified as the most healthful, age-resistant, high-energy-sustaining and fat-free metabolic types.

## *Dietary Zones*

HTMA reports refer to a specific macronutrient zone, usually expressed as a 40/40/20 ratio (for certain slow I metabolic rate/types) or (40% of calories from proteins/40% of calories from carbohydrates/20% of calories from fat). In certain slow and fast metabolic rate/types who demonstrate a protein catabolic pattern, a 50/25/25 may be indicated, or in certain fast and slow types a 33.3/33.3/33.3 ratio can be called for, and there are times for other ratio combinations as well. Your test-given Zone will help you to promote the fastest, most efficient metabolism at this particular moment in time as determined by laboratory research. The Zones can change as your body favorably responds to the Targeted Nutrition Therapy recommended in your latest report.

Arranging these macro Zones into a daily meal plan consists of three condensed steps:

*Step 1* Organizing foods into precalculated calorie amounts according to weight or portion size.

248

It's best to use weight measures at first—ounces or grams—in order to organize foods into proper proportions. (I know that a lot of people hate to weigh things but two weeks of doing this is all you need for the rest of your life. For the sake of science and best health, you'll be able to quickly drop weight and eye portion size quite easily.)

*Proteins* 1 oz. of low-fat protein = 7g of protein. Low-fat protein is protein which has approximately 2-3 grams of fat or less in it. If there is more fat in the protein, this will add calories. Obviously, it is desirable to have low-fat protein when keeping calories down. **For example,** extra-lean ground beef is considered to be approximately 7% fat, whereas lean ground beef is considered to be 15% fat, and regular ground beef is usually somewhere between 25 to as high as 30% fat. So it follows that the fattier meats possess more calories and provide less protein than leaner meats.

For ease of application consider the following list as your low-fat proteins, (taken from the Food-families chart above) which equal about 7g of protein and 2 to 3 g of fat, max, and about 55 calories per 1 oz. serving:

*Bovid Family:* extra-lean beef, lamb, goat, bison, venison, nonfat or very low-fat cheese, skim milk, nonfat yogurt
*Bird Family:* chicken, turkey, duck, goose, cornish hen, pigeon, quail, pheasant, ostrich, egg whites
*Swine:* pork, ham
*Crustaceans:* crab, crayfish, lobster, prawn, shrimp
*Mollusks:* abalone, clam, squid, mussel, oyster, scallop, snail
*Saltwater Fish:* bass, cod, flounder, roughy, sole, swordfish, tuna
*Freshwater Fish:* bass, catfish, perch, whitefish, trout, tilapia, salmon*
*Salmon is considered to be low-fat protein, but it is also a high purine fish which must be used sparingly by slow metabolic types or until metabolism accelerates adequately.

The following represents higher fat proteins, which are those that at 1 oz. contain approximately 6 g of protein and 4-5 grams of fat, and add up to about 84 calories.

*Bovid Family:* high-fat-content cuts of beef, (such as filet mignon), or any milk product with regular fat content—except for soft cheeses (brie, Camembert), cream and egg yolk, which are considered to be a different category
*Swine:* tenderloin, sausage

*Saltwater Fish:*   halibut, sea herring, anchovy, mackerel
*Freshwater Fish:*   sturgeon, herring, some cuts of salmon

When it comes to *carbohydrates* we have 5 types to consider:

*Dense starches:* complex vegetable carbohydrates which contain the greatest amount of calories; 1 oz. = 30 usable calories = 7 grams of digestible or net carbs

*High fiber/low starches:* complex vegetable carbohydrates which contain fewer calories than dense starches due to a higher indigestible fiber content; 1 oz. = 15 usable calories = 3.5 grams of digestible or net carbs plus 3.5 grams of unusable carbs (fiber)

*Super high fiber/micro starches:* complex vegetable carbohydrates which are predominantly fiber and contain very little starch, if any; 1 oz. = 7 usable calories = 2 grams of digestible or net carbs plus 5 grams of unusable carbs (fiber)

*Simple sugars:* some vegetables like carrots but mostly fruit, which predominantly contain sugar as fructose with varying degrees of fiber; 1 ounce = 30 usable calories = 7 grams of digestible or net carbs

*Refined/concentrated sugar:* the least desirable of all carbs; 1 ounce = 45 usable calories = 12 grams of digestible carbs with no fiber whatsoever

The following represent food families, according to the type of starch that is characteristic of them.

### *Dense starches*

| | |
|---|---|
| **Sweet Potato/Yam** | wheat, triticale, corn, oats, barley, pumpernickel, rye, all rices |
| **Pea/Legume** | peas, lima beans, black-eyed peas, black-brown-pinto-navy-red-dry beans, soybeans |
| **Potato** | all potatoes, no matter what color |
| **Buckwheat** | all buckwheat, kasha, amaranth and greens not considered wheat |

## *High fiber/low starches*

| | |
|---|---|
| **Mustard** | turnip, all cabbages, broccoli, cauliflower, brussels sprouts, kraut, rutabaga |
| **Beet** | beets, swiss chard and all chards |
| **Mallow** | okra |
| **Potato** | tomato, eggplant |
| **Melon (gourd)** | all gourd type of squashes or those with hard shells such as butternut squash |
| **Aster** | artichokes |
| **Lily/Onion** | onion, garlic, asparagus, leeks |
| **Olive** | any kind of fresh olives |

## *Super high fiber/micro starches*

| | |
|---|---|
| **Mustard** | watercress, collards, kale, kohlrabi |
| **Sweet potato/Yam** | sorghum, bamboo sprouts |
| **Grass** | parsley, aster |
| **Fungus** | mushrooms |
| **Parsley** | celery, parsley, coriander, cumin, celeriac |
| **Beet** | spinach, lambs quarters (greens) |
| **Melon (gourd)** | all squashes not contained in gourds such as zucchini |
| **Aster** | all lettuces, including chicory, endive, escarole, romaine |

## *Simple Sugars*

| | |
|---|---|
| **Plum** | plum, peach, apricot, nectarine, wild cherry |
| **Blueberry** | blueberry, huckleberry, cranberry, wintergreen |
| **Citrus** | orange, lemon, grapefruit, lime, tangerine, kumquat, citron |
| **Banana** | banana, plantain, arrowroot (Musa) |
| **Palm** | date |
| **Grape** | all grape varieties |
| **Pineapple** | pineapple |
| **Rose** | strawberry, raspberry, blackberry, dewberry, loganberry, youngberry, boysenberry, rosehips |
| **Melon** | all melons including watermelon and cantaloupe |
| **Apple** | apple, pear, quince |
| **Mulberry** | fig, breadfruit |
| **Gooseberry** | currant |

### *Refined/Concentrated Sugar*

Any concentrated sugar (from any food source including fructose, sucrose, dextrose, maltose, glucose, etc.)

*Fats* can be categorized into 2 basic groups:
saturated fats
unsaturated fats
They both have different properties but have the same caloric value, which is 1 gram = 9 kcal, and given that 1 teaspoon of concentrated fat such as olive oil = 45 calories which = approx. 5 grams or about 1/5 of an ounce. Here are the food sources:

### *Saturated Fats*

| | |
|---|---|
| **Laurel** | avocado |
| **Red Meat** | lamb, pork,sausages or filet mignon or tenderloins, |
| **(Bovid mostly)** | very soft cheeses, butter, and cream |
| **Nuts** | macadamia, hazelnuts, cashews, walnuts, chestnuts, almonds, pecans; all have a significant amount of saturated fat in them along with unsaturated fat |

### *Unsaturated Fats*
(All nuts listed above) plus:

| | |
|---|---|
| **Pea** | peanuts and groundnuts |
| **Birch** | filberts |
| **Conifer** | pine nuts |
| **Subcaya** | brazil nuts |
| **Oil** | corn oil, bird/fowl family oils (such as chicken fats for soup), soybean, peanuts, cottonseed, safflower, sunflower canola, flaxseed |
| **Seeds** | flaxseed, pumpkin, sunflower, psyllium |

### *Quickly Compute Calories*

I.   Take out your calculator—you must estimate your BMR first.
     Males burn 1.0 calories per kilogram of body weight per hour, which equals 24 calories per kilogram of body weight per day. Females burn 0.9 Calories per kilogram of body weight per day, which equals 22 calories per kilogram of body weight per day.

So take your weight in pounds and divide by 2.2 (pounds per kilogram).

A) Your weight_____ divided by 2.2 = _____Kgs.

B) Your weight_____multiplied by 22 or 24 = _____calories/day.
(Multiply your weight in kilograms by 24 for males and 22 for females.)

Note: Subtract 10% of this figure (BMR) if you are over 40 years of age and/or you have a slow metabolism; add 10% of this figure (BMR) if you are under 21 years of age and/or have a fast metabolism.
Also, Kcal = Calories

II. Next you must calculate your Daily Physical Activity Need (DPAN) by choosing one of the following categories:

| | | |
|---|---|---|
| _____ Bed rest | = 0 Kcals or Calories | |
| _____ Very light activity or sedentary (Light work, no formal exercise) | = 1/4 BMR (25% of BMR) 0.25 multiplied by BMR | |
| _____ Light activity **(Light-duty job** combined with 30 minutes of exercise 3–4 days/week) | = 1/3 BMR (30% of BMR) 0.33 multiplied by BMR | |
| _____ Moderate activity **(Light-duty job** combined with 5 to 9 hours of exercise/week or **moderate duty job** combined with 2–5 hours of formal exercise per/week) | = 1/2 BMR (50% of BMR) 0.50 multiplied by BMR | |
| _____ Moderately heavy activity **(Light-duty job** combined with 10 to 15 hours of exercise/week or **moderate duty job** combined with 5 to 10 hours of exercise/week) | = 3/4 BMR (75% of BMR) 0.75 multiplied by BMR | |
| _____ Heavy activity **(Heavy-duty job** combined with 5 or hours of exercise/week— armed forces recruits or national and professional athletes, 15 or more hours of exercise/week) | = 1 BMR (1 full BMR) 1 multiplied by BMR | |

*Light-duty job*—very light activity such as a sitting or standing with minimal walking as in a desk job or light housework

*Moderate-duty job*—moderate activity where one is moving or lifting most of the time as in a waitress or warehouse type job

*Heavy-Duty Job*—heavy activity where one's on one's feet most of the time and has to constantly carry heavy objects as in trades such as construction or masonry

Note: Except for professional athletes, most of my patients fall into the first four categories of DPAN. Aerobics Instructors should fit into DPAN categories on the basis of how many hours they teach per week (usually moderate to heavy activity or 50–100% & of BMR).

> **Example:** Your hypothetical category is moderate activity which = 1/2 BMR
>
>    Your BMR (plus) DPAN   =  _____

III. Last, you must add in your Specific Dynamic Activity (SDA). To calculate SDA: Take 6% of your combined BMR and Daily Physical Activity Need (DPAN) measurements:

> Your SDA equals: BMR + DPAN = _____Kcal
> .06 X _____Kcal          = _____Kcal          .
>               SDA      = _____ Kcal
> Then ADD all together:
> BMR___+ DPAN___ + SDA___ = TCND (Total Caloric Need Per Day)___

This last figure represents your energy need per day. The next step is to make a decision about whether you want to lose, gain, or maintain weight. To maintain weight, do not change the Total Caloric Need Per Day figure (TCND). To gain weight healthfully, add 500 Kcal to this figure. To lose weight efficiently, subtract 500 Kcal from this figure to determine your Target Calorie Level (TCL):

IV. Your TCND + or - 500 = _____Kcal = Target Calorie Level or TCL

**Note**: This 500 caloric addition or subtraction/day translates into a 3,500-calory gain or loss per week or 500 Kcal multiplied by 7 days = 3,500 Kcal. Since, 3,500 Kcal is equivalent to 1 pound of fat, you will lose approximately 1 pound of fat/week on a weight loss program (negative calorie balance). On weight gain programming (positive calorie balance), you will gain approximately 1 pound of mostly muscle if you exercise hard enough, although some of this gain may be from fat as well. To not risk any fat gain whatsoever, it is best to stay on a neutral calorie balance which is your Total Caloric Need per Day and let the exercise program harden up your body by building muscle as your body naturally reduces its body fat composition concurrently. Those under 18 years old should add 300 calories (if weighing under 150 pounds) or 500 calories (if weighing over 150 pounds) in to their Total Calorie Need per Day to allow for normal growth patterns if they are exercising regularly.

Now that you know your Target Calorie Level (TCL), we must compute your macronutrient balance based on each macronutrient calorie percentage scientifically recommended for good health:

EXAMPLE as a Slow I from your test:

| | |
|---|---|
| Protein | 40% |
| Carbohydrate | 40% |
| Fat | 20% |

**YOUR** ZONE I PERCENTAGES if not a Slow I:
     Protein___Carbohydrate___Fat___

Now that you know the ideal calorie percentages, these calories can be converted into food weight so that you can precisely measure food intake. The Atwater Coefficients presented previously in chapter 8, are used to accomplish this where 1 gram of protein or carb = 4 Kcal., 1 gram of fat = 9 Kcal. and 1 gram alcohol = 7 Kcal.

(In your case, substitute your own figures)     *Your Case*
(TCL)    ____ *multiplied by .40 (40% protein)*    = *Kcals protein* _____
          ____ *multiplied by .40 (40% carbs)*    = *Kcals carbs* _____
          ____ *multiplied by .20 (20% fat)*     = *Kcals fat* _____

The above equals the TCL for each macronutrient.

**VI.** Now convert percentages of food weight (in grams):
___ (Kcals protein) divided by 4 Kcals (per gram)= ___ grams of protein/day
___ (Kcals carbs) divided by 4 Kcal (per gram) = ___ grams of carbs/day
___ (Kcals fat) divided by 9 Kcals (per gram = ___ grams of fat needed/day

The above macronutrients must then be spread out over 3 meals/day.

Now we must obtain the right amount of protein, carbohydrate and fat from real foods. Here is a basic food-grouping chart to help you to understand where to obtain these foods (see Best and Worst Foods for Rebalancing Your Metabolism from earlier in this chapter and Basic Food Family Spread sheet Later in the chapter).

### Sample Diet Formatting

*Step 2* Choosing the foods that your report findings recommend.

*Step 3* Placing those foods into a daily meal that is calorie correct for your special metabolism.

### Hypothetical Statistics

1,500 calories at 40% calories from protein, or 137 g-(600 divided by 4.35 calories per gram of protein); 40% calories from carbohydrates, or 144 g-(600 divided by 4.15 calories per gram of carbohydrate); 20% calories from fats, or 33 g-(300 divided by 9 calories per gram of fat).

1,500 divided by 3 meals = approx. 500 calories or slightly less per meal to allow for a snack of about 120 to 150 calories; approx. 40 g of protein, 40 g of carbohydrate, and 11 g of fat per meal as follows:

### Breakfast

*Protein* – 41g. or 180 calories
3 egg whites (an extra-lean protein) – 12 low-fat protein grams
1 whole egg (a high-fat protein) – 8 high-fat protein grams
3 oz. lean smoked turkey breast deli slices – 21 low-fat protein grams

*Carbohydrate* – 42g. or 175 calories
2 slices of whole-grain bread (a dense starch carbohydrate) – 30 carbohydrate grams
1 tablespoon low-carb fruit spread (sucralose sweetened) – 2 (net) carbohydrate grams
one medium-sized orange (a simple sugar carbohydrate) – 10 carbohydrate grams
12 oz. licorice tea flavored with Splenda = 0 calories/protein/carbohydrate/fat

*Fat* – 9g. or 81 cal.
1 egg yolk (a very high-fat protein) – 4 saturated fat grams
2 slices whole-grain bread – 2 unsaturated fat grams
3 oz. turkey breast – 3 unsaturated fat grams

(TOTAL – 436 calories)

256

### Snack
1 whey-based protein bar

*Protein* – 15 low-fat protein grams

*Carbohydrate* – 15 simple carbohydrate grams

*Fat* – 5 saturated fat grams, 4 unsaturated fat grams

(TOTAL – 150 calories)

### Lunch
**Protein** – 38 g. or 165 calories
6 oz. solid white tuna in water – 38  low-fat protein grams

*Carbohydrate* – total 36 g. or 148 calories
6 oz. lettuce/greens (super high fiber/micro starch) – 12 carbohydrate grams
1/4 cup (2 oz.) carrots (simple sugar) – 6 carbohydrate grams
1/2 cup (4 oz.) cucumber (super high-fiber carb.) – 6 carbohydrate grams
1 tomato (high fiber/low starch) – 6 carbohydrate grams
1/8 cup onions (1 oz.) (high fiber/low starch) – 6 carbohydrate grams
16 oz. iced green tea (decaffeinated)—sweetened with Splenda or stevia = 00

*Fat* – total 8 g. or 72 calories
1 teaspoon olive oil –7 unsaturated fat grams
6 tablespoons vinegar –1 unsaturated fat gram

(TOTAL – 385 calories)

### Dinner
*Protein* – 42 g. or 185 calories
6 oz. (extra lean – 7 % fat) grilled beef burger – 38 low fat protein grams
1 teaspoon grated Parmesan cheese – 2 high-fat protein grams

*Carbohydrate* – 36 g. or 150 calories
1/2 small or 3 oz. sweet potato (dense starch) – 10 carbohydrate grams
1 cup steamed zucchini (super high fiber starch) – 16 carbohydrate grams
1 small apple (simple sugar) – 10 carbohydrate grams
16 oz. lemon water
*Fat – Fat* – 10 g. or 90 calories
fat from burger – 8 saturated fat grams
2 tablespoons of butter buds (for sweet potato)—0

(TOTAL – 425 calories)

*Actual Total Calories  = 1,400 allowing 100 calories for miscalculations or hidden values*

## MACRONUTRIENT QUALIFICATION
## RATIOS WE CONSIDER

### BASIC FOOD FAMILY SPREAD SHEET

| Proteins | Complex Carbs (cal dense) | Complex Carbs (cal dilute) | Simple Carbs | Fats/Oils |
|---|---|---|---|---|
| 1ounce (or oz.) or 1 gram | 1 oz. or 1 gr. | 3oz./gr. | 2 oz./gr. | 1/4 oz./gr. |
| Salt W. Fish | Yam/Sweet Pot.* | Aster/Daisy (all lettuces) | Plum/Peach | Laurel/Avocado |
| Fresh W. Fish | Pea/Legumes/ Beans | Mustard/Cabbages/ Cruciferous | Blueberry | Cream/Butter |
| Crustaceans | Corn | Fungus/Mushr. | Papaw | Fatty Cheeses |
| Mollusks | Artichokes | Parsley/Celery | Citrus | Egg Yolk |
| Bovid | Jicama | Spinach/Goosefoot | Banana | Protea/Macad. |
| Cheese/Milk | Br. Rice | Broccoli | Palm | Birch/Filberts |
| Bird | Wheat/Oats* | Spinach | Rose/Berry | Flaxseed |
| All liver | Rye/Millet/Barley | Squashes (Gourd) | Pineapple | Conifer & Sunflower seeds |
| Tofu | Buckwheat | Herb | Melon | Cashews |
| Bison/Venison | Potato/ Nightshade | Lily/Onion/ Asparagus | Mulberry | Brazil Nuts/Cashews |
| Raw Milk | | Mallow | Apple/Pear | Almonds |
| Eggs | | Alfalfa Sprouts | Gooseberry | Peanuts |
| Lamb | | Mung Sprouts | Mango | Soybeans |
| Ham (non-cured), Pork, etc. | | | Guava | Walnut/Chestnut /Sesame |
| Lamb/Goat | | | Pomegranates | *All Oils |
| Snake Meats | String Beans | | Raw Coconut | Coconut Oil |
| Escargot | Horsegram | Cucumbers | Blackberries | |
| Gar Fish | Raw Roots | Seaweed | | |
| Turtle | Raw Tubers | | Tangerines | *Safflower Oil |
| Insects | White Mshrms. | | | *Sesame Oil |
| | White Rice | | Rhubarb | Processed Meat |
| High Purine Meats*** | White Bread | Eggplant | Apricots | |
| | | Peppers | Cantaloupe | |
| | Field Beans | Tomatoes | | |
| | Tora-Beans | Kelp | | |

*shared family members
***High purine proteins include: liver, kidney, heart, tuna, shellfish, sardines, mackerel, salmon, sturgeon, herring and anchovy.

### *Rule of Thumb Zones by Metabolic Type/Rate*

**Using the chart on previous page:**

*Most Slows* 40/40/20 = 1(gr. or oz.) protein to 1/3 (gr. or oz.) complex high-calorie carbs. to 1/3 low-calorie complex carbs to 1/3 simple carbs to 1/4 fats/oils. Or in rounder numbers, 3 parts protein or 3 gr./oz. to 1 part complex (high-calorie) carbs or 3 gr./oz. to 1 part complex (low-calorie) carbs or 3 gr./oz. to 1 part simple carbs to 1 part fats/oil or 1/4 gr./oz.

*Simply put,* protein and carb amounts (carbs are divided up evenly between the 3 types of carbs listed above) that are very much the same while fat is kept to a minimum

*Most Fasts* 2 parts high purine-proteins to 2 parts milk products to 1 part low-calorie complex carbs to 1/4 part high-calorie carbs to 1/4 part simple carbs to 1/2 part fat/oil

*Simply put,* lots of purine-rich and all meats/fish/fowl, dairy proteins with smaller amounts of carbs; especially high-calorie complex carbs which are held to a minimum in favor of low-calorie fibrous carbs and some fruit

These above ratios or zones should always be calorie corrected for best results. Once the above is put into action and your first HTMA retest is taken, the lab will compare results and refine the program further. This is the time to study your own body's response by examining the before and after status of your biochemistry and re-answering the same questions we had on the first test as a comparative such as: 1-What's my new rate of metabolism – slow 1, 2, 3, 4, or fast 1, 2, 3, 4? 2- What are my new nutrient mineral levels? 3 - What are my new symptoms of mineral imbalances? 4 - What are my new general dietary suggestions indigenous to metabolic rate and number classification? etc. Then recompute BREAKFAST, LUNCH, DINNER, and when a new test is advised, or if another type of test is called for because of a poor response, etc.

Note: At this point, unless you have your first HTMA retest in hand, it's impossible to tell which other test(s) you may need. For some people who are highly stressed or still have not lost a satisfactory amount of weight due to a total lack of adrenal response as demonstrated by their first HTMA retest, an Adrenal Stress Indication or, ASI, test might be indicated next to more closely examine the biochemical function of that gland. This would yield certain, even more specific target nutritional/adaptogenic therapies that could help accelerate imbalance correction as a synergistic complement to the HTMA program. A digestive function study might be indicated because a gas problem did not completely go away and the minerals related did not change significantly on the retest.

Perhaps energy levels did not climb high enough so that an organic acid analysis is called for. On the retest, other mineral relationships that show a breakdown in protein metabolism might indicate the need for an amino urinalysis test, which can then be undertaken and which then will customize a crystalline amino acid therapy program to accelerate the changes in this nonresponsive, weakened area of metabolism. Or a blood spot allergy test might be necessary because a certain food or two recommended from the original program by retest time still does not go down well. This could be investigated further and a special food rotation implemented as a result. Or, as in most cases, the retest shows obvious changes and a very satisfactory response and the patients is extremely happy with their results, both from a symptomatic and biochemical standpoint.

Because the results can vary greatly and optional test indications can vary as well, I've included questions that need to be answered for any of these other tests and then used to refine the nutrition plan and supplements further when it's required.

### GUIDE FOR ORGANIC ACID ANALYSIS
Please answer the following questions taking the information from the tests you have taken:
1. Which organic acids are too high or too low?_____
2. What corrective food and nutrition supplement sources does my test suggest are necessary? _____
3. What does my report say about toxins? _____

### GUIDELINES FOR INTERACTIONAL HORMONE TESTS
Please answer the following questions taking the information from the tests you have taken:
1. Which hormone compounds are excessive or deficient in my body? _____
   _____
2. What nutritional and/or environmental sources do my tests suggest are contributing to my body's hormone imbalances?_____
3. What does my report say to do to rid my body of imbalances? _____
   _____

### *GUIDELINES FOR VITAMIN ANALYSIS*

Please answer the following questions taking the information from the tests you have taken:

1. Which vitamin compounds are too high or low in my body? _____

2. What nutritional and/or environmental sources do my tests suggest are contributing to my body's imbalances? _____

3. What does my report say to do to correct the problems found? _____

### *GUIDELINES FOR AMINO ACID ANALYSIS*

Please answer the following questions taking the information from the tests you have taken:

1. Which amino acid compounds are too high or low in my body? _____

2. What nutritional and/or environmental sources do my tests suggest are contributing to my body's amino acid imbalances? _____

3. What does my report say to do to correct the problems found? _____

### *GUIDELINES FOR FATTY ACID ANALYSIS*

Please answer the following questions taking the information from the tests you have taken:

1. Which fatty acid compounds are too high or low in my body? _____

2. What nutritional and/or environmental sources do my tests suggest are contributing to my body's imbalance of these compounds? _____

3. What does my report say to do to correct the problems found? _____

### *GUIDELINES FOR LIPID PEROXIDES AND HOMOCYSTEINE*

Please answer the following questions taking the information from the tests you have taken:

1. Which of these compounds are too high in my body? _____

2. What nutritional and/or environmental sources do my tests suggest are causing a buildup of these compounds?_____

3. What does my report say to do to correct the imbalances found?_____

## GUIDELINES FOR DIGESTIVE EFFICIENCY

Please answer the following questions taking the information from the tests you have taken:

1.  What part of my digestion is not working properly? (protein, carbs, fat)
    _____

2.  Any toxic accumulation present? Please list._____
3.  What nutritional and/or environmental sources do my tests suggest are contributing to my body's weakened digestive process?_____
4.  What does my report say to do to correct the problems found?_____

## GUIDELINES FOR TOXIC ACCUMULATION

What can be done about heavy metal toxicity has demonstrated in my reports? The four cardinal rules to heavy metal detoxification as found in greater detail in Chapter VI are:

1.  Avoid exposure.
2.  Reduce absorption (reminder: a nutritional plan replete with a good variety of fiber is healthfully beneficial). The following foods are particularly useful in reducing the absorption of toxic metals and should be worked into the diet as much as possible.
    *   All kinds of beans—use them as liberally as you can, according to report findings.
    *   Most cooked vegetables—use liberally where possible.
    *   Whole grain breads—use liberally.
    *   Whole grain cereals and especially oatmeal (which heads the list)—use liberally.
    *   Most fresh fruits including apples and quinces, along with red wine, most helpful for uranium retention problems.
    *   Special supplements which can bind heavy metals such as bentonite, activated charcoal, and algal extracts which will be outlined by the close of the program.
3.  Increase elimination of toxins. There are a number of chelation therapies available depending on each case. The following are commonly used:
    *   Methionine
    *   Ascorbic Acid
    *   Lipoic Acid
4.  Ingest more of the most competitive nutrient elements as part of the principal of IAND or Interactive Antagonistic Nutrient Displacement. The customized supplements come in particularly handy here because they help to accelerate detoxification rates due to their potency than food alone. (Refer to Chapter 6 for a list of most commonly used toxic metal antagonists)

Please answer the following questions taking the information from the tests you have taken and the tables in Chapter 6:

1.  Which toxic compounds are in my body, and what nutrient minerals are they

competing against?_____
2. How much of each toxin is in my body according to the test results? _____
_____
3. What nutritional and/or environmental sources do my tests suggest are contributing to my body's burden of these toxins?_____
4. What does my report say to do to rid my body of these toxins including antagonists and chelation agents, if any?_____

### GUIDELINES FOR GENETIC EVALUATION
1. Which genes were found to be improperly functioning?_____
2. What weaknesses were the single nucleotide polymorphisms demonstrative of?_____
3. What corrective suggestions did the test make to help my body improve its metabolic functions?_____

*pH* If one is found to be to acidic or alkaline, the following is a reference table that we can use to quickly correct the problem as correlated with the results of the HTMA test.

If you are too acidic, consumption of the following foods will help rebalance your system, provided they are not least healthy for your type as demonstrated on your other tests.

| FRUITS/SUGARS | VEGETABLES | PROTEINS | NUTS & GRAINS |
|---|---|---|---|
| Apricots | Avocados | Cottage Cheese | No grains except for |
| Apples | Alfalfa | Cheese (white) | Kasha; no nuts |
| Bananas | Artichokes | Dairy Products | except for peanuts |
| Berries (all types) | Beans (string) | Milk | and brazil nuts; |
| Cherries | Beans (wax) | | pumpkin seeds and |
| Currants | Carrots | | squash seeds. |
| Dates | Cucumbers | | |
| Fits | Corn | | |
| Grapes | Cauliflower | | |
| Honey | Celery Knobs | | |
| Pumpkin | Greens (all types) | | |
| Persimmons | Kohlrabi | | |
| Rhubarb | Leeks | | |
| Syrup (maple) | Lettuce | | |
| | Okra | | |
| | Parsley | | |
| | Spinach | | |
| | Squash | | |
| | Sweet Potatoes | | |
| | White Potatoes | | |
| | Yams | | |

If you are too alkaline, eat more of the following foods that are not incompatible with your type.

| FRUITS/SUGARS | VEGETABLES | PROTEINS | NUTS & GRAINS |
|---|---|---|---|
| Grapefruit | Asparagus | All Meat, Fish | Chestnuts |
| Lemons | Beans (brown or white) | and Fowl | Barley |
| Oranges | Cabbage | | Grains (almost all |
| Peaches | Chickpeas | | grains, including |
| Plums | Eggplant | | wheat, rye, oats |
| Prunes | Lentils | | Etc.) |
| Raisins | Olives | | Pasta |
| Tangerines | Sauerkraut | | Rice |
| | Sprouts (brussels) | | Tapioca |
| | Tomatoes | | |

The general rules of thumb to either acidify or alkalize your body chemistry to achieve a more optimum pH balance are to use the above foods only for three days in a row and then retest pH from saliva and urine three days in a row until correction is achieved.

### Finally Taking Full Control: Balancing Mineral Ratios

Balancing mineral proportions is the most overlooked aspect of conventional nutrition yet is the most important variable of all. The relationship of one mineral to the next as synergism or antagonism, sedation or stimulation, yin or yang, acid or alkaline, has to be taken into account. Too much calcium in your system depresses the absorption of iron, which in turn increases the body's need for copper and so on. If one's heavy metal accumulation, like lead or aluminum, is found to be high, then increasing other mineral intake such as calcium, zinc, and iron can rid these killers from the body in combination with proper prevention measures. Many solvents are connected to toxic metals as well. Once the intake of minerals as food and supplements is corrected to actual body needs, the other variables of a perfect nutrition program can be fit into place harmoniously. This is why HTMA is so crucial to the process of personalized nutrition. If nothing else, it's important to memorize the following:

Which minerals do you have an absolute deficiency of?_____
Which minerals do you have a relative deficiency of and what are their ratio numbers? _____
Which minerals do you have an absolute excess of?_____

Which minerals are being antagonistic to one another?_____

Which minerals are most synergistic?_____

The lab-recommended programs will correct the above problems. It's helpful to think of the keynote foods which reverse these imbalances. As an example, a person may have a very high calcium to potassium ratio; that is, way too much calcium in the system relative to potassium. Strawberries reverse this ratio most directly not only because they contain primarily potassium and only a trace of calcium but also because they contain a phytonutrient, phytic acid, which literally leeches the calcium out of your soft tissue where it doesn't belong in the first place. Becoming a "strawberry-aholic" temporarily serves to accelerate rebalancing results. Those individuals that have this type of information make fewer mistakes. It pays to know yourself in these orthomolecular ways.

What drug/herb/homeopathic/mineral or nutrient interaction do I potentially have? (Check Appendix B for details)_____

### *Synergizing Vitamin Proportions*

Strategizing vitamin intake is based on a lab-simplified system of do's and don'ts specific to your test findings and in relation to vitamin-to-vitamin and vitamin-to-mineral synergies and antagonisms. If a test shows that you have a vitamin A deficiency, then vitamins C, E, B1, B2, B3, and B6 must be increased in order to increase vitamin A absorption, as well as increasing A intake from foods and supplements. Add too much E into the mix and you'll antagonize A utilization and depress the other vitamins synergistic to A. Your A deficiency may be caused by deficiencies of zinc, potassium, phosphorous, selenium, magnesium, and manganese, which showed up in your mineral tests. Balancing these nutrient chemicals and all others according to test results "bulletproofs" your body against metabolic breakdown.

### *Equalize Protein Intake*

After further testing amino acid profiles, it's time to proportion protein, food, and certain amino acid supplements in order to correct any imbalances found. Perhaps a given test reveals that your personal amino acid retention is low in the amino acid methionine, which is typical of overweight people and vego-vegetarians. To rectify this, simply consume more methionine-rich foods such as chicken, pumpkin seeds, and fish in order to compensate for the metabolic imbalance and to stimulate weight loss in conjunction with an L-methionine crystalline supplement in order to accentuate even faster results. Sulfur-rich aminos such as cysteine can be taken individually to draw heavy metals such as mercury out of the body when necessary. Other aminos layer into the nutrient customization process in total biochemical synergy when applied according to test results.

### *Proportion Fats*

If your test results reveal any fatty acid imbalances or disorders, highly specific foods and supplements can rectify the problem directly. A good example of this that I encounter frequently is deficiencies of Omega-6 fats as discussed in *The Zone* by Barry Sears, PhD. Omega-6 problems are remedied by a greater consumption of sunflower seeds, flax, certain other vegetable oils, and borage oil supplements in conjunction with balancing the minerals, vitamins, proteins, sugar, and glands tested.

### *Balancing the Sugar Equation*

Setting the ratio of one sugar to the next within the carbohydrate interzone is metabolically critical. Sugar intolerance reveals itself in nutritional sensitivity and mineral tests. Knowing about this biochemical criteria allows us to balance metabolism precisely by using sugar as high-energy-efficient metabolic fuel instead of as an antagonistic metabolic irritant. Easy-to-follow do's and don'ts simplify this process. It's fundamentally best to utilize the lowest glycemic foods (in the following tables) whenever possible in order to minimize hypo and hyperglycemic rebounds highly characteristic of many imbalanced metabolisms, especially the numerous slow metabolic rate/types 1, 2, 3 and 4 which are very sensitive to fast-blood-sugar releasing also known as high glycemic index foods.

As a reminder, GI or Glycemic Index is a number-based system designed to reflect the rate at which a given carbohydrate triggers an increase in circulating blood sugar. The higher the number, the more dramatic the increase in blood sugar levels, and the greater the insulin need to control ("insulin rebound" by a healthy pancreas). In the case of Type I diabetes m (mellitus), where the pancreas doesn't function properly to produce enough insulin, this phenomenon can lead to death if exogenous (from outside the body) insulin is not given to control blood sugar. In Type II diabetes, this same type of blood sugar phenomenon can take place but with one significant difference: the pancreas produces ample insulin but in spite of this, blood sugar levels can still rise dramatically due to an impairment of insulin receptors found on cell membranes. Dysfunctional receptors won't allow the sugar in blood to enter the cell, which otherwise would lower blood sugar levels before they reach health-threatening levels. In either case of diabetes, consuming low-GI foods reduces the likelihood of physiological damage to the body. Eating foods that have low glycemic indexes also reduce the chance for developing diabetes insipidus, whereby an overproduction of insulin (due to a heightened pancreatic response by a sensitive pancreas) drops sugar levels in blood to dangerously low levels (hypoglycemia). Altogether, Type I, II, Diabetes M and Diabetes Insipidus are much easier to prevent and control when low-GI foods are used in the personalized nutrition program. Generally, higher-fiber foods have lower GIs while more sugar/starch-dense foods are higher on the list. A low GI is classified as 55 or less, a medium GI is 56 – 69, a high GI is 70 or more.

Another helpful metabolic sugar impact measurement is known as the GL or Glycemic Load. GL is a mathematical value that reflects another dimension of food beyond the GI. Where GI demonstrates how quickly a given carbohydrate turns into sugar, GL rates this food property on the basis of how much of this same given carbohydrate is in a particular food. Using watermelon as an example, its GI is a high 72 plus while it's GL is very low at 4 (on a scale where 1–10 is considered low, 11–19 = medium, 20+ = high). Since GL is low for this food, it can be concluded that watermelon (per serving) has very low body-available carbohydrate to raise blood sugar levels. The remainder of what's found in watermelon per serving (not counting minerals, vitamins, aminos, water, fats, toxins, and pro-hormones) is termed "body-unavailable" substances, better known as indigestible fiber. In effect, we encounter a sugar content in watermelon that theoretically should rapidly turn itself into high blood sugar levels when eaten—but thanks to an indigenously high fiber content we'd have to eat a much larger serving of watermelon to cause a problem, as compared to foods with both high GIs and GLs which in effect will upset blood sugar levels significantly. The table below reflects GI ranges for some select foods. Those with an * are desirable as both low GI and GL foods. Use asterisked (*) foods whenever possible as suggested by your testing specifications. An expanded list is available from Angel Mind Publishing, Inc.

## GLYCEMIC INDEX RANGES

|  | LOW | HIGH |
|---|---|---|
| **Some Bakery Products** | | |
| Cake, Banana | 46 | 67 |
| Pizza with cheese | 60 | 86 |
| Muffins | 62 | 88 |
| | | |
| **Beverages** | | |
| Soy Milk | 30* | 43 |
| Orange Cordial | 66 | 94 |
| Most soft drinks | 68 | 97 |
| | | |
| **Breads** | | |
| Burgen Soy-Lin | 19* | 27 |
| Burgen Oat Bran & Honey | 30* | 43 |
| Burgen Mixed Grain | 34* | 48 |
| Barley Kernel Bread | 39* | 55 |
| Burgen Fruit Loaf | 43* | 62 |
| Rye Kernel Bread | 46 | 66 |
| Fruit Loaf | 47 | 67 |
| Oat Bran Bread | 47 | 67 |
| Mixed Grain Bread | 48 | 69 |
| Pumpernickel | 50 | 71 |
| Bulger Bread | 53 | 75 |
| Linseed Rye Bread | 55 | 78 |
| White Pita Bread | 57 | 82 |
| Rye Flower Bread | 64 | 92 |
| Oat Kernel Bread | 65 | 93 |
| Barley Flour Bread | 67 | 95 |
| High Fiber Wheat Bread | 68 | 97 |
| Wholemeal Flour, Wheat | 69 | 99 |
| Gluten Free Wheat Bread | 90 | 129 |
| | | |
| **Breakfast Cereals** | | |
| Rice Bran | 19* | 27 |
| Kellogg's All Bran Fruit-Oats | 39* | 55 |
| Kellogg's Guardian | 41* | 59 |
| All Bran | 42 | 60 |
| Bran Buds | 53 | 75 |
| Special K | 54 | 77 |
| Oat Bran | 55 | 78 |
| Muesli | 56 | 80 |
| Porridge (Oatmeal) | 61 | 87 |
| Cheerios | 74 | 106 |
| Corn Bran | 75 | 107 |
| | | |
| **Cereal Grains** | | |
| Pearled Barley | 25* | 36 |
| Rye | 34* | 48 |
| Wheat Kernels | 41* | 59 |

| | LOW | HIGH |
|---|---|---|
| **Cereal Grains (cont.)** | | |
| Instant Rice | 46 | 65 |
| Bulgur | 48 | 68 |
| Parboiled Rice | 48 | 68 |
| Cracked Barley | 50 | 72 |
| Quick Cooked Wheat | 54 | 77 |
| Buckwheat | 55 | 78 |
| Sweet Corn | 55 | 78 |
| Brown Rice | 55 | 79 |
| Wild Rice | 57 | 81 |
| White Rice | 58 | 83 |
| Couscous | 65 | 93 |
| Rolled Barley | 66 | 94 |
| Millet | 76 | 109 |
| Quick Cook Brown Rice | 80 | 114 |
| **Cookies** | | |
| Oatmeal | 55 | 79 |
| Rich Tea | 55 | 79 |
| Shredded Wheatmeal | 62 | 89 |
| Shortbread | 64 | 91 |
| Arrowroot | 67 | 95 |
| **Crackers** | | |
| Jatz | 55 | 79 |
| High Fiber Rye Crispbread | 65 | 93 |
| Breton Wheat Crackers | 67 | 96 |
| Rice Cakes | 77 | 110 |
| **Dairy Foods** | | |
| Low Fat Yogurt – Art. Sweet | 14 | 20 |
| Choc. Milk – Art. Sweet | 24 | 34 |
| Milk | 27* | 39 |
| Skim Milk | 32* | 46 |
| Low Fat Yogurt – Fruit | 33* | 47 |
| Choc. Milk w/ sugar | 34* | 49 |
| Yogurt | 36* | 51 |
| Yakult (fermented milk) | 45 | 64 |
| Low Fat Ice Cream | 50 | 71 |
| **Fruit and Fruit Products** | | |
| Cherries | 22* | 32 |
| Grapefruit | 25* | 36 |
| Dried Apricots | 31* | 44 |
| Pear | 37* | 53 |
| Apple | 38* | 54 |
| Plum | 39* | 55 |
| Apple Juice | 41 | 58 |
| Peach | 42 | 60 |
| Orange | 44 | 63 |

|  | LOW | HIGH |
|---|---|---|
| ***Fruit and Fruit Products (cont.)*** | | |
| Canned Pear | 44 | 63 |
| Grapefruit Juice | 48 | 69 |
| Orange Juice | 52 | 74 |
| Kiwi Fruit | 53 | 75 |
| Banana | 54 | 77 |
| Mango | 56 | 80 |
| Apricots | 57 | 82 |
| Pawpaw | 58 | 83 |
| Cantaloupe | 65 | 93 |
| Pineapple | 66 | 94 |
| Watermelon | 72 | 103 |
| | | |
| ***Legumes*** | | |
| Canned Soybeans | 14* | 20 |
| Soybeans | 18* | 25 |
| Red Lentils | 25* | 36 |
| Dried Beans | 28* | 40 |
| Lentils | 29* | 41 |
| Kidney Beans | 29* | 42 |
| Green Lentils | 29* | 42 |
| Butter Beans | 31* | 44 |
| Yellow Split Peas | 32* | 45 |
| Lima Beans | 32* | 46 |
| Garbanzo Beans | 33* | 47 |
| Kidney Beans | 34* | 49 |
| Navy Beans | 38* | 54 |
| Pinto Beans | 39* | 55 |
| Black-eyed Peas | 42* | 60 |
| Canned Pinto Beans | 45 | 64 |
| Romano Beans | 46 | 65 |
| Canned Baked Beans | 48 | 69 |
| | | |
| ***Pasta*** | | |
| Protein-Enriched Spaghetti | 27* | 38 |
| Fettuccine | 32* | 46 |
| Vermicelli | 35* | 50 |
| Whole Meal Spaghetti | 37* | 53 |
| Star Pastina | 38* | 54 |
| Durum Ravioli | 39* | 56 |
| Boiled Spaghetti | 36* | 52 |
| White Spaghetti | 41* | 59 |
| Durum Spirali | 43* | 61 |
| Capellini | 45* | 64 |
| Macaroni | 45* | 64 |
| Linguini | 46* | 65 |

270

|  | LOW | HIGH |
|---|---|---|
| **Root Vegetables** | | |
| Yam | 51* | 73 |
| Sweet Potato | 54 | 77 |
| White Potato | 56 | 80 |
| Carrots | 49 | 70 |
| Rutabaga | 72 | 103 |
| Baked Potato | 85 | 121 |
| **Soups** | | |
| Tomato | 38* | 54 |
| Lentil | 44* | 63 |
| Split Pea | 60 | 86 |
| Black Bean | 64 | 92 |
| Green Pea | 66 | 94 |
| **Sugars** | | |
| Organic Agave Nectar | 10* | 14 |
| Fructose | 22* | 32 |
| Lactose | 46 | 65 |
| Honey | 58 | 83 |
| **Vegetables** | | |
| Dried Peas | 22* | 32 |
| Dried Marrowfat | 39* | 56 |
| Green Peas | 48 | 68 |
| Sweet Corn | 55 | 78 |
| Lima Beans | 36* | 51 |

Other questions that the tests have answered for you are important to remember at this time as they have much to do with an imbalanced sugar mechanism:

Which proteins am I deficient in at this time? (Poor quality proteins are turned into sugar very easily at an undesirable metabolic cost.) _____

Which sugars do I have excesses of?_____

Which sugars do I have deficiencies of?_____

Which sugars are in antagonistic proportions?_____

What drug/herb/homeopathic/sugar or nutrient interaction do I potentially have?

**(Refer to appendix B.)** _____

### Applying Food Rotation and Detoxification

Please refer to Chapter 6 for the three phases of allergenic correction from which you can set up your own simplified charts as follows or simply follow the reports which should do this automatically for you. Laboratory tests reveal your hidden nutrition sensitivities and toxic accumulation, now it's up to you to systematically use the food rotation suggested and healthy results will be forthcoming:

## FOOD ROTATION CALENDAR

| WEEK 1 | |
|---|---|
| DAY | FOODS |
| 1 | |
| | |
| | |
| | |
| 2 | |
| | |
| | |
| | |
| 3 | |
| | |
| | |
| | |
| 4 | |
| | |
| | |
| | |
| 5 | |
| | |
| | |
| | |
| 6 | |
| | |
| | |
| | |
| 7 | |
| | |
| | |
| | |

## *Albert Einstein's New World*

From the theory of relativity to the relationship of body to mentality to spirit, the most celebrated scientist of the millennium and his followers have allowed for the organization of the human body into a quantum model of nutritional cause and effect. This model defines human life on the terms this book has been predicated. Genetically corrected, metabolically measured, individualized nutrition is an Einsteinian concept. In fact, Dr. Einstein became a vegetarian type of eater based upon his interest in this subject (as did Hitler, by the way). Profiling is a result of Dr. Einstein's most fundamental scientific efforts.

Your new world of wellness begins with a nutrition test, and thanks to countless researchers who've developed the scientific principles of orthomolecular medicine, the necessities of nutrition perfection can fall into place very efficiently and conveniently.

# Chapter X

## Your Personal Life of Wellness

*When we change the way we look at things,*
*the things we look at change.*
—Wayne Dyer

Taking back control over the nutrients that go into our bodies and then measuring exactly how they are utilized by the body is the most potent and personal life actualization mechanism for radiant health that we can employ. It takes the guesswork out of setting our bodies up for the greatest disease-resistant, longest, healthiest, most energetic, leanest life possible while it actually helps us to guard against inappropriate health and nutrition practices that we would otherwise be susceptible to without this personalized nutrition process in place. Its prevention potential is almost unlimited.

The knowing that comes from these insights provides us with the most potent tool we could have against the onslaught from those who promote and provide unnecessary, wrongful, unaccountable, dangerous and overpriced products and services. With our own tests in hand, we can't be talked into just anything anymore by sell-happy people in corporations whose private mandate is to attempt to take advantage of our ignorance and who don't care about our well-being, just our pocketbooks. Thanks to personalized nutrition, we can enjoy feeling younger and vital once again, with far fewer obstacles to the most productive life possible. It's literally a method of self-love based on the fact that when you love your body, it will love you back with better performance. You can finally know yourself better inside and out in ways you never thought possible. While there are those who disregard this advantage, by not taking this historical research and information to heart and acting on it, we who do are able to place ourselves way ahead.

*What to Expect—Final Considerations*

From the very start of this book we've outlined exactly how to make better use of the external environment in order to optimize your internal environment, or body chemistry. In this regard, we need to mention a couple of important wellness points that are first and foremost in many people's minds these days.

### *The Eicosanoid Connection or*
### *Not Getting Sick*

Achieving a balanced state of metabolism from the implementation of nutrition testing done right automatically includes systematically optimizing the occurrence of health-promoting eicosanoids. They are referred to in ***The Zone*** by Dr. Barry Sears, in books and articles by Dr. David Horrobin (the Godfather of essential fatty acids), in *Fats That Heal - Fats That Kill* by Dr. Udo Erasmus, PhD and in the Nobel Prize award of October 11, 1982 to two Swedes and a Briton (Sune Karl Bergstrom, PhD, Ingeman Samuel Berg, PhD and Robert John Vane, PhD). Although eicosanoids are in effect breakdown products of fatty acids formed inside of the body, which we in effect put under the microscope with testing, the topic warrants further discussion because of its importance to health.

*Eicosanoids* are considered to be the super hormones of the body. They are manufactured by every living cell in the human body. These fatty-acid-derived compounds arise, effect a physiological response, and then break down, all in mere seconds. There are literally hundreds of these compounds that are known about and perhaps thousands we don't know about yet. They impact on all of the body's regular hormonal systems, and each target cell, and also further exert control on just about every vital physiological function which sustains life. We know most about eicosanoids in regard to helping sustain and control the immune system, cardiovascular system, nervous system, respiratory system, and reproductive system. These compounds are believed to be involved in the control and function of every system of the body to some extent—in ways still not totally defined and understood. Ongoing orthomolecular research continues to reveal the hidden secrets of these essential-to-life molecular body constituents. Eicosanoids are a family of biological chemical compounds which include prostaglandins, prostacyclins, leukotrienes, lipoxins, hydroxylated fatty acids, and thromboxanes. They are derived from two dietary unsaturated fatty acids (Omega-6 and-3) which are considered as essential fatty acids, and one nonessential activated fatty acid known as gamma-linolenic acid which can be made by the body or found in dietary sources. The Omega-6 essential fat is chemically called cis-linoleic acid and the Omega-3 essential fat is called alphalinolenic. The Omega-6 is found mostly in vegetable oils and the Omega-3 is found primarily in fish oil. A related nondietary essential fat is called arachidonic acid and is found in red meats or manufactured by the body. Arachidonic acid is considered essential only in its ability to progressively convert into certain classes of eicosanoids but isn't necessary to be taken in from dietary sources. Eicosanoid production proceeds through a series of enzyme-mediated desaturation and elongation biochemical steps from the initial dietary forms of Omega-6 and Omega-3 fats. Eicosanoid production depends on the initial presence of the dietary 3s and 6s (called substrates in enzymology), the concentration and availability of all involved enzymes and their coenzymes (cofactors or vitamin/minerals), the proportion of the opposite-effect sugar-control hormones glucagon and insulin to each other and the actual concentration of products (eicosanoids and related products) already created by this metabolic subsystem. These variables all affect the efficiency and the outcome of the eicosanoid's step by step enzymatic building process. Just like any enzyme system, these particular biochemical pathways have a check and balancing feature which can either work for you or against you depending upon your diet and exposure to the strongest inhibitors of efficient eicosanoid metabolism.

When this system is working efficiently within itself and within its connection to the overall process of metabolism, more of the so-called anti-sickness eicosanoids will be present with all of their health-promoting benefits. If this system is inhibited in any way, or out of balance for any reason, it automatically forms a greater concentration of sickness eicosanoids which then adversely affect the overall metabolic balance and consequently the entire health status of the body. Many diseases and diseases have already been linked to an abnormal balance of sickness eicosanoids to anti-sickness eicosanoids within the body and brain. The anti-sickness eicosanoids and sickness eicosanoids have completely opposite effects to one another (much like the sugar-controlling "opposite" hormones insulin and glucagon or calcium controlled by one's parathormone and calcitonin). If one "good anti-sickness" eicosanoid opens up blood vessels to decrease blood pressure, its corresponding "bad sickness" eicosanoid does the exact opposite by closing the same blood vessels to increase blood pressure. Below is a simplified table of some of the known actions of eicosanoids:

**TABLE V:** *EICOSANOIDS: THE GOOD, THE BAD and (THE UGLY)*

| GOOD EICOSANOIDS (Anti-Sickness Effects) | BAD EICOSANOIDS (Sickness Effects) |
|---|---|
| Resists inflammatory processes | Promotes inflammatory processes |
| Inhibits blood platelet aggregation | Promotes platelet aggregation (clots) |
| Promotes vasodilation | Promotes vasoconstriction |
| Inhibits cellular proliferation | Promotes cellular proliferation |
| Decreases pain transmission | Increases pain transmission |
| Stimulates immune response | Depresses immune response |

The eicosanoidal submetabolic system, just like the overall metabolism at large in all of its manifestations throughout the body, is always in a dynamic state of balance between opposing forces—one force being construed as "good" (or health-promoting) while the other as its opposite is "bad" (or nonhealth-promoting). Proper balance is achieved when the good forces significantly outweigh the bad forces. The perfect balance of good versus bad is highly specific to each individual's biochemical individuality. This person-specific overall metabolic balance is, of course, the same for eicosanoid submetabolism. The check and balance effect of metabolism is exceedingly easy to see when you understand the nature of eicosanoid production and its dietary controlling forces. Given that our most fundamental goal in life is (or at least ought to be) the promotion of anti-sickness or well-being, from which all positive experiences in life flow, then our immediate objective is to demonstrably increase the concentration of "good" eicosanoids over "bad" in the body. **Table V above,** Eicosanoids: The Good, The Bad and The Ugly, lists a few of the good and bad things eicosanoids do.

First, we have to locate and eat enough in the proper combination of the two most primary essential fats in nature (cis-linoleic or Omega-6 fat and alphalinoleic or Omega-3 fat) as itemized by your personalized nutrition testing program. These two front-line dietary fats provide the raw product (or substrate) which ensures the manufacture of the best eicosanoids within the body. In order for things to work well, these fats must not only be present within the diet in high enough amounts in and of themselves, but also provide a synergistic dominance in their relation-ships to nonessential fats ( such as saturated fats) in order to provide an abundance of optimal good eicosanoid benefits. Unfortunately, the majority of people don't realize that they can't guess this just right with-out proper orthomolecular intervention.

Today, most people are so busy blindly cutting fat from their diets for the sake of weight loss and cholesterol reduction, that they unintentionally create their own dietary deficiency of the most essential fats. In fact, sta-tistically more than 70% of deaths in the U.S. are related to fat deficien-cies, imbalances, and excesses (think of heart disease, for one). Therefore, in any nutrition program we must properly balance all fats in the diet by proportioning PUFAs, MUFAs and SAFAs into a person-specific intra-macronutrient fat zone. For best results, we also have to properly desig-nate the intermacronutrient Zone I (carb-protein-fat connection) to indi-vidual specifications. Too many of the wrong carbohydrates (high glycemic index and/or high acid-forming carbs, depending on metabolic type/rate) in relation to essential and non-essential fats can harmfully increase insulin production which then depresses production of good eicosanoids, while hastening the development of bad eicosanoids. Too many carbohydrates in general, and in relation to interproportional fats, can seriously inhibit good prostaglandin production. Additionally, imbal-ances of intraproportional (Zone V) carbohydrates, specifically simple and refined high-glycemic index/load sugars enhance bad eicosanoid pro-duction through constantly elevating insulin activity. Then there's the proper level and type of each protein you must take for proper eicosanoid balance. Because protein in general inhibits insulin production, enough protein must be in the diet proportionate to carbohydrate, and actually eaten simultaneously with it (carbohydrate) for best results, and again specific to an individual's testing profile. This can occur when protein and carbs, and protein and fat, are in synergistic balance.

Protein and fat proportions are also critical because many fats are present in protein sources and therefore must be accounted for in this regard— such as the fat present on a steak—and then proportioned properly with-in one's personal zones. The (intra/inter) macronutrient proportions of protein, carbs and fat all have a synergistic/antagonistic balancing effect on one another in relation to eicosanoid metabolism. Again, a properly personalized nutrition program automatically determines this for each individual metabolic type/rate and is especially discernable from fatty

acid fingerprint tests. Proper food/supplement proportioning complements the process to ensure optimal eicosanoid balance. Since specific
diet/supplement balance exerts so many effects upon eicosanoid balance,
we must consider the effects of super-heated fats. Super-heated fats (such
as those created from frying) are in a chemically deranged form called
"trans fats" versus the natural or "properly arranged" chemical state of
"cis" fats. Cis fats are in their natural state and are therefore utilized by
the body most efficiently. Trans fats, however, are not metabolically
received as nourishment by the body and in fact ultimately inhibit the
production of good eicosanoid formation. Therefore it's wise to avoid
fried fatty foods whenever possible no matter what type,rate, or profile of
nutrient retention you possess, in order to minimize the harmful intake
of trans fat.

Our next concern when it comes to promoting the optimum production
of eicosanoids is regarding the balanced intake of all micronutrients as
found in the master list of essential nutrients mentioned previously
(coenzyme/cofactors/minerals/vitamins/amino acids, etc.), which most
strongly stimulate the particular enzymes that expedite the formation of
only good eicosanoids. Remove any one or all of these stimulating coenzymes (minerals, vitamins, etc.) and the whole eicosanoidal system of
metabolism becomes completely undermined and dysfunctional. The
most necessary, most enzyme-stimulating cofactors include the antioxidants beta carotene, vitamin C complex, vitamin E (d-alpha tocopherol
only) and the enzyme catalysts vitamin B3, B6, minerals zinc and magnesium, and less directly iron, copper, manganese, melatonin, essential
amino acids, cadmium, calcium, phosphorus, and other B vitamins due
to their interconnected relationships with enzyme stimulators which
automatically allow them to be available to the enzymes in the first place.
It is obvious, therefore, that the overall balance of vitamins, minerals and
other vitamin-like substances is critical to a good anti-sickness
eicosanoid production level because of their metabolic necessity to be
available at the right time and in the right amounts. Cofactor availability in turn is dependent on dietary presence (within the foods and supplements you eat), in conjunction with efficient digestion, assimilation,
and elimination. These factors in turn are dependent on all related personalized nutrition procedures to ensure optimum bioavailability for
good eicosanoid production in the first place. One thing is connected to
the next—and that is how the body works, even when it comes to super
hormones. *One-size-fits-all or guesswork* practices only serve to under-

mine good eicosanoidal metabolism, whereas the specificity in personalized nutrition automatically optimizes this function every time. Tests
and retests keep this process on track.

Thirdly, in the eicosanoid producing biochemical system (as in all
enzyme systems), there's always that one sluggish enzyme (known as the
rate-limiting enzyme) that all other chemical reactions have to wait for
before they can happen. In this particular biochemical system, it is delta-
6 desaturase that's our "bottleneck" or stopgap. D6DS's capacity to function at peak efficiency, allowing the rest of the system to function efficiently, is highly susceptible to a number of factors. These enzyme antag-
onizing factors, when present, always hasten the production of bad over
good eicosanoids because they suppress delta-6 desaturase. These enzyme
blockers include:

- all/any dietary imbalances including essential fat imbalances and the presence
  of too much trans fat and red meat containing arachidonic acid (an undesirable fatty acid)
- aging prematurely
- reductions in energy production due to slowing metabolism, disease infiltration (especially viral infections), stress-related hormones (such as endogenous)
  cortisone and adrenaline (exogenous), pharmaceutical and recreational drugs
  which specifically depress immune function such as corticosteroids found in
  prescription and non-prescription drugs or heroine
- regular use of/exposure to tobacco, caffeine, alcohol, all toxins and poisons,
  aspirin, hydrogenated fats like those found in margarine (a concentrated
  source of trans fat), excess saturated fats, tartrazine
- obesity
- continued too high or too low blood cholesterol levels

There are a few personalized nutrition, good eicosanoid-forming tricks that
we can systematically apply to speed up the body's response to a personalized nutrition program. These tricks involve manipulating the therapeutic
application of concentrated/activated essential fatty acids not only through
customized diet, but also through customized supplementation procedures. Activated essential fatty acids such as gamma-linolenic acid (GLA)
and eicosapentaenoic acid (EPA) are those which are produced by enzymes
in the body through normal eicosanoid synthesis which can also be found
in certain foods and provided for in supplements that we consume. The
gamma-linolenic acid found in mother's milk, evening primrose and borage seed oil are good examples, where they apply. Another good example is

that of EPA and DHA found mostly in fatty fish like mackerel, sardines, and salmon. Taking EPA and GLA directly and in concentrated amounts from diet and supplements can help bypass any faulty enzyme metabolism in the body which converts Omega-6 fat to GLA and Omega-3 fat to EPA. In this way, a greater concentration of GLA and EPA is attained directly without interference from enzymatic efficiency breakdowns. Using this trick method, we can successfully exert a more direct influence on good eicosanoid balance by forcing another eicosanoidal enzyme delta 5 desaturase or D5DS, to automatically inhibit the formation of arachidonic acid. Arachidonic acid, when present, immediately converts into only bad eicosanoids. More GLA and EPA in combination with lower insulin levels and higher glucagon levels (from eating lower GI and GL sugary foods) greatly suppress delta 5 desaturase activity which in turn chokes off the production of arachidonic acid. Furthermore, keeping arachidonic-acid-containing red meat intake in balance by proportioning intra- and inter-macro- and micronutrient proportions, according to metabolic testing information, also complements this process. Personalized nutrition does so by accounting for meats' presence in the diet and within the body and balancing it accordingly.

A properly planned custom diet and supplement plan automatically takes the process of eicosanoid metabolism into full account in combination with all other components of metabolism both directly related and indirectly related to eicosanoids on a highly individualized basis. This ensures a more perfect balance with optimal levels of eicosanoids and all other related health-promoting/anti-disease metabolites.

### *The Permanent Weight Loss Solution*

Part of feeling better in your future wellness scenario, beyond establishing an unbreakable defense against becoming sick, is looking great: radiant, lean, and toned. This is something that you should actually expect to happen as you follow through on your personalized nutrition program closely. Realize that out of 200 people who go on any diet, only ten lose all the weight they set out to lose. Out of those ten dieters, only one keeps it off for any reasonable length of time. This is a failure rate of 99.5% reported the **Washington Post** (as reprinted in the **Houston Chronicle** by Arthur Frank). I believe this to be one of the saddest commentaries on the futility of *one-size-fits-all* weight loss. What's even worse is that this statistic is very typical.

Probably the most common physical and psychological annoyance among Americans is the unwanted, progressive deposition of body fat. Most people consider excess body fat unsightly and attempt to deal with it on the basis of its appearance-robbing effects. Just how good you look on the outside has a lot to do with how people treat you and is a clue to upsets on the inside, both physical and emotional. Literally hundreds of billions of dollars are spent on cosmetic control of fat and wrinkles. The health-robbing effects of excess body fat, however, go much further than what is merely observed on the outside. People with excess fat accumulation usually experience certain states of disease and sub clinical (just-not-feeling-well, nothing-too-serious-at-the-moment), symptomatic syndromes that automatically accompany unsightly appearance. A lower effective energy level, feeling less than one's best overall and experiencing more strain on the feet, legs, and spine are common over-fat subclinical experiences. Being over-fat in combination with the predisposing causative slowed metabolic state that typically accompanies it and continues to preserve its excesses has much further-reaching implications than most people would like to admit. From an orthomolecular scientific standpoint and finally now from common knowledge, we've acknowledged that being over-fat is a major risk factor in all disease and for all subclinical dis-ease (discomfort), not to mention being a complicating factor in all surgery and child delivery. A state of "over-fatness" ensures a fundamental resistance factor which can only serve to inhibit complete metabolic balance. Fat's excessive presence mirrors the fact that there is metabolic imbalance in the first place. Excess body fat deposition is easily one of the most observable signs of metabolic imbalance. Excessive body fat accumulation is a potential imbalance which can plague any body rate/type if not addressed. Some rate/types typically gain weight more readily than others but in some types this unwanted tendency can actually be an advantage for greater longevity and superior athletic achievement when controlled properly. The accumulation of excess body fat has different ramifications and consequences for each body chemistry type, which has a different health and fitness tolerance for fat. Five excess pounds to one type of body can be more like 15 pounds to another depending on physical and biochemical characteristics. In effect, suffice it to say that some body types are genetically designed to carry more fat than others even when in a state of total metabolic balance. So when someone says they weren't (genetically) designed to be "that thin" or "that fat," there may be some truth to this statement (whether they know it or not).

It is our aim to reduce body fat levels into an acceptable range specific to each individual and their individually specified body design objectives (such as getting ready for an athletic contest, a movie role, fitting into a dress for a reunion, etc.). On a naturally slimmer type of body-build, excess fat's health-reducing effects are much greater than on a naturally rounder type of body-build. In other words, on a naturally thinner body type excess fat accumulation, pound for pound, seems to have a more degenerative effect than pound for pound gains on rounder types. Ultimately, working within the phenotypic framework of each rate/type is the all-encompassing key to restore low fat metabolic balance. Two researchers, William Sheldon and Carl Jung, categorized phenotypic body types on the basis of fat distribution and personality for comparison purposes. The associations that they have made between mind and fat distribution are interesting.

From a generalized standpoint, the most common causes of excess fat accumulation are:

- Eating too much for the rate/type of body and lifestyle one has
- Consuming/retaining the wrong balance of macro- and micronutrients for one's specific type, and especially too much calcium and other sedative nutrients
- Eating infrequently, or at non-fixed and variable times in the daily routine
- A lack of regular exercise in combination with the 3 points above
- Aging without proper dietary and lifestyle modifications to synchronize with this process
- Certain disease states and drugs which foster fat accumulation
- Certain glandular imbalances which inhibit the efficient metabolism of food
- Toxin accumulation which provides resistance to metabolic efficiency and balance (This includes drug-induced metabolic inconsistencies that lead to fat accumulation)
- The combination of any and all factors mentioned in factors 1 through 8

It should be obvious that all of the previous fat fostering factors can only result from one not fully understanding his or her given rate/type and what lifestyle modifications are most directly called for in order to rebalance metabolism and reduce fat. Any fat loss program designed without utilizing personalized nutrition can be exceedingly dangerous to one's health—and statistically doomed to failure. Becoming fatter simply leads to more illness and goes much beyond mere calorie reduction in its remedy. The latest statistical success figure for those who lose weight but fail to keep it off for very long is less than 2%. That means that at least 98% of those who lose weight at first fail to reach their target weight level and also fail to keep the fat off because they eventually rebound into an oftentimes fatter state than ever before, or what is called *the yo-yo diet* effect. What's even worse is that most weight loss programs have little to no emphasis on building better health accountably while weight loss proceeds. This oversight results in people who perhaps weigh less but who actually become less healthy than when they started losing weight. This is due to far too much guesswork, too much desperation, too many shortcuts and too many extremes taken—not to mention no scientific regard for biophysiological uniquenesses. Therefore, the net effect in the overwhelming majority of attempted fat loss is temporary weight loss and usually some health loss to go with it! Just losing weight alone doesn't guarantee better health. Eating less food on a *one-size-fits-all* fat loss mode can further worsen existing nutrient deficiencies and metabolic inconsistencies severely, undermining one's health. And, there's no real nutrition-related health accountability of body chemistry whatsoever (other than a few pounds lost).

I've had patients who've undergone typical *one-size-fits-all* weight loss programs and who have lost a good portion, if not all, of their hair in the process. Hair loss during weight loss is an extreme sign of health loss. You'd think people would figure that out or at least wonder about it. A couple of my own patients reported that their weight loss counselor/adviser (untruthfully) actually told them that the hair loss was from detoxing just to keep them on the program. If your hair is quickly graying and/or disappearing on a fat-loss program, this is a sure sign that your health is fading fast. If you're losing a lot of muscle, bone, electrolytes, vitamins and minerals, water and other body essentials, something's wrong. In fact, fat may account for the least of what you've lost in terms of overall health when this happens. I don't think that losing your hair or health from an inappropriate weight loss scheme was ever in your particular vision of life, or anybody's, for that matter. So, we have:

## Reality Check #13
**Don't be fooled into thinking that weight loss is automatic health gain. One-size-fits-all weight loss doesn't work this way.**

Watch out for advice given from some of our so-called fat loss authorities. Fat loss guru Richard Simmons, as an example, during an appearance on the Maury Povich talk show some years ago, openly admitted to losing all of his hair when he first dieted to lose weight. Why do you think this happened? Probably because Mr. Simmons practices *one-size fits-all-fat loss* and consequently damaged his health, which he must have initially sacrificed for some quick weight loss. When this type of thing happens, you need to think to yourself, "Why should I take weight loss advice from this guy (or anyone) who lost all of his hair when he/she dieted?" That's like going to the same cardiologist for heart/health advice who ends up suffering from a heart attack him/herself. This kind of ridiculous contradiction is very commonplace and happens all the time; we take health advice from people who don't fully practice or understand what they preach. Unfortunately, MDs statistically don't outlive their patients. We tend to make the same *one-size-fits-all* mistakes that they're all making and subsequently duplicate their failure to know and do for ourselves.

So, when Maury Povich asked Mr. Simmons exactly why he lost all of his hair from dieting, from under his wig he replied "That was before I knew how to diet properly." A true political coverup. The obvious implication here is that he knows how to diet properly now. But when Maury opened up Mr. Simmons' refrigerator and spied all of the partially eaten sweet treats, he again was startled. Mr. Simmons quickly assured Maury that "nobody's perfect" and that if you exercise and eat right most of the time you can sneak treats without fatty consequences. We can all agree somewhat. But it is quite possible that Mr. Simmons' need for sweet treats (like chocolate Hagen Dazs) was because of nutrition imbalances which when corrected would partly or perhaps completely eliminate these cravings? Without belaboring the point, it's always wisest to listen to somebody who sets a good example, who truly practices what he/she preaches, although that *still* might be wrong for you because of individuality differences. Additionally, I've never seen much muscle tone overall on Mr. Simmons or many of our so-called health/fat loss and fitness gurus of today. Do you think that you could ever find your abs after listening to those who don't even find their own by following their advice? Guess again. The point I would really like to make here is a noteworthy observation of *one-size-fits-all* fat loss ineffectiveness. I'm referring to the part where, despite all of the discomforts of dieting, there's still that last bit of fat that just never seems to come off no matter how hard one tries. That lumpy fat that just seems to hang on no matter how hard you struggle, no matter how much your skin sags, no matter how much good health you lose and no matter how many unnecessary wrinkles you've collected in your *one-size-fits-all* quest for rapid weight loss. Precisely rate/typing yourself should completely eliminate that last stubborn fat deposit and protect you from the health loss which predisposes you to sags and wrinkles typical of improper weight loss techniques. A freshly achieved and maintained optimal metabolic balance will prevent yo-yo fatness rebounds; minimize or completely eradicate food cravings; restore appetite balance; ensure optimal health and fitness; and provide a long, satisfying, low fat-life span.

To attempt permanent and healthy fat loss without personalized nutrition is suicidal at best because it robs you of vitality, "killing you softly" on a most subtle physiological basis and can simultaneously doom you to future fat loss failure replete with all of the psychological sufferings and aggravations typically associated with overweight states. Attempting fat loss without the benefits of orthomolecular science is like taking a shower in a raincoat. In effect, you go through the motions of taking a shower but without taking off the raincoat and getting the soap and water on your skin, you'll never fully realize the cleansing benefits of the shower. Personalized nutrition closely adhered to will always promote the balance of your unique biochemistry so that you can once and for all rid the body naturally of something it was never designed to have in overt excess in the first place—fat.

### The Super Athlete

The fundamental goal of all soft- or hard-core athletic fitness and training is to improve the conditioning effect to the body and therefore increase overall performance. To do this at peak energetic efficiency, we must more specifically feed and train the body into a state of hyper-functional metabolic balance. This in effect is an advanced-capacity metabolic state wherein all body and mind adaptations to a given sport/conditioning stimulus have efficiently taken place, maximizing the development of continuous free energy used to hasten workout recovery and push the body beyond its previous limitations of performance. It should be obvious that personalized nutrition is just what the athlete ordered because it provides the science to more effectively individualize nutrition, training, and performance-enhancing synergistic combinations in the achievement of a higher physiological capacity for work. This "ergogenic" or energy-producing advantage effectively brings one closer to his or her biological potential for fitness development than by any other means. A metabolically unbalanced athlete is truly a physically handicapped one and will not go as far as possible in his or her performance achievements as a more balanced athlete.

An athlete's metabolism that (initially) is in a state of disarray only provides unchecked resistance to free energy production, which in turn limits performance potentials drastically. Even athletes with the best genetic predispositions to their given sport still cannot fully liberate their biological potential without more individualized nutrition. These genetically gifted athletes may still surpass those who possess fewer genetic advantages but still won't individually achieve all that is physically and mentally possible in their given sport or physical endeavor. A fully worked up athlete has a profound advantage over athletes not utilizing personalized nutrition in all of the fitness-related parameters of the physical and mental challenge their sport provides. From enhanced injury protection to greater endurance and strength development, to a more concentrated performance focus and positive attitude and to the duplication of peak performance, personalized nutrition wins out over all else. I advise this as an experienced athlete myself. Being a specialized sports medicine health practitioner, I have always utilized personalized nutrition enhancements for my athletic and fitness-minded patients, whether world class or weekend warrior.

I agree in principle with Dr. Joel Wallach, D.V.M., N.D., when he (over) states that "exercise without supplementation is suicide." But I would add that any exercise- or sports-related physical undertaking without proper nutritional testing is foolhardy at the least, and may not cost you your life, as Dr. Wallach implies, but may inevitably cost you the thrill of victory in exchange for the agony of defeat. You may give up access to a body that could look better and feel better. A large amount of world-class and pro-level sports teams currently use elements of orthomolecular science in order to maximize their athletes performance levels, with much success. We have many testimonials on file to this effect with before and after tests which when compared to one another, over time, always demonstrate a reduction of deficiencies, excesses and imbalances overall as performance increases—no matter what nutrition or toxic measurements were taken. It is only due to orthomolecular science that world records continue and will continue to be broken without the use of illegal substances such as steroids to enhance performance levels.

*More Youthful Life Out of Life*

Life extension is a topic that seems to be very heated these days. An increase in life expectancy is desirable as long as the quality of life maintained is as high as possible. This really equates with staying younger longer and having much more energy to meet the demands of daily life. This is an area of focus for orthomolecular medicine: *when you maintain more nutrition in balance you secure a younger life longer.* Old age really is a metabolic slowdown process. Youth is about faster metabolisms. Keeping one's own metabolism as efficient as possible, as long as possible, provides the key element in any youth extension scenario.

UCLA predicted 166 years of life when commenting on the ideal lifestyle/diet/environment created for the researchers in the Arizonian Biosphere II. The university researchers actually measured and calibrated a slowdown in the aging process which clearly aided in a prediction of 166 years of life. In my own clinical experience, it seems like my older clients are in much better shape than their contemporaries when given medical workups. Muriel is 80 years old and was worked up for physiological age using various formulas and testing and was calculated to be in the top 15th percentile of good health for 40-year-olds. This should not seem unusual inasmuch as knowing exactly what nutritional state your body is in and really doing something about it on the most specific levels provides an incredibly terrific advantage over the aging process. Staying younger longer and increasing life expectancy is something you can expect when you pursue the personalized nutrition process. It's clearly a good idea to get started as soon as possible and not wait until you already are a geriatric, although we do have one more reality check to mention here:

# Reality Check #14
## It's never too late to get started on a personalized nutrition program

No matter what age you are, what shape you're in, what drugs you are taking, what golden life you have, there is no time sooner than the present to get started on having a longer, healthier life, with much more control and many fewer health surprises, if any.

*Better Sex*

It should be relatively evident that if in fact your body works better thanks to superior nutritional input, your ability to have sex will improve. This works for both men and women whose hormone levels can be deranged prematurely due to poor nutrition, too many drugs, and not enough physical activity.

I had an interesting clinical case whereby the patient brought in medical tests which demonstrated a slightly lowered testosterone level which he claimed was interfering with his sexual performance. We worked him up using several nutrition tests and an interactional hormone test, finding multiple measurements out of balance. After instituting a law of opposites type of nutrition program for him, 23 of his original symptomatic complaints had shrunk to only one by the end of six months. I received a call from his wife, thanking me for making her husband more "frisky," as she put it. When I asked the patient about this he reported that he was getting much more enjoyment out of sex and was very satisfied. In other standard medical tests given at approximately that same time, it was revealed that an actual increase in the testosterone level took place. Finding this a geriatric rarity, the doctor actually asked the patient if he was taking steroids, which of course he wasn't. This is why we say the nutrient comes before the hormone like the chicken versus the egg controversy, and why I always insist on nutrient replacement therapy before hormone replacement therapy is undertaken. Better sex is a welcome benefit to better nutrition.

*Better Memory—Faster Thinking*

Since the body and mind are inseparable, it only logically follows that as the health of the body improves so does mental function. Better cognition is something people can look forward to on a more scientifically personalized nutrition program. This brings us to:

## Reality Check #15
*In life, the mind and body are inseparable;*
*what hurts one hurts the other,*
*what helps one helps the other,*
*and superior nutrition helps them both*

You simply cannot think straight when your body's not well and your body suffers when you cannot use your brain properly. Countless numbers of my clients report improvements in body and mind easily observed in test by retest. The reverse never happens, that if test measurements worsen, people report more benefits and fewer symptoms. It just doesn't work that way, unless someone's being untruthful. This brings us finally to:

## Reality Check #16

**Biochemical improvements as demonstrated in nutrition tests and retests always correlate with feeling better, fewer symptoms, performing better physically and mentally, living longer, looking better, having more energy and enjoying a better life**

### *A Word about Our Human Tribe:*
### *We're All in This Together, No Matter Who You Are*

In modern times, it's very difficult to find "pure" societies which have changed little or not at all in the last 40,000 years and still have the majority of their given environment intact. A book called *The Paleolithic Prescription* was written by scientists who were able to locate a group of untainted hunter-gatherer societies and study them extensively. This revealing information has been added to the wealth of information scientists have compiled about the Hunzas, Soviet Georgians, Tibetan tribes, the Titicaca tribe, Armenians, Abkhazians, Azerbaijani, Vilcabamba Indians, Amazonian tribes and many others. Examining this material gives one a genuine look at how life used to be for all of us when we were in our most primal environments, living off the land and learning how to work together at the most fundamental survival levels.

This rapidly diminishing group of pure, unadulterated, unmodernized hunter-gatherer, fisherman, and agrarian societies are still exactly matched to the environments which spawned their genetic makeup (until, of course, civilization invades and disrupts everything in the name of progress). These simple-living people are still practicing the same eating, exercise, and lifestyle habits that their ancestors practiced thousands of years ago. Be reminded that our ancestors were in a similar setting at one time, practicing the same type of habitual rites of life, generation after generation. An interesting movie to watch regarding tribes is *The Emerald Forest* which portrays a good idea of what we're referring to. Today, in our "anything goes" society, we are living completely outside of our most fundamental environments, as well as the natural patterns and order of life, and as statistics show, it's killing us. Keep in mind that *scientific research regarding these unchanged ancient tribes demonstrates an absolute lack of diet-related disease and expected longevity well over 100 years for most individuals* not dying from accident or infection. Based upon his studies on these tribes and his own clinical experience, Joel Wallach, D.V.M., N.D., believes our rightful lifespan to be 130 to 140 years if our diets are right for us. To reiterate, the researchers living in the Arizonan Biosphere under ideal conditions were given over 160 years of life from UCLA computer predictions. When closely examining these long-living primal tribes, researchers have found that their peoples simply don't seem to suffer much from osteoporosis, heart disease, diabetes, obesity, allergy syndromes, arthritis, cancer or many of the other across-the-board diet-related diseases. In fact, the vast majority of these tribal people are energetic, active, productive, and disease-free up until the day they die, which is just about always from natural causes (old age). Interestingly, the popular "40-30-30 zone" classifications of diet do not fit these people squarely.

A large amount of these tribal individuals do pass away due to ever-so-slight nutrient deficiencies that finally catch-up with them well into their 100s. An example of this phenomenon is typified by the bone tuberculosis that has taken the lives of some Hunzas (well into their 100s by the way). This disease is blamed on an ever-so-slight protein deficiency manifested over hundreds of years. Imagine. To think the average American only lives to be 75.4 years old and our medical doctors only about 68 years old. In reality, the majority of that seemingly acceptable 68 to 75 years of life is still plagued by a host of varying diseases and medication/surgical dependencies, obesity, low energy, and various routine symptoms from headaches to constipation to fatigue to indigestion to joint pains and so on. While your average Hunzan is out in the fields, able to work ten to twelve hours a day consistently and well is naturally thin, optimistic and energetic, your average "old" American can barely get out of their chair to go to the restroom. While Soviet Georgians are reaching their sexual peak well into their 40s, 50s, and beyond, by comparison, the average middle-aged American regards complete sexual fulfillment as a pleasant memory at best or needs drug-induced, pill-mediated virility and/or libido to get by. At this point, the question begs to be asked about our approach to health care, "What are we thinking?"

You may think to yourself, "To be healthy I'll have to move to Lake Titicaca and do as the Titicacans do." In fact, it does not work this way. The disease-free and longevity success of these primal tribes should confirm the need for us to do as our personal ancestral roots dictate. Of course, there may be nothing left of your ancestors to speak of, at least in a tribal society under ideal environmental conditions. If you did move to Lake Titicaca to live better, it still may not improve upon your own wellness status due to one problem: Your genometabolic type does not match that of the Titicacans because your tribal ancestry follows a line of people who lived in an entirely different environment under entirely different gene-affecting circumstances than your ancestors, who have genetically formed *your personal life* constitution accordingly. Much more important than that information is what's really being retained inside your specific body at this moment; even though your primal tribe may have been carni-vegan type eaters who subsisted on completely different foods than a more vegetarian Titicacan would. However, if you are a genuine Titicacan who left the tribe to become a lawyer in New York City for the past fifteen years and then moved back home due to your brand new set of society-imposed, diet-related illnesses, you would be happily rewarded with optimum health again in a very short period of time. You'd be back in your primal element doing what your genes were designed to do. For the rest of us, testing and correcting more scientifically, more personally is what is needed. In these modern times we all cannot realistically return to our tribes or even countries of origin, so we must better utilize nutrition testing and individualized correction to reveal the essence of how our bodies function and what they specifically require to operate at peak efficiency no matter what we're doing or where we are in the world or what kind of genes we possess. When we know our nutrient/toxic retention we can so much more efficiently organize our personal diets (and lives) very close to reality and perhaps with a more similar dose of what our ancestors thrived upon—those same individuals who rarely strayed from their tribes of origin or countries and who typically practiced life in harmonious synchronicity with their natural environment.

Outside of the U.S., many countries fare much better when it comes to overall health status. Japan, for instance, is one of the 10 healthiest countries in the world, and for good reason: Even with all of the health-inhibiting factors of modern civilization like stress, pollution, drug dependence, etc., the Japanese adhere closely to the ritualistic living patterns of their ancestors. This is true for many Asian countries where tradition reinforces the diet and lifestyle practices of their country's past. In essence, these peoples are doing more of what their specific body type was designed to do and have the absence of most diet-related disease to show for it. This health-sustaining phenomenon is fading fast due to the never-ending ravages of modernization, specifically, the introduction into these societies of the Western style of life – TV, fast food, and drugs. Subsequently, for prevention purposes, nutrition testing is fast-becoming a Japanese trend (according to the testing labs who do business in that country).

### Genotype Abstract
### The Eskimo versus the Indian

A dramatic metabolic individuality contrast is evident when you consider the differences between the Eskimo's and the East Indian's dietary patterns. Traditional Eskimos ate as much as ten pounds of very fatty meat per day, thrived physically, and were able to successfully survive the harshest climate on earth. Historically, their overall incidence of diet-related disease was miniscule, with little to no traces of cardiovascular disease or cancer until only recently, with the advances of Western civilization encroaching on their lifestyles (progressive dental decay is a new phenomenon that modern mankind has given the Eskimos, with the introduction of refined sugars into their lifestyles). During countless previous generations, the Eskimos' physiological constitution became perfectly suited to their environment through natural adaptation and mutation (phenotyping). Their bodies became progressively more efficient at metabolizing the types of food naturally occurring within their harsh living environments. In essence, the Eskimos developed a genetic need for high protein and high fat in their diets in order to healthfully survive. Without fatty meats, their health and survival would rapidly deteriorate. The East Indian vegetarian diet offers the most vivid contrast on earth to the Eskimos carni-vegan diet adaptation (Eskimos are almost pure carnivores, as are the Masai tribes in Africa and South American Gauchos). East Indians have an opposite food need of mostly vegetables, grains, and fruits, with no animal meats or fat. If either group completely switched to the other's typical diet, both groups would suffer an overwhelming dietary-disease plague that potentially could end the existence of both races very rapidly. Interestingly, many paleontologists blame changes in the food chain many millions of years ago for both dinosaur mutations and their eventual extinction. Isn't it conceivable, when you think about it, that man may suffer the same fate as the dinosaurs from changing his dietary patterns too quickly for the necessary phenotypic adaptation to keep metabolic pace? Man potentially could bring on his own extinction by altering his nutrition too drastically in too short a period of time. vata, pitta, kapha, etc., spawned in India isn't going to healthfully sustain a carnivorous Eskimo. In fact, Ayurvedic practices may actually doom him or her instead. Our only protection from accidental food-related extinction is to pay closer attention to our body-specific nutritional requirements and not take any drastic leaps into incompatible nutrition plans. There is simply no other way out of this personal reality.

### *Don't Expect Much in the Food,*
### *the Soil is Nutritionally Deficient*

The last 50 years or so has been a time of extreme change for the farming industry. Prior to this time period, most farms in the U.S. were small and primarily managed by the families who lived on them, sometimes for several generations. These agrarian or farming families tended their own gardens and lived off the land growing potatoes, corn, and other assorted vegetables and grains. Typically, they had a flock of chickens, some dairy cows, a few hogs, a horse or two and perhaps apple, pear, or plum trees and some blueberry or raspberry bushes. What these farmers did not consume themselves they sent to local markets for sale to the public. These same farmers ate fish occasionally and other wild foods that they either fished, picked, or hunted, like trout, berries, wild turkeys, or deer. They routinely took shavings, peelings, leftovers, and other natural organic garbage and used it as compost by plowing it back into the soil as fertilizer. These agrarians also collected their cow, horse, chicken, and pig manure and plowed it back into the soil. Through this continuous ecological process, the soil was constantly being recycled so that all of the nutrients originally found in the soil remained there. Crops were rotated for the express purpose that some crops deplete certain elements of soil more than others, while others actually help to synergistically recharge certain elements found in soil. In this way, the soil was kept in a state of nutrient balance and yielded healthy crops from within its own natural ecosystem with few outside influences. This was all part of farming tradition.

During wintertime, the soil rested and all of the microorganisms, worms, and bugs in the soil would continue to interact and ultimately break nutrients down into forms most usable by plants. This winter "rest and recycling" period increased the concentration of nutrients bio-available for next year's crops. The lowland fields near streams and rivers were naturally flooded through winter's thaw and rainy seasons and experienced large-scale flooding every one to three years, which served to bring in new layers of silt. These layers of silt from the surrounding mountains and highlands brought in even more minerals and nutrients to the farming soils. This was a period in American farming history when chickens would be free to roam around eating whatever bugs and seeds appealed to them, and the typically "small udder" dairy cows free were to roam the fields and sample whatever elements of nature they chose. Collectively, this natural feeding process resulted in food that looked, felt, smelled, and tasted much different than our mass-production foods of today. Eggshells and egg yolks defied breaking and milk was thick and tangy versus the brittle eggs and watery milk (from hybridized, mass-produced "big udder" cows) of today.

This was a time in history when vegetables had deep, tangy flavors and whole grain breads were dark and heavy to satisfy our appetites versus the waxy tasteless vegetables and crumbly, air-filled breads of our modern, mega-supply chain. It is obvious to anyone who is old enough to remember or to those who have been fortunate enough to be able to tend their own private gardens through the years that food in the grocery stores is totally different now. The modernization changes applied to our agribusiness farming system began with the emergence of gigantic, big-profit farms which progressively replaced the status quo of small farms in America. These large farms were measured in square miles instead of mere acres like their small farm predecessors. The shift from small into large farming operations was exceedingly widespread throughout the U.S. and Canada in the race to produce more food. The new gigantic farms were extremely productive, turning out huge surpluses of grains, dairy products, vegetables, and livestock on a magnitude never seen before. This potent agricultural force became the backbone of U.S. supremacy in the world as a superpower. In a land of such great abundance, we go so far as to pay our farmers not to produce (subsidies) and either give away or practically give away food for the political manipulation of other countries in the world. Is this charity or politics? In our mass-production world of super-productive agribusiness farming, the soils are pushed well beyond their limits of natural ecological balance.

Many of these same soils where one crop per year previously was grown are now subjected to two or three (and even more) crops per year with no rest in between. This holds especially true for the warmer climates in the U.S. (the Sunbelt) where there is a continuous year-round harvest.

The typical, large-scale, modern corporate farm uses powerful insecticides to kill bugs and deadly herbicides to destroy unwanted plants. These powerful poisons are dropped from the air by planes, from the undersides of tractors, and in some cases by hand to contain agricultural pests. Unfortunately, these poisons also tend to destroy beneficial bugs, worms, and microorganisms needed in the soil to keep it nutrient-rich—not to mention getting directly into the food we eat. Rivers which used to follow their natural courses are now dyked and dammed to prevent flooding. The minerals they used to carry in from the surrounding highlands and distant mountains to deposit as silt over agricultural top-soils are now whisked directly out to sea and lost forever. The growing soils of today are pushed to the limit, highly toxic with deadly poisons and wholly miss out on the majority of nutrient-recycling phenomena common just fifty years ago. Our modern soils are no longer replenished within the fundamental ecology of nature. Instead, man has brought in billions of tons of artificial chemical fertilizers to help enrich the soil for purely productivity purposes, *not* ecological balance. In effect, these specific fertilizers are put into the soil only to keep crop yields up and *not* to restore the natural ecological balance of the soil and all that grows on it and feeds on it. Crops produced today can look reasonably good (even without artificial colors which may be used to optimize food appearance). Corn still looks like corn and may even grow to 12 feet tall (if it's not prematurely cut), strawberries and melons look good, lettuce, tomatoes, carrots, and potatoes all look colorful, juicy, full and well shaped. Looks are deceiving and when you get down to the finer science of what's actually in our food (and ends up in our bodies) something major is missing.

Plants construct themselves from out of about seventy to eighty different elements provided that should be available in the soil as the plants grow. Commercial growing fields are continuously overused and the chemical fertilizers added to maintain productivity does not replace nutrients adequately that the plants have been extracting from the soil. Typically, the most common synthetic fertilizers are composed of only three to five different elements such as nitrogen, potassium, phosphorus, and calcium.

These few elements are isolated and used because they are the only ones that are needed to make the plants grow big and appear healthy. Unfortunately, these few elements are not all a plant needs to have the greatest nutrient capability. Plants by nature need about 70 or so different elements as sustenance for optimum life. But these natural elements just aren't in the soil anymore, as they were even 30 years ago. All that is left in the soil in dense amounts are potassium, phosphorus, nitrogen, and calcium. The other necessary plant nutrients are found few and far between, if at all, in our modern soils. This nutrient deficient soil crisis has affected our food in many ways for more than 50 years, but in particular has undermined the nutrient qualities of food drastically. We are paying a personal price with the health of our bodies. According to the *Firman E. Bear Report* published by Rutgers University, variations in the mineral content in foods vary by hundreds to even thousands of percent in some cases. Please see Appendix C, "Variations of Mineral Content In Vegetables" for more details.

According to Dr. Erwin L. Gemmer on his audiotape, *Who Stole America's Health?* at the turn of the century "wheat was 40% protein, now its 9%. If two slices of bread were to give you a certain amount of food value in 1900, now you may have to eat ten slices to get the same nutrition." Also according to Dr. Gemmer, "In 1948, spinach had 150 mg of iron per 100 grams. In 1965, spinach had 27 mg of iron per 100 grams. In 1973, spinach had 2.2 mg of iron per 100 grams." Dr. Joel Wallach, D.V.M., N.D., 1991 Nobel prize nominee in medicine, in his tape, "Dead Doctors Don't Lie," echoes his serious concerns about the state of soil depletion which is undermining the mineral content of our growing soils, which in turn is compromising the mineral density of our foods. Dr. Wallach grew up on a farm and worked with plants and livestock for many years.

From my personal experience, having had access to my grandparents' vegetable garden which covered about half an acre, I was always delightfully spoiled by the rich flavors, crisp freshness, and complete appetite satisfaction I experienced with our home-grown foods as compared to the supermarket produce which didn't look, taste, smell, or satisfy my appetite as well. So far, in my professional research I have seen many similar statistics to Dr. Gemmer's wheat and spinach reports in relation to other foods as assayed by consumer groups, government agencies, and from other professional publications including research work done by

Michael Colgan, PhD. These statistics demonstrate a wide array of varying nutrient densities in foods usually far below the values you'd expect. Imagine oranges with only a trace of vitamin C left (today we need to eat six oranges to get the same nutrients that we would get from one orange 30 years ago) and other produce completely devoid of selenium and other vital minerals we're seriously counting on for our good health. Plus, we have a new host of toxic residues in food from pesticides, herbicides, and other mass production, storage and refinement aftereffects. Meats are full of fat, antibiotics, and steroids, milk is pasteurized and homogenized to compensate for dirty cows as well as toxic from hormone injections to produce more milk per cow, and our meats are deficient in nutrients not apparent in livestock feeds or supplements. (Yes, even farm animals need many supplements, as humans do, because their foods are not up to par either.) Scientists have developed new genetic food hybrids (plants and animals) aimed at increasing the quantity of yields but not necessarily the quality of nutrient density. It all tastes different and affects us differently than food in the "good old days."

This disturbing and commercially based hit or miss phenomenon of the varying nutrient and toxin density in our foods is only one more reason why we all need to be properly tested. We should not leave our foundation of good health to chance with such questionable farming methodologies and subsequent food chain abnormalities.

### Food is Good or Bad

After considering the reality of our biochemical individualities, is it fair to think of any food as good or bad? Any given food in and of itself cannot really be considered either good or bad unless it's riddled with toxins or spoiled. A given (unspoiled) food is good or bad relative only to its effect on a specific individual. Is whale blubber compatible with an East Indian's metabolism? I doubt it, just as much as a whole grain rice dish is not compatible to a tribal Eskimo's metabolism. "Compatible" is a better word than good or bad in reference to foods. Is a food compatible with you? Only personalized nutrition can tell you for sure. This is the crucial basis and foundation for your personal life.

There is a category of generically bad or incompatible food in existence and no matter what body rate/type you possess, this bad food simply is not really compatible with human beings. I'm referring to highly processed, heat-treated, chemical-laden, nutrient- and nutrient/enzyme-dead overcooked foods. By nature, these foods undermine the health of all individual types because of their toxin-laden and nutrient-scarce nature. Organically grown, fresh, and simple foods are more nutrient alive and are generically preferred over synthetically altered, highly processed, mass-produced foods in every case. Do not expect good results on any nutrition program from "dead" foods, no matter how many supplements you take.

### New Food?

There is a whole new breed of food known as "super nutritious food" developed because of those who wish to resist the widespread use of sub-standard food. It contains an even greater nutrient density and less toxic accumulation than our best standard organically grown foods. Expect to see more super nutritious food make an appearance on the market—and use it when you can.

### A New You

A new you begins with your first orthomolecular nutrition test and continues throughout your life. Superior wellness, fitness, and leanness are automatically built into your life when these very special tests and customized diet/supplement therapies are used as guidelines. Science has worked extremely hard to deliver this wellness system. Enjoy the benefits for your personal life.

# Dr. Greg Tefft

## Man of 100,000 Nutrition Tests
## A Personal Note

Very early on in life I trusted too much. I was surrounded by very trust-worthy people—family and friends who never hurt me in any way, and therefore I assumed that just about everyone else was like them, which as you know in today's world is simply wishful thinking. I also trusted in authority. That is, if you were a doctor, I thought you automatically knew what you were talking about. The same was true for a lawyer or teacher or any other authority figure. I had no reason to believe other-wise excepting for occasional dirty deeds that appeared on television, which seemed to only happen to a small minority of other people. Therefore, I trusted fearlessly.

In fact, I never actually was "taken" financially until I was 37. The loss only involved about $4,000; I was cheated by my business partner. Even after this shocking experience, I still did not learn my lesson and lost a much larger sum later on before I finally wised up.

However, when it came to medical and health authority, I did begin to trust less and question more much earlier on in my life. As with most adolescents who go through stages of general rebelliousness, my version became more focused on people either socially perceived as health and fit-ness authorities such as the family doctor or physical education teachers or self-anointed health/fitness authorities such as some of my opinionat-ed classmates and athletic competitors. One high school coach in partic-ular provided a turning point in my life in this regard.

An incident with Coach M set me off in a new direction. At this moment in my life, I had just been named athlete of the month by the school newspaper because of my extensive swimming competition victories and the Olympic hopeful status that circled around me. Meandering into Coach M's morning phys-ed class, eyes bloodshot, hair still a little wet, a few minutes late due to a morning swim practice that went slightly overtime, Coach pointed his finger at me and demanded I come up to the front of the class, which was in the middle of stretching at that moment. He put his hands on his hips and said he did not want to hear any excuses, and then pointing his finger to the ground, told me to give him 50 pushups. As I was taking up my position, I couldn't help but stare at his beer belly literally shake up and down and side to side as he went through these body language motions. He was quite overweight. I thought to myself, "What a fat slob," and with defensive anger blurted out "Why don't you give yourself 50? You need it more than I do!"

As you would expect, all hell broke loose and he took me by the shirt to the principal's office and just about everybody in authority had at me. Coach F, the swimming coach, quickly came to the rescue and turned what could have been a suspension into what I considered a blessed event. Because I was the "celebrity swimmer," it put me in a good place of leverage and the whole incident backfired on Coach M, who was accused of overreacting since I had a legitimate reason for being late. He did not want to hear it. All that was needed was an apology to him for snapping back as I did. Coach F took me out in the hall and said, "Son, when you're right, you're right. This was Coach M's mistake for not letting you explain, but you were at fault for challenging his authority at a time when you were most vulnerable."

The more I thought about this incident, the more it stuck out in my mind as something that was just so narrow-minded and hypocritical. Here was a fat guy trying to tell me how to stay in shape in the first place as my teacher, who then punishes me with the same exercise that he's supposed to be teaching me to love, and because of his authority was free to demand from me almost anything, no matter what I really thought of him as a professional or fellow human being. There was no concern for the reality of my moment, or the truthfulness of the circumstance. I felt like I was part of a machine, where authority was priority and reality was of secondary importance and politics—my swim team coach—could get you off the hook due to his special interests because in his mind, I was a somebody. Without that special leverage I would have been doomed.

This shed a new light on my dealings with the family doctor who himself was a physical wreck, had a large beer belly, thought he knew everything and was always right and who practiced the philosophy "do as I say, not as I do." He told me not to smoke or eat too many eggs or fat, not to drink or do drugs. At a family party, there he was, smoking a cigarette, drinking, eating deviled eggs all night and I discovered he was addicted to pain pills. This is a man of higher learning whom we should all trust and respect? This was maximum hypocrisy. On the other hand, I always had perfect medical tests and even when I developed asthma he couldn't find anything wrong with me through his tests and examinations other than breathing difficulties, for which he referred me to other specialists. In one incident of defiance when I was in college, soon after he told me how important it was to keep my cholesterol as low as it always was, I ate a about dozen eggs every day on average, because I didn't believe him and other athletes encouraged me to eat more protein. On my next cholesterol test, my levels were even lower than they were previously. When I told Dr. H. about this, he simply didn't believe me and actually accused me of doctoring the truth just to give him a hard time. By this time we had developed a love/hate relationship because of my incessant questioning and resistance to what I considered medical hypocrisy. Ultimately, it fostered an attitude whereby I did not like trusting doctors when it came to health and fitness advice and I learned to question, not blindly accept what I considered the limitations of others and their instruments.

The shortcomings of the medical community became crystal clear when I came down with acute asthma, as mentioned previously in the "Clinical Case Studies," and all the medical doctors could do was tell me that the asthma was incurable and systematically load me up with a series of inhalers and pills, after concluding with standard medical testing that I was allergic to cat hair, chicken feathers and dust. Then I heard the radio program with Dr. Carlton Fredericks, where he directed me to a clinic which performed all the other types of tests (nutrition/toxic tests) and which discovered that I was allergic to 78 out of a hundred different foods, along with a huge chlorine poisoning (from the pools) as well as a vast array of nutritional imbalances. One and a half years later, after adhering to a special rotation diet, target-chlorine detoxification and a synergistically customized supplement program, the asthma was gone for good. Additionally, I had an incredible athletic comeback.

Is it any wonder that since that time, I have championed the Hippocratic method set forth in 2400 B.C. by Hippocrates, "in all disease look to the spine first...thy food shall be thy remedy...treat the individual not the disease...and physician do ye no harm"? Early on, I decided that conventional medicine was limited to the test or exam that was given and the people giving the tests and that foodnutrients were the most potent weapons against disease, as I concluded in my complete recovery from asthma. This was also supported in my graduate studies with Dr. Bob Haslam on athletes where we manipulated and measured vitamin B and protein intake and utilization to increase athletic performance. I learned from Dr. Bob that there is no such thing as an average person, bell curves are a joke and that you cannot presume a thing about any body—especially when it comes to nutrition. Talk about going against one-size-fits-all, averaged statistic, standard routine medical and scientific logic and insight.

Subsequently, in clinical practice I emphasized nutrition testing for everybody from day one to every patient who I could get to do it as part of their overall treatment. To me, I just could not be as therapeutically effective without the use of more precise nutrition to expedite the healing process by correcting any problems found in conjunction with other therapy that I practiced upon them. Test by nutrition test, now over 100,000 strong, more than any other health care practitioner, I can tell you that each person, each body is unique. There are no two test results that are the same. I can also tell you that I've witnessed in case after case, health, wellness, and fitness improvements that most people (doctors included) simply find hard to believe can be as simple as eating exactly the right foods and supplements for their specific body. I can also tell you that the labs and researchers that specialize in these tests are the unsung heroes of the truest, most natural, and unadulterated medical healing arts in history. I can also tell you that I've never been more well or felt or looked better by practicing what I preach over all my years and when I demand that you to get down to give me "50," believe that I'm there alongside, doing the work with you.

# Tables, Charts and Graphs

# *APPENDIX A*

Drugs deplete valuable nutrients from the body. The following represents a list of the most researched interactions between drugs and nutrients for your perusal. Remember, personalized nutrition will help to overcome these antagonisms.

### *COMMON DRUG-to-NUTRIENT DEPLETIONS*

| *PRESCRIPTION DRUGS* | *NUTRIENT DEPLETION* |
|---|---|
| Female Hormones | B2, B6, B12, Folic Acid, C, Zinc, Magnesium |
| Diuretics | B1, B6, Magnesium, Potassium, Sodium, Zinc |
| Cholesterol-Lowering Drugs | CoQ10, A, D, E, K, B12, Beta carotene, Folic Acid, Fat |
| Anticonvulsants | D, Calcium, Folic Acid, B12 |
| Anti-inflammatory Drugs | Folic Acid, Calcium, D, Potassium, Selenium, Zinc, Beta carotene, B12 Sodium, Folic Acid, C, Amino Acids, Iron |
| Antibiotics | Acidophilus, Bifidus, All B Complex Vitamins, C, Calcium, K, Magnesium, Zinc, E, Nitrogen, Sodium, Iron, A |
| Antidiabetic Drugs | CoQ10, B12 |
| Ulcer Medications | B12, Folic, D, Protein, Iron, Zinc |
| Heart Medications | Calcium, Magnesium, CoQ10, B2, B12 |
| Chemotherapy Drugs | Most nutrients |
| Theophylline | B6 |
| Coumadin | K |
| Zidovadine, Perovir AZT | Copper, Zinc |
| *NONPRESCRIPTION DRUGS* | *NUTRIENT DEPLETION* |
| Aspirin | C, Folic Acid, Potassium, Zinc |
| Laxatives | A, D, E, K, Beta carotene, Calcium, Potassium |
| Antacids | Calcium, Magnesium, Phosphate, Copper, Iron, Potassium, Zinc, Proteins |
| Ulcer Medications | Folic Acid, B12, D, Zinc |

# APPENDIX B

## DRUG, FOOD, COFACTOR, AND
## HERB INTERACTION GUIDE

Adverse reactions can take place between the following drugs and supplements that can create antagonism within the chemical equilibrium of the body, allowing for advanced degeneration and a general weakening effect if not taken into account. Personalized nutrition helps to correct these antagonisms but care must be taken not to incorrectly mix the following chemicals improperly.

| ANTAGONISTIC SUBSTANCES | |
|---|---|
| ACE Inhibitors | Potassium |
| Abciximab | Any form of vitamin E/tocopherols |
| Acarbose | Niacin, supplemental enzymes |
| Acetaminophen | L-methionine, Mo |
| Acetyl Cystine | Carbamazepine, Nitrates, Nitrites |
| Acitratin | Vitamin A |
| Activated Charcoal | Most drugs, food, herbs, and nutritional supplements (take approx. 2 hours apart) |
| Alcohol | GHB, B6 |
| All Trans Retinoic Acid | Vitamin A |
| Allium Sativum | E, Garlic, Borage Oil, EPA, EPO, Fish Oil, Flaxseed Oil, Parrilla Oil, Tocotrienols |
| Alpha Adrenergic Blockers | Inositol, B2 |
| Alpha Cerotene | Phytosterols |
| Alpha Galactosidase Enzyme | Prebiotics |
| Alpha Lipoic Acid | Antidiabetic Drugs |
| Alprazolam | DHEA |

This is a partial representation of this full chart. To order a complete version send an e-mail to: Chart@Angelmind.net with a description of the chart you'd like to order.

# APPENDIX C

## VARIATIONS OF MINERAL CONTENT IN VEGETABLES

Average phosphorus and minor nutrient content of snap beans and tomatoes and lowest individual values for these and three other vegetables. P is listed by percentage and minor elements by parts per million dry matter.

| Snap Beans | | | | | | | |
|---|---|---|---|---|---|---|---|
| | P | B | Mn | Fe | Mo | Cu | Co |
| Georgia | 0.27 | 14 | 24 | 83 | 0.5 | 12 | 0.02 |
| S. Carolina | 0.27 | 17 | 9 | 110 | 0.4 | 13 | 0.05 |
| Virginia | 0.28 | 12 | 21 | 68 | 0.1 | 17 | 0.05 |
| Maryland | 0.22 | 12 | 30 | 75 | 0.2 | 11 | 0.12 |
| New Jersey | 0.25 | 25 | 7 | 88 | 0.6 | 14 | 0.03 |
| New York | 0.23 | 16 | 20 | 74 | 0.5 | 9 | 0.06 |
| Ohio | 0.27 | 15 | 14 | 77 | 3.0 | 16 | 0.06 |
| Indiana | 0.24 | 20 | 7 | 130 | 5.0 | 14 | 0.03 |
| Illinois | 0.25 | 19 | 7 | 129 | 3.4 | 30 | 0.05 |
| Colorado | 0.26 | 16 | 4 | 130 | 4.3 | 24 | 0.06 |
| **Highest** | **0.36** | **73** | **60** | **227** | **8.1** | **69** | **0.26** |
| **Lowest** | **0.22** | **10** | **2** | **10** | **0.1** | **3** | **0.00** |
| Tomatoes | | | | | | | |
| Georgia | 0.25 | 8 | 6 | 107 | 0.1 | 10 | 0.03 |
| S. Carolina | 0.27 | 10 | 4 | 119 | 0.1 | 11 | 0.06 |
| Virginia | 0.27 | 7 | 3 | 59 | 0.2 | 21 | 0.01 |
| Maryland | 0.19 | 10 | 5 | 97 | 0.1 | 16 | 0.04 |
| New Jersey | 0.24 | 9 | 7 | 113 | 0.2 | 20 | 0.08 |
| New York | 0.23 | 11 | 2 | 87 | 0.1 | 26 | 0.04 |
| Ohio | 0.27 | 20 | 3 | 96 | 0.3 | 12 | 0.02 |
| Indiana | 0.29 | 12 | 4 | 52 | 0.5 | 14 | 0.06 |
| Illinois | 0.30 | 12 | 2 | 179 | 2.0 | 27 | 0.03 |
| Colorado | 0.25 | 13 | 4 | 265 | 0.5 | 24 | 0.11 |
| **Highest** | **0.35** | **36** | **68** | **1,938** | **1.3** | **53** | **0.63** |
| **Lowest** | **0.16** | **5** | **1** | **1** | **0.0** | **0** | **0.00** |

Other extrapolations from this extensive study showed highest and lowest nutrient densities as follows:

| Cabbage | | | | | | | |
|---|---|---|---|---|---|---|---|
| Highest | 0.38 | 42 | 13 | 94 | 24.1 | 48 | 0.15 |
| Lowest | 0.22 | 10 | 2 | 20 | 0.0 | 0.4 | 0.00 |
| Spinach | | | | | | | |
| Highest | 0.52 | 88 | 117 | 1,584 | 5.6 | 32 | 0.25 |
| Lowest | 0.27 | 12 | 1 | 19 | 0.0 | 0.5 | 0.20 |
| Lettuce | | | | | | | |
| Highest | 0.43 | 37 | 169 | 516 | 4.5 | 60 | 0.19 |
| Lowest | 0.22 | 6 | 1 | 9 | 0.0 | 3 | 0.00 |

| Cabbage | | | | | |
|---|---|---|---|---|---|
| | Ash | Calcium | Magnesium | Potassium | Sodium |
| Highest | 10.38 | 60.0 | 43.6 | 148.3 | 20.4 |
| Lowest | 6.12 | 17.5 | 15.6 | 53.7 | 0.8 |
| Spinach | | | | | |
| Highest | 28.56 | 96.0 | 203.9 | 257 | 69.5 |
| Lowest | 12.38 | 47.5 | 46.9 | 84.6 | 0.8 |
| Lettuce | | | | | |
| Highest | 24.28 | 71.0 | 49.3 | 176.5 | 12.2 |
| Lowest | 7.01 | 16.0 | 13.1 | 53.7 | 0.0 |

Ash values are given in percentages and other mineral cations (positively charged minerals) in milliequivalents per 100 grams dry water.

Source: Firman E. Bear Report from Rutgers University, 1937. Contributing researchers include Steven J. Toth, Arthur L. Prince, and Arthur Wallace.

308

# APPENDIX D

*Malibu Quick Check* is the Old School non-laboratory-mediated step that we use to help you match your physical, intellectual, personality, ethnic, and religious characteristics as closely as possible to your primary metabolic type. *Quick-Geno-Check* helps you to recognize one's genotrophic category (or metabolic type) to better clarify how your body and mind work. It reflects how your ancestral environment has shaped you and indicates your ideal environment and lifestyle.

It would be so much simpler if we could just identify you or me as a Hunzan tribesperson, for example, with a pure genotrophic category that has not been historically impacted by other people's cultural and genetic influences or man-made environmental changes. Then we could send you to your homeland or at least simulate its living conditions in order to optimize your wellness level. Unfortunately, this is rarely possible in this day and age, so instead we have to compile your personal data into a metabolic profile from which we can match your nutritional, environmental, and lifestyle needs. The end result is what the Hunzans already know—100 plus years of quality (disease-free) life.

There are eight generalized genetic patterns that I encounter regularly although there are many more including sensory types, exocrine types, somatypes etc. Because there are so many genotypes, the complexity is too high to utilize in clinical practice, while its value is too little in the face of orthomolecular analysis. I used to utilize the *Quick-Geno-Check* typing system which features Super Quick Check, Dead Giveaways, No Doubt About It (flow chart), Typing At A Glance, and Super Duper Quick Check which I have condensed due to space limitations. These systems would quickly and easily identify primary dominant patterns and any secondary patterns that relate to you as well. Your blood type is matched to a basic food profile, while your endocrine gland balance as determined in *Quick-Geno-Check* refines this information further and also outlines special supplemental needs and ranges.

On a side note, there are many more types than the eight basic ones presented here such as exocrine types, sensory types, nerve types, oxidation types, somatotypes, constitutional types, etc. But these were considered to be of secondary (or lesser) incremental importance to the controlling primary essence metabolic types presented here. These eight types are in effect based solely upon the most powerful biochemical-physiological-psychological regulators of the body, and not the secondary or tertiary ones. In other words, the metabolic types presented here represent the *essence* of one's genetic/metabolic design, which sets the pattern from which the other types as mentioned above (really minor subtypes) manifest over time. The functional distinctions of these other significant minor subtypes is covered only for the most discriminating typer but in light of testing accomplishes very little any more.

For now, do not concern yourself with the smaller details. Rather, if you can, fit yourself into your metabolic types as described in the following pages. There is a chart and a table that are included which will minimize any chance for mistakes. The goal of the **Quick Check** System is to take what would otherwise be an even more complicated procedure and simplify it so that anyone can find his or her type quickly.

In order to properly type yourself, you must first scrutinize your body and mind closely. For some this may seem the hardest part because your awareness of self is put to the test. It's time to face up to what you look like and who you really are.

First you need to find out what your blood type is from your doctor, a blood test, or relatives. Your blood type is a must because it helps identify your basic **theoretical** food pattern as a meat eater, vegetarian derivative or omnivore. Are you blood type O, A, B, or AB? Are you Rh negative or positive?

Next, you must obtain your height in feet and inches in bare feet. For typing purposes tall men are considered to be six feet and over, tall women are considered to be five feet seven inches and over. Average height for men is considered to be five feet seven inches to five feet eleven inches, for women, five feet three inches to five feet seven inches. Short men are less than five feet seven inches while short women are considered to be short at five feet three inches or less in height.

Your body shape, fatness, hairiness, and muscularity must also be characterized. Are you round, fatty with very soft muscles? Are you long, thin with average-looking musculature? Are you naturally muscular with an athletic appearance such as toned muscles and a very sturdy look to you? Ladies, do you have an hourglass figure with large breasts and/or hips, soft muscles and cellulite tendencies when you gain a few pounds? Gentlemen, do you have a barrel type chest with abundant hair and/or extra large shoulders, small hips, and average to better than average muscle tone? Do you have a large prominent forehead or a large round occiput (rear of skull)? Or are you one of those rather rare individuals who is just symmetrical – the human average – not particularly fat, tall, short, overly muscular, round, square, triangular, voluptuous, hairy, and with no features that are seemingly out of proportion?

Two easily identifiable psychological traits also need to be characterized. Are you only happy when you are the leader or when in front of an audience? Are you extremely charismatic? Are you highly sensitive and intuitive to the point of being a psychic or clairvoyant? Think about it.

One word of warning: do not make the typing process more complicated than it really is by over rationalizing your descriptors. Simplicity is the key. Pick your blood type first, then obtain your height, then visualize your shape, and next consider your personality in terms of being a leader or highly sensitive/intuitive. The rest will fall into place as typing and testing proceeds further.

### *Super Quick Check*

**About forty percent of the civilized world is blood type O.** This is the oldest of the blood types. If you are a blood type O there is only one of four primary metabolic types that you can be. The metabolic types are named after the strongest functioning gland in the body (except for the balanced type, where all is equal). For "O" blood these types are:

1. Gonadal Type – Gonads are the sexual glands
2. Pancreatic Type – Pancreas controls blood sugar/digestion
3. Thymic Type – Thymus effects growth/immune system development
4. Pituitary Type – Pituitary is the master gland over all others

***Dead Giveaways*** – To quickly discover which metabolic type you may be based on blood type O, match yourself up with the four physical and/or psychological descriptions listed for each of the types below:

| | | |
|---|---|---|
| <u>Gonadal</u> -<br>(sexy) | *Women:* | Curvaceous, hourglass type figure (large breasts/hips)<br>Cellulite tendencies and sexy voice<br>Up to 5'7" tall (rarely over 5'7")<br>Slight weight gain tendency |

|  |  |  |
|---|---|---|
| | *Men:* | Male pattern baldness<br>Barrel chest/pot-bellied over time<br>Hairy body, especially chest, deep voice<br>Up to 5'11" (rarely over 5'11") |
| Pancreatic -<br>(overweight) | *Women:* | Always overweight or obese since childhood<br>Chubby features/very round body and face<br>Can be big eaters, fat and sugar-aholics<br>Any height |
| | *Men:* | Always overweight or obese since childhood<br>Chubby features/round body and face<br>Can be big eaters, fat and sugar-aholics<br>Any height |
| Thymic -<br>(tall) | *Women:* | Taller than average, usually 5'7" or more<br>Long limbed/linear body<br>Long face shape<br>Knobby joints and/or large rib cage |
| | *Men:* | Taller than average, usually 6' or more<br>Long limbed/linear body<br>Long face shape<br>Knobby joints and/or large rib cage |
| Pituitary -<br>(leader) | *Women:* | Large prominent forehead in terms of width, depth, height<br>Slightly receding frontal hairline<br>Has to be the leader in a group<br>Extremely charismatic and outspoken |
| | *Men:* | Large prominent forehead in terms of width,<br>depth, height<br>Slightly receding frontal hairline<br>Has to be the leader in a group<br>Extremely charismatic and outspoken |

**The second oldest of the blood types is blood type A.** If you are a blood type A, there is only one of four metabolic types you can be. These types are:

1. Thyroid Type  – Thyroid controls metabolic and oxidation rate
2. Pineal Type  – Pineal sets wake/sleep hormone cycles
3. Thymic Type  – Thymus effects growth/immune system development
4. Balanced Type (this only applies to men) – No dominant gland

***Dead Giveaways*** – To quickly discover which metabolic type you may be based on blood type A match yourself up with the four physical and/or psychological descriptions listed for each of the types.

| Thyroid -<br>(thin & quick) | *Women:* | Always on the thin side<br>Up to 5'7" in height<br>Small bones/delicate features<br>Move quickly and/or restless |
|---|---|---|

|  |  |  |
|---|---|---|
| | *Men*: | Always on the thin side<br>Up to 5'11" in height<br>Small bones/delicate features<br>Move quickly and/or restless |
| Pineal -<br>(intuitive) | *Women*: | Large occiput (rear skull area)<br>Usually thin, sometimes frail/soft-spoken<br>Extremely aware/sensitive/intuitive<br>Any height |
| | *Men:* | Large occiput (rear skull area)<br>Usually thin, sometimes frail/soft-spoken<br>Extremely aware/sensitive/intuitive<br>Any height |
| Thymic -<br>(tall) | *Women*: | Taller than average, usually 5'7" or more<br>Long limbs<br>Long face shape<br>Knobby joints and/or large rib cage |
| | *Men:* | Taller than average, usually 6' or more<br>Long limbs<br>Long face shape<br>Knobby joints and/or large rib cage |
| Balanced -<br>(average) | *Men:* | No overpowering physical characteristics<br>Medium body shape and features<br>5'6" to 5'11" |

**Blood type B is the next-oldest blood pattern which occurred from a genetic mutation allowing for better milk digestion.** These types are:

1. Adrenal Type – Adrenals control amount of oxidation and metabolism
2. Thymic Type – Thymic effects growth/immune system development
3. Balanced Type (primarily women) – No dominant gland

**Dead Giveaways** – To quickly discover what metabolic type you may be based on blood type B, match yourself up with the four physical features listed under each of these types:

|  |  |  |
|---|---|---|
| Adrenals -<br>(muscular) | *Women*: | Prominent muscles/stable weight<br>Good muscle tone<br>Strong, dense bones<br>Any height but usually 5' to 5'8" |
| | *Men:* | Prominent muscles/stable weight<br>Very good muscle tone<br>Strong, dense bones<br>Any height but usually 5'2" to 6' |

Thymic -      *Women*:    Taller than average, usually 5'7" or more
(tall)                     Long limbs with above-average muscle tone
                             Long face shape
                             Knobby joints and/or large rib cage

                 *Men:*    Taller than average, usually 6' or more
                             Long limbs with above-average muscle tone
                             Long face shape
                             Knobby joints and/or large rib cage

Balanced -    *Women*:    No overpowering physical characteristics
(average)                    Medium body shape and features
                             5'3 to 5'7"
The statistical human average: 1% to 3% of world population

**Blood type AB is the newest and rarest of the blood types which mutated approximately 1,000 years ago from blood type B and blood type A interbreeding, according to geneticists.** If you are a blood type AB there is only one of two primary metabolic types that you can be. These types are:

1. Balanced Type (men and women) – No dominant gland
2. Thymic Type – Thymus affects growth/immune system development

***Dead Giveaways*** – To quickly discover what metabolic type you may be based on blood type AB, match up with the four physical descriptions listed:

Balanced -    *Women*:    No overpowering physical characteristics
(average)                    Medium body shape and features
                             5'3 to 5'7"
The statistical human average: 1% to 3% of world population

                 *Men:*    No overpowering physical characteristics
                             Medium body shape and features
                             5'6" to 5'11"
The statistical human average: 1% to 3% of world population

Thymic -      *Women*:    Taller than average, usually 5'7" or more
(tall)                     Long limbs with above-average muscle tone
                             Long face shape
                             Knobby joints and/or large rib cage

                 *Men:*    Taller than average, usually 6' or more
                             Long limbs with above-average muscle tone
                             Long face shape
                             Knobby joints and/or large rib cage

## *No Doubt About It Flow Chart*

| BLOOD TYPE O | | | |
|---|---|---|---|
| *T4 | T5 | T6 | T7 |
| Gonadal Type | Pancreatic Type | Thymic Type | Pituitary Type |
| F: Curvy, to 5'7" | M&F: Round and overweight | F: Long, over 5'7" | M&F: Huge forehead |
| M: Balding, to 5'11" | | M: Long, over 5'11" | Leader mentality |
| **BLOOD TYPE A** | | | |
| T1 | T1A | T6 | T3 |
| Thyroid Type | Pineal Type | Thymic Type | Balanced Type |
| F: Small features, under 5'7" | M&F: Lrg occiput, frail, intuitive | F: Long, over 5'7" | M: 5'6" –5'11" |
| | | M: Long, over 5'11" | Human average |
| M: Small features, Under 5'11" | | | Medium features |
| **BLOOD TYPE B** | | | |
| T3 | T6 | T2 | |
| Adrenal Type | Thymic Type | Balanced Type | |
| M&F: Muscle tone, athletic appearance | M&F: Muscle tone, long limbs | F: Med. features, human average | |
| F: 5'0" – 5'8" | F: 5'7" plus | F: 5'3" – 5'7" | |
| M: 5'2" – 6' | M: 6'0" plus | | |
| **BLOOD TYPE AB** | | | |
| T6 | T3 | | |
| Thymic Type | Balanced Type | | |
| M&F: Long limbs | M&F: Med. features, human average | | |
| F: Over 5'7" | | | |
| M: Over 5'11" | F: 5'3" – 5'7" | | |
| | M: 5'7" – 5'11" | | |

**\*T4, T5 etc. are abbreviations**

If any confusion exists at this point, do not fret; you can still make your metabolic connection by contacting info@RealPNC.com for the full report so that you can "OLD SCHOOL" Type yourself fully if so desired.

Reminder – the nutrition tests and their recommendations take full precedence over "Pure Typing" which is considered purely hypothetical unless you are known to be a "Modern Day Primitive" tribal member. That is why this process is considered obsolete and is not of primary concern in determining your most critical needs up-to-the-moment.

# GLOSSARY

**absorption** - the physiological process by which the body takes in through the digestive mucosa the smallest individual components left after the digestive process is completed

**Actual Daily Calorie Consumption (ADCC)**— the actual amount of calories that you're taking in per day; when this figure is higher than your TCND figure, you gain weight. If it is lower, then you'll lose weight; if they are both the same, you'll stay the same weight

**anabolism**—the building up phase of metabolism

**ancestral (or tribal) typing**—using the science of genealogy to trace one's phenotypic origins during the process of determining biochemical individuality

**assimilation**—the process by which the body utilizes the nutrient compounds provided by digestion and absorption for metabolism

**autonomic nervous system**—controls your overall response to stress; that part of the nervous system concerned with regulating the activity of cardiac muscle, smooth muscle, glands and other involuntary functions

**balascopy**—patented perceptual technology with a cascade of 15 methodologies devised for the detection, extraction, quantification, assessment, and mapping of multiple relationships within a given system (in this case, human metabolism)

**Basal Metabolic Rate (BMR) (expressed as calories)**—the daily rate at which your body consumes calories in a resting state to sustain life (as if you were to lie in bed 24 hours); males burn 24 Kcal/Kg of bodyweight per day; females burn 21.9 Kcal/Kg of bodyweight per day

**biochemical**—any chemical compound found within the body which is involved with the vital processes and physiological chemistry of life

**biochemical individuality**— a phenomenon of personal uniqueness where no two people are exactly alike in the way their bodies and minds

are structured and function and therefore in the precise needs of their bodies and minds for overall wellness

**blood typing**—using the chemical groupings and subgroupings of blood to help delineate metabolic types to further distinguish individual biochemical identity

**calorie deficit (negative calorie balance)**—a lower calorie intake or fewer calories than the body needs to maintain itself at its present weight; the body is forced to come up with missing food calories from fat storage because it's not receiving enough calories from the diet to maintain its current weight level

**calorimetry**— specific scientific procedures which measure the amount of heat given off as measured in calories by a living individual or for measuring the potential energy in food. All heat measures are given in calories or their equivalent

**carni-vegan**— person with a type of diet containing red and white meats and mostly low starch, alkaline vegetables and fruits

**carnivorous**— pure meat-eater (over 70% of calories in diet from animal and fish sources). Traditional Eskimos are considered pure carnivores

**catabolism**—the breaking-down phase of metabolism

**catalyst**—any substance that increases the velocity of a chemical reaction or process which in itself is not consumed in the net chemical reaction or process

**clinical nutritionist**— a highly trained professional nutritionist with degrees in nutrition, biology or physiology with thousands of hours of professional school in the basic and clinical sciences, including every basic and clinical knowledge parameter from cadaver dissection to treating diet-related illnesses in the clinical environment; is addressed as "Doctor" and uses physical examination and laboratory procedures in nutritional work-ups

**coefficient of activity**—the measurable level of the sum total of all biochemical processes in relation to the process of ionization which forms the nature of one's metabolism

**coenzymes**— also known as cofactors, vitamins, and minerals, all of which stimulate enzyme action

**Daily Physical Activity Need (DPAN, also known as the energy level of physical activity)**—the caloric energy needs of your body as a result of getting out of bed, moving around and exercising

**deductive reasoning**—reasoning from the general to the specific

**desaturase**—any enzyme that catalyzes the desaturation of a fatty acid

**desaturation**—chemical process of introducing a double bond between the carbon atoms of a fatty acid

**detoxification**—process of removing the health-damaging effects of a toxic substance

**digestion**—chemical process by which the body breaks apart all of foods' nutrients into their smallest individual components

**drug** – any chemical that can create symptomatic relief, but that is not already part of or derived from the body's chemical structure or essential needs, i.e., vitamin C is not a drug because the body becomes sick without it; Prozac is a drug because it doesn't occur naturally within the body nor is essential to the body's life processes

**ectoderm**— the outermost of the 3 primary embryonic germ layers which form the skin and nervous system, the predominance of which in a given body relates to the high-strung, highly intelligent, lean or seemingly underweight ectomorph type

**ectomorph**— an individual having a type of body in which tissues derived from the ectoderm predominate: preponderance of linearity and fragility, with large surface area, thin muscles and subcutaneous tissue, low body fat, and slightly developed digestive viscera (digestive systems)

**ectotonia**—psychological state of being centered on privacy, self-restraint and a highly developed self awareness

**eicosanoids**—"super hormones" manufactured by every living cell of the human body as derived from essential fatty acids within the diet

**electrochemical resistance**—the effect produced when atomic particles of varying energy potentials encounter one another and release energy

**elimination**—the process by which the body rids itself of residual chemical waste products produced by the body as a result of metabolism

**elongation**— the chemical process of increasing the length of a molecule

**endocrine glands**—organs that secrete hormones directly into the circulatory system influencing metabolism and other bodily processes including behavior

**endocrine typing**—using the strength and weakness hierarchy of the body's endocrine glands to group people into body types, metabolic types, or constitutional types to help delineate individual biochemical identity

**endoderm (aka entoderm)**— the innermost of the 3 primary germ layers of the embryo from which is derived the digestive tract and linings of the pharynx, respiratory tract, bladder, and urethra

**endogenous**—made within the body

**endomorph**— an individual who has a body build predominately composed of tissues from the endo or entoderm; possesses a preponderance of soft roundness throughout the body with large digestive viscera and fat accumulation, large trunk and thighs, and tapering extremities

**endotonia**— psychological state of being demonstrated by the love of relaxation, comfort, food, and people

**energy (human)**—the electrochemical force that sustains life released through the biochemical processing of nutrients, air, and water

**enzyme**—a cellular protein capable of accelerating the chemical reaction of a substance into a product without being destroyed or altered during the process

**exogenous**—from outside of the body

**food assay**— qualitative and quantitative analysis of the nutrient and nonnutrient composition of food

**Forced Feeding Incompatibility Syndrome (FFIS)**—a phenomenon where *one-size-fits-all* symptom relief marketing promoters encourage unsuspecting consumers to risk their health by eating foods which are either generically unhealthy or specifically incompatible with an individual while they promise to relieve the symptomatic consequences that one will suffer from eating these foods with their special symptom-blocking wonder drug

**free energy**—the life force available to the body above and beyond that which is being consumed to counteract resistance within the body and mind

**genotype**— reflection of the entire genetic constitution of a person which distinguishes his or her physical appearance

**health index**—the degree of metabolic balance reflected by the mathematical ratio of energy to resistance expressed as a factor of probability

**homeostasis**—the mechanism of the body that keeps it in life-sustaining balance; a tendency toward stability in the normal body states (internal environment) of an individual achieved by a system of control mechanisms activated by negative feedback

**inductive reasoning**—reasoning from the specific to the general

**ionization**—the metabolic process by which nutrients are moved from one place to another by ions or dispersed as ions internally

**ions**—positively or negatively charged particles; elemental minerals are all ions with either positive or negative charges until neutralized as salt or chelation compound

**laboratory testing/typing a.k.a. Profiling**—that component of the overall typing process which utilizes human specimens (blood, urine, feces, saliva, hair, etc.) to help determine biochemical identity by measuring nutrient and toxin states in the body

**macronutrients**—basic nutrients which we need to consume as humans on a daily basis in "larger than gram" amounts; they consist of proteins, fat, carbohydrates, water, and air and each have their own caloric and metabolic value; ethanol is considered a nonessential macronutrient

**megadoser**—someone who takes in too much of anything (usually foods, drink, supplements, drugs, or exercise)

**mesoderm**—the middle layer of the 3 primary embryonic germ layers which form the connective tissue and muscles and is therefore associated with the typically muscular mesomorph type

**mesomorph**—an individual whose body build is characteristic of mesodermal predominance: possesses a preponderance of muscle, bone, and connective tissue usually with a hard, heavy physique and with rectangular or squarish appearance

**mesotonia**—psychological state of being which focuses on being assertive and on a love of action

**metabolic balance**—when the chemistry of the body is working at peak efficiency and follows the relative path of least resistance for energy production

**metabolic map**—a graphic representation of both balanced and imbalanced metabolic relationships between body chemicals as demonstrated through the phenomenon of metabolic networks; metabolic maps can also be considered metabolic patterns

**metabolic network**—a network of metabolic relationships which reflect metabolic function as an integrated whole and not as a list of isolated variables

**metabolic typing (patterning)**—process of categorizing certain constitutional elements of the body into their own unique subgroups to help determine biochemical identity; includes all aspects of typing short of lab-mediated profiling

**metabolism**—the total profile of all biochemical activity required to maintain life

**micronutrients**—essential nutrients your body needs in "less than gram" amounts, e.g. vitamins, minerals, and vitamin-like substances

**MUFA (Monounsaturated Fatty Acids)**—nutritional fats with a characteristic single open molecular bond per carbon chain

**negative feedback**—an inhibitory (resistive) controlling effect on the output of a system. Example: the buildup of acids in the blood from anaerobic exercise triggers an increase in bicarbonate output by the kidneys to buffer the acids and restore pH balance

**nerve typing**—using the sympathetic/parasympathetic dominance hierarchy to help delineate metabolic types and to further distinguish individual biochemical identity

**novice nutritionist**—self-proclaimed nutritionist who does not have years of study nor the necessary degrees to fully understand the body's inner workings and the clinical application of precise nutritional science to optimize body function; may possess a correspondence degree or some minor degree of schooling

**nutrient**—any naturally occurring essential substance that provides or catalyzes energy production for the functional growth and maintenance of the human organism

**nutrition**—the measurable process by which nutrients maintain the life of the body and mind

**omnivore**—person who can eat all types of foods

**omnivorous**—able to eat all types of foods for efficient metabolism

**overfat**—a specific amount of body fat accumulation which when reached creates resistance to overall metabolic balance and is characteristically different for each body type and each individual as measured by the science of typing/profiling

**oxidation (biological)**—the enzymatic process by which food is metabolized using oxygen, resulting in the release of energy

**oxidation typing**—using oxidation rates and amounts as the basis to delineate metabolic types in the quest to distinguish biochemical identity; used in conjunction with nerve typing and endocrine typing as a secondary distinguishing feature of metabolism

**parasympathetic nervous system**—controls the alkaline cells or basophils which is that part of the nervous system that has a calming effect on the body including digestion

**phenotype**—body classification which reflects the entire physical, biochemical, and physiological makeup of an individual as determined both environmentally and genetically

**phytonutrients (aka phytochemicals)**—nutrient compounds found in vegetables and fruits including vitamins, minerals, enzymes, and other compounds

**piecemealer**—someone who takes a little bit of this and a little bit of that of food and supplements (not knowing if they really need them or not) to try to make a complete diet and supplement plan

**profiling**—see **laboratory typing**

**psychological typing**—using patterns of personality in the quest to determine biochemical identity

**pseudonutritionist**—self-proclaimed nutritionist with absolutely no formal training in nutritional sciences whatsoever

**PUFA (Polyunsaturated Fatty Acids)**—nutritional fats with characteristic open molecular bonds throughout the carbon chain mostly from plant sources particularly grains, seeds, and vegetables; includes the body's essential fatty acids: cis-linoleic and alpha linolenic acids

**pure typing**—using only those typing procedures not directly involving laboratory procedures of specimen evaluation except for blood type

**purine**—by-product of nucleic acid (genetic material) breakdown in red meat which forms uric acid; found in high concentrations in red meats; can cause gout in people who are biochemically susceptible or have certain mineral deficiencies

**ratio**—proportion of one nutrient to the next construed as either synergistic or antagonistic in terms of physiologic response

**resistance**—(overall) the electrochemical inhibition of "free energy" production within the body due to the presence of inadequate nutrition, pathological (disease) states, physical degeneration (including premature aging), and/or the spiritual condition of the individual

**SAFA (Saturated Fatty Acids)**—nutritional fats with characteristic closed molecular bonds predominantly from animal sources

**shotgunner**—someone who takes a huge variety of nutrients and supplements thinking that they are going to cover all of their metabolic needs

**somatyping**—using the predominate pattern of primal derm distribution when categorizing metabolic types

**Specific Dynamic Activity (SDA)**—the calorie energy required for the process of digestion and reflexive fat thermogenesis after eating

**state of health**—the continuing variable adaptation of the biochemistry of metabolism between the internal environment and the external environment of a living organism relative to its coefficient of activity

**submetabolic**—a small profile of biochemical activity which contributes in some part to the total profile of metabolism

**substrate**—a substance upon which an enzyme acts

**sympathetic nervous system**—the part of the autonomic nervous system which controls acid cells known as acidophilus and which is that part of the nervous system which prepares our bodies for fight or flight

**thermogenesis**—heat production by the body. About 75% of the energy liberated by the human body is given off as heat, the rest is converted into ATP

**Total Caloric Need per Day (TCND)**—the amount of calories your body needs to maintain itself at a constant weight without a net gain or loss of weight

**toxic overload**—when the presence of toxins internally stresses the process of metabolism beyond its capacity to neutralize the deteriorative effects of the toxins

**toxin**—any substance present internally or externally that increases resistance or stress to the metabolic process

**typing**—the science and art of determining a person's unique biochemical identity utilizing all aspects of metabolic typing (endocrine, blood, psychological, body shape and features, nerve, oxidation, laboratory assessment, quantification and qualification)

**yo-yo diet**—a dietary syndrome of rapid weight loss followed by rapid weight gain which can repeat itself many times over

**zeta potential**—mathematical basis for the physical chemistry governing the stability of liquid-solid systems; in more biological terms, the maintenance of fluidity within the aqueous (water-based) systems of both plant and animal life based upon inherent ionization properties

# Index

# *Bibliography*

Abravanel, Elliot, D., M.D. *Dr. Abravanel's Bodytype Diet*. New York: Bantam Books, 1983

Bajusz, E., M.D. *Nutritional Aspects of Cardiovascular Disease*. London: Crosby, Lockwood, and Son, 1965

Balch, James F., M.D. and Balch, Phyllis A., C.N.C. *Prescription For Nutritional Healing*. New York: Avery Publishing Group, 1990

Beach, Rex. "Modern Miracle Men," United States Government Printing Office Washington, 264 (1936)

Beasley, J.D., M.D. and Swift, Jerry, M.A. *The Kellogg Report: The Impact of Nutrition & Lifestyle on the Health of Americans*. New York: Annandale-On-Hudson, 1989

Beddoe, A.F. *Biologic Ionization As Applied To Human Nutrition*. Grass Valley, CA: Agro-Bio Systems, 1990

Bieler, Henry G. and Block, Maxine. *Food Is Your Best Medicine*. New York: Random House, 1965

Bland, Jeffrey, PhD. *Trace Elements in Human Health and Disease*. Bellevue; Washington: Northwest Diagnostic Services, 1979

Bralley, Alexander J., PhD, C.C.N., and Richard S. Lord PhD. *Laboratory Evaluations in Molecular Medicine*. Norcross, Ga.: The Institute For Advances in Molecular Medicine, 2001

Braly, James, M.D. *Dr. Braly's Food Allergy & Nutrition Revolution*. New Canaan, Connecticut: Keats Publishing, 1992

Brody, Jane. *Jane Brody's Nutrition Book*. New York: Bantam Books, 1981

Bucci, Luke R., PhD, C.C.N., C(ASCP). "Role of Individualized Convenient Assessment," *CCA Journal*, 19:3 (March, 1994)

Cass, Hyla, M.D. and Patrick Holford. *Natural Highs,* New York: Avery 2002

Cheraskin, E., M.D., D.M.D., et al. *Diet and Disease*. New Canaan, Connecticut: Keats Publishing, 1977

Colgan, Michael, PhD. *Your Personal Vitamin Profile*. New York: William Morrow & Company, 1982

Collin, Jonathan, M.D. "Food and Drug Insider Report," *Townsend Letter For Doctors*, 108 (July, 1992)

Colt, George Howe. "Heal Me," *Life Magazine,* (September, 1996)

Communications Research Machines, Inc. *Biology Today*. Del Mar, California: CRM Books, 1972

Crawford, Michael, PhD and Marsh, David, PhD. *The Driving Force - Food, Evolution and The Future*. New York: Harper & Row, 1989

Cummings, Stephen, M.D. and Dana Ullman, M.P.H. *Everybody's Guide to Homeopathic Medicines*. New York: Putnam, 1991

D'Adamo, James, N.D. "ABO Bias May Signal Innate Differences In Natural Immunity," *Journal of Naturopathic Medicine*, 2:1 (1991)

D'Adamo, James, N.D. *One Man's Food*. Madrid, Spain: Everest, 1980

D'Adamo, Peter, N.D. *Eat Right For Your Bodytype*. New York, New York: G.P. Putnam's Sons, 1996

Chopra, Deepak, M.D. *Quantum Healing: Exploring The Frontiers of Mind-Body Medicine*. New York: Bantam Books, 1989

Chopra, Deepak, M.D. *Perfect Health*. New York: Harmony Books, 1991

DeGowin, Elmer L., M.D. and DeGowin, Richard L., M.D. *Bedside Diagnostic Examination*. New York: Macmillan Publishing Company, 1981

DeRoeck, Richard E., D.C. *The Confusion About Chiropractors*. Danbury, Connecticut: Impulse Publishing, 1989

Eaton, S. Boyd. M.D. *The Paleolithic Prescription*. New York: Harper & Row, 1988

Erasmus, Udo, PhD *Fats That Can Heal, Fats That Can Kill*. B.C., Canada: Alive Books, 1996

Feuer, Elaine. *Innocent Casualties: The FDA's War Against Humanity.* Pittsburgh: Dorrance Publishing Co., 1996

Galsey, Alan R., M.D. "Literature Review and Commentary," *Townsend Letter For Doctors,* 108 (July, 1992)

Gelb, Barbara Levine. *The Dictionary of Food and What's In It For You.* New York: Ballantine Books, 1978

Gittleman, Ann Louise, M.S., C.N.S. "A New Year, A New You," *Healthy Talk,* Premier Issue (1996)

Gittleman, Ann Louise, M.S., C.N.S. *Your Body Knows Best.* New York: Pocket Books, 1996

Goldfinger, Steven, E., M.D., ed. "Unkind Milk," *Harvard Health Letter,* 18:12 (October, 1993)

Goldfinger, Steven E., M.D., ed. "By The Way, Doctor," *Harvard Health Letter,* 19:10 (August, 1994)

Goldfinger, Steven E., M.D., ed. "Food Allergies That Stretch To Latex," *Harvard Health Letter,* 19:5 (March, 1994)

Goodhart, Robert S., M.D., D.M.S. and Shils, Maurice E., M.D., Sc.D. *Modern Nutrition in Health and Disease.* Philadelphia: Lea & Febiger, 1980

Guthrie, Helen Andrews. *Introductory Nutrition.* Saint Louis: C.V. Mosby Company, 1971

Guyton, Arthur C., M.D. *Textbook of Medical Physiology.* Philadelphia: W. B. Saunders Company, 1981

Hausman, Patricia and Hurley, Judith Benn. *The Healing Foods.* Emmans, Pennsylvania: Rodale Press, 1989

Hendler, Sheldon, PhD, M.D. and Daniel Rorvic, M.S., *PDR for Nutritional Supplements.* Montvale, New Jersey: Medical Economics Company Inc., 2001

Herbert, Victor, M.D. "What You Should Know About Vitamins - The Case Against Supplements," Bottom Line, 15:23 (December, 1994)

Horrrobin, David, M.D., PhD. *Clinical Uses of Essential Fatty Acids.* Montreal - London: Eden Press, 1982

Jacobsen, Michael, PhD, ed. "Pumping Immunity," *Nutrition Action Health Letter,* 20:3 (April, 1993)

Jacobson, Michael, PhD, ed. "Short Takes," *Nutrition Action Health Letter,* 20:10 (December, 1993)

Jacobsen, Michael, PhD , ed. "Viva La Difference: Aspirin," *Nutrition Action Health Letter,* 22:2 (March, 1995)

Jung, Carl. *Psychological Types or The Psychology of Individuation.* New York: Pantheon Books, 1923

Jung, Carl. *Psychological Types.* California: Princeton University, 1976

Kennedy, Charles C., M.D., ed. "Beta Carotene Supplements - Do They Prevent Or Promote Lung Cancer?" *Update Mayo Clinic Health Letter,* April 14, 1994)

Kennedy, Charles C., M.D., ed. "Second Opinion," *Mayo Clinic Health Letter,* 12:8 (August, 1994)

Kennedy, Charles C., M.D., ed. "Breakfast Cereal," *Mayo Clinic Health Letter,* 12:9 (September, 1994)

Kennedy, Charles C., M.D., ed. "Herbal Supplements," *Mayo Clinic Health Letter,* 12:6 (June, 1994)

Klafs, Carl E., PhD, F.A.C.S.M. and Arnheim, Daniel D., D.P.E., F.A.C.S.M., F.A.C.T.A. *Modern Principles of Athletic Training.* Saint Louis: C.V. Mosby Company, 1973

Kreutler, Patricia A., PhD. *Nutrition In Perspective.* New Jersey: Prentice-Hall, Inc., 1980

Langman, Jan, M.D. PhD. *Medical Embryology.* Baltimore: Maryland, 1981:

Matthews Larson, Joan, *Depression-Free, Naturally,* New York, NY: The Random House Group,1999

Liebman, Bonnie, M.S. "Sneak Previews," *Nutrition Action Health Letter,* 20:1 (January/February, 1993)

Liebman, Bonnie, M.S. "Non-Trivial Pursuits: Playing The Research Game," *Nutrition Action Health Letter,* 21:8 (October, 1994)

Liebman, Bonnie, M.S. "Just The Calcium Facts," *Nutrition Action Health Letter*, 22:4 (May, 1995)

Liebman, Bonnie, M.S. "Quick Studies: Trans Wreck," *Nutrition Action Health Letter*, 22:4 (May, 1995)

Liebman, Bonnie, M.S. "Fish Oil Flops," *Nutrition Action Health Letter*, 20:6 (July/August, 1993)

Liebman, Bonnie, M.S. "Coffee Lovers," *Nutrition Action Health Letter*, 21:3 (April, 1994)

Liebman, Bonnie, M.S. "Short Takes," *Nutrition Action Health Letter*, 21:3 (April, 1994)

Liebman, Bonnie, M.S. "Antioxidants: Surprise, Surprise," *Nutrition Action Health Letter*, 21:5 (June, 1994)

Liebman, Bonnie, M.S. "M.D. = Mediocre Diet?" *Nutrition Action Health Letter*, 21:3 (April, 1993)

Liebman, Bonnie, M.S. "Tea For 250 Million?" *Nutrition Action Health Letter*, 21:9 (November, 1994)

Lipton, Bruce, PhD The *Biology of Belief*, USA: Fountain of Love/Elite Books, 2005

Luciano, Dorothy S., Vander, Arthur J., and Sherman, James H. *Human Function and Structure*. New York: McGraw-Hill Book Company, 1978

Malter, Rick, PhD. "Trace Mineral Analysis and Psychoneuroimmunology," *Journal of Orthomolecular Medicine*, 9:2 (1994)

Margolis, Simeon, M.D., ed. "Drugstore Aisle," *John Hopkins Health After 50 Medical Letter*, 6:6 (August, 1994)

Margolis, Simeon, M.D., ed. "Our Readers Ask," *John Hopkins Health After 50 Medical Letter*, 6:8 (October, 1994)

Margolis, Simeon, M.D., ed. "Weighing The Latest Cancer Risks," *John Hopkins After 50 Medical Letter*, 6:10 (December, 1994)

Margolis, Simeon, M.D., ed. "Tamoxifen: Cancer Cause or Cure," *John Hopkins Health After 50 Medical Letter*, 6:8 (October, 1994)

Marion, Joseph B. *Anti-Aging Manual – Encyclopedia of Natural Health*. Connecticut: Information Pioneers, 1996

Mathews, Donald K. and Fox, Edward L. *The Physiological Basis of Physical Education and Athletics*. Philadelphia: W. B. Saunders Company, 1976

McCance, Katherine, R.N., PhD and Sue E. Huether, R.N., PhD. *Pathophysiology*. St. Louis: Mosby, 1994

Mein, Carol, D.C. *25 Body Types—25 Diets*.

Meir, Edith C., PhD, et al. *An Evaluation of Research in the United States on Human Nutrition: Report No. 2: Benefits from Nutrition Research*. Washington D.C.: U.S. Department of Agriculture, 1971

Mendelsohn, Robert, M.D. *Confessions of a Medical Heretic*. New York: Warner Books, 1979

Metropolitan Life Insurance Company Statistical Bulletin, July–September 1992

Monte, Tom. *World Medicine*. New York: Perigee Books, 1993

Napier, Christine, K. "What Is A Good Checkup?" *Harvard Health Letter*, 20:3 (January, 1995)

National Center for Health Statistics, First Health & Nutrition Examination Survey, DHEW Pub No. (PHS), U.S. Public Health Services, 1984

National Center for Health Statistics, Data from the National Health Survey, Series II, No. 231, Department of Health & Human Services, 1984

National Academy of Sciences Recommended Dietary Allowances, 9th Edition, National Academy of Press, Washington, D.C., 1980

Nussbaum, Bruce. *Good Intentions*. New York: Penguin Books, 1990

Oppenheim, Michael, M.D. *The Complete Book of Better Digestion*. Emmaus, Pennsylvania: Rodale Press, 1990

Page, Melvin E., M.D. *Your Body Is Your Best Doctor*. New Canaan, Connecticut: Keats Publishing, 1972

# Bibliography

Pataki, Ladislov, PhD and Holden, L. *Winning Secrets.* U.S.: Pataki and Holden, 1989

Pauling, Linus PhD. *How to Live Longer and Feel Better.* New York: HarperCollins, 1986

Pennington, J.A. and Young, B.E. "Nutritional Elements in U.S. Diets: Results From The Total Diet Study, 1982 - 1986," *Journal of the American Dietary Association,* 89:659 (1989)

Perlmutter, David, PhD. *The Better Brain Book.* New York: Riverhead Books, 2004

Personal Health Response, *"The Metabolic Health Map - Professional's Guide."* San Francisco, California, The Human Technologies Group, Inc. and Personal, 1996

Power, Richard T., PhD and Power, Laura, B.A. *Metabolic Typing: Old and New Systems.* *Maryland:* self-published, 1982

Rath, Matthias, M.D. *Eradicating Heart Disease.* San Francisco, California: Health Now, 1993

Reams, C.A., PhD and Dudley, Cliff. *Choose Life or Death.* Tampa, Florida: Holistic Laboratories, 1990

Rector-Page, Linda G., N.D., PhD. *Healthy Healing: An Alternative Healing Reference.* 9th edition, California: Healthy Healing Publications, 1992

Riddick, Thomas. *Heart Disease: A New Approach To Prevention and Control.* Vermont: International Study Group For Research In Cardiac Metabolism, 1970

Riddick, Thomas. *Control of Colloidal Stability Through Zeta Potential.* New York: Zeta Meter, Inc., 1968

Robb, Jay., C.C.N. *The Fat Burning Diet.* USA: Jay Robb, 1994

Robbins, Stanley, M.D. and Cotran, Ramzi S., M.D. *Pathologic Basis of Disease.* Philadelphia: W.B. Saunders, 1979

Rogers, Sherry A., M.D. *The High Blood Pressure Hoax,* Sarasota, Florida: Sand Key Co., 2005

Sanders, T. A. B. "Essential and Trans-Fatty Acids In Nutrition," *Nutrition Research Reviews,* 1 (1988)

Schardt, David. "Phytochemicals: Plants Against Cancer," *Nutrition Action Health Letter,* 21:3 (April, 1994)

Schardt, David. "Pumping Immunity," *Nutrition Action Health Letter,* 21:3 (April, 1993)

Schwartz, Bob, PhD. *Diets Don't Work.* Houston, Texas, 1996

Sears, Barry, PhD. *The Zone.* New York: HarperCollins, 1995

Segarnick, David, PhD and Rotrosen, John, M.D. "Essential Fatty Acids, Prostaglandins, and Nonsteroidal Antiinflammatory Agents: Physiological and Behavioral Interactions," *Alcoholism: Clinical and Experimental Research,* 11:1 (January/February 1987)

Selye, Hans, M.D. *The Stress of Life.* New York: McGraw-Hill, 1956

Sheldon, William H., PhD. *Varieties of Human Physique.* New York: Harper, 1940

Sica-Cohen, Robban, M.D. "What You Should Know About Vitamins," Bottom Line, 15:22 (November 15, 1994)

Silver, Helene. *The Body-Smart System.* Sonora, California: Bantam Books, 1994

Solomon, Graham, T.W. *Organic Chemistry, Second Edition.* New York: John Wiley & Sons, 1980

Stern, Mark, M.D. "Clinical Applications of the Metabolic Urine Study," A report compiled by the Utilization Review Associates for Personalized Nutrition

Tefft, Gregory H., N.D., D.C. *For Your Body Only,* St. Paul MN: Dragon Door Publications, 2002

VINIS: Vitamin Nutrition Information Service (2:2). New Jersey: Hoffman-LaRoche, Inc., 1981

Wallach, Joel D., B.S., D.V.M., N.D. "Exercise Without Supplementation is Suicide," *Health Consciousness*, 15:3 (February, 1995)

Walker, N.W., Sc.D. *Fresh Vegetable and Fruit Juices: What's Missing In Your Body.* Prescott, Arizona: Norwalk Press, 1970

Watson, George, PhD. *Nutrition and Your Mind.* New York: Harper & Row, 1972

Watts, David, DC, PhD, C.C.N. *Trace Elements in Other Essential Nutrients.* USA: D.L. Watts, 1995

Weil, Andrew, M.D. *Spontaneous Healing.* New York: Alfred A. Knopf, 1995

Williams, Roger J., PhD *Alcoholism: The Nutritional Approach.* University of Texas Press, 1959

Williams, Roger J., PhD. *Nutrition Against Disease.* New York: Bantam Books, 1971

Williams, Roger J., PhD. *Biochemical Individuality.* New York: Wiley & Sons, 1956

Williams, Roger J., PhD. *The Wonderful World Within You: Your Inner Nutritional Environment.* Bio-Comm. Press, 1987

Williams, Roger J., PhD. and Lansford, Edwin M. *The Encyclopedia of Biochemistry.* New York: Reinhold, 1967

Williams, Roger J., PhD. *A Physician's Handbook on Orthomolecular Medicine.* Keats, 1979

Williams, Roger J., PhD. *You're Extraordinary.* New York: Random House, 1967

Wilson, George, PhD. *Personality, Strength, Psychochemical Energy.* New York: Harper, 1979

Wilson, George, PhD. *Nutrition and Your Mind: The Psychochemical Response.* New York: Harper, 1972

Wolcott, William L. *The Metabolic Typing Diet.* New York: Doubleday, 2000

RealPNC.com


KPNCradio.com


PUBLISHED BY

New Media for an Emerging World

# Angel Mind

*Angelmind.net*